Healing
Foods

Healing Foods

Eat your way to a healthier life

LONDON, NEW YORK, MELBOURNE, MUNICH, AND DELHI

US Consultant Kate Curnes Ramos
US Editor Constance Novis
US Senior Editor Rebecca Warren

DK UK
Editor Susannah Steel

Project Editor Shashwati Tia Sarkar
Senior Art Editor Tessa Bindloss
Editorial Assistant Christopher Mooney
Managing Editor Dawn Henderson
Managing Art Editor Christine Keilty
Senior Jacket Creative Nicola Powling
Jacket Design Assistant Rosie Levine
Producer, Pre-Production Raymond Williams
Senior Producer Jen Scothern
Art Director Peter Luff
Publisher Peggy Vance

DK INDIA
Senior Editor Chitra Subramanyam
Senior Art Editor Balwant Singh
Editor Ligi John
Art Editor Prashant Kumar
Assistant Art Editor Tanya Mehrotra
Managing Art Editor Navidita Thapa
DTP/CTS Manager Sunil Sharma
DTP Designer Anurag Trivedi
Photo Research Aditya Katyal

This paperback edition published in Canada in 2013

Dorling Kindersley is represented in Canada by
Tourmaline Editions Inc., 662 King Street West, Suite 304
Toronto, ON CANADA M5V 1M7

13 14 15 16   10 9 8 7 6 5 4 3 2 1
001–187277–Sept/13

DISCLAIMER See page 352

ISBN 978-1-55363-229-0

DK books are available at special discounts when purchased in
bulk for sales promotions, premiums, fund-raising, or
educational use. For details, contact: DK Publishing Special
Markets, 345 Hudson Street, New York, New York 10014 or
SpecialSales@dk.com

Color reproduction by Opus Multimedia Services, India
Printed and bound in China by South China (DK)

Discover more at **www.dk.com**

CONTENTS

RECIPES THAT HEAL 146

KEY TO ICONS

These icons are used throughout to signpost you to dietary benefits for different health areas.

 HEART AND CIRCULATION

 DIGESTION

 URINARY

 RESPIRATORY

 DETOX

 METABOLIC BALANCE

 IMMUNE SUPPORT

 ENERGY BOOST

MUSCLES AND JOINTS

SKIN AND HAIR

MIND AND EMOTIONS

EYE HEALTH

MEN'S HEALTH

WOMEN'S HEALTH

ABOUT THE AUTHORS

Susan Curtis has practiced as a homoeopath and naturopath since the mid-1980s and is the Director for Natural Health for Neal's Yard Remedies. She is the author of several books, including *Essential Oils*, and co-author of *Natural Healing for Women*. Susan has two grown-up children and is passionate about helping people to eat well and live a more natural and healthy lifestyle.

Pat Thomas is a journalist, campaigner, broadcaster, and passionate cook. She is the author of several books on health and environment, and has worked with leading campaign organizations to outline sensible strategies for healthy and sustainable eating. She is a former editor of *The Ecologist* magazine and was the director of Paul McCartney's "Meat Free Monday" campaign in the UK. She currently sits on the Council of Trustees of the Soil Association—the UK's premier organic certification body —and is the editor of Neal's Yard Remedies' natural health website, *NYR Natural News*.

Dragana Vilinac, medical herbalist, comes from a family with a long lineage of traditional herbalists. Her life's purpose is the exploration of the healing dynamics between plants, the planet, and people, and educating others in the subject. She has worked in the field of western, Chinese, and traditional Tibetan (Bhutanese) medicines since the 1980s, and has been a consultant on international development projects related to herbal medicines in Europe and Asia. She has co-authored books with the theme of plants as food and medicine. Dragana is the Chief Herbalist for Neal's Yard Remedies.

INTRODUCTION

"LET FOOD BE THY MEDICINE
AND MEDICINE BE THY FOOD"

HIPPOCRATES

THE FOOD WE EAT HAS AN OVERREACHING EFFECT ON OUR HEALTH AND **WELL-BEING**, WHETHER WE ARE CONSCIOUS OF IT OR NOT. BECOMING MORE AWARE OF YOUR DIET AND THE **HEALING PROPERTIES** OF FOOD WILL HELP YOU TO MAKE NECESSARY ADJUSTMENTS TO MEET THE NEEDS OF **YOUR BODY**—AND IT WILL DO AN ENORMOUS AMOUNT TO MAINTAIN AND IMPROVE YOUR **HEALTH**.

THE PROTECTIVE POWER OF FOOD

Nutritional science has shed much light on the importance of "whole food": we now understand that nutrients in our food work synergistically to promote health—and that processed food, denuded of many of its intrinsic nutrients, can promote disease. We also know of 50 or so essential vitamins, amino acids, minerals, and essential fatty acids that we need to get on a regular basis from our diet, and more than 1,200 phytonutrients found in fruits, vegetables, beans, grains, and animal products.

A RAINBOW OF PHYTONUTRIENTS

Phytonutrients are the bioactive compounds in plants ("phyto" means plant) that supply their color and flavor. Although not essential to life in the way that vitamins and minerals are, they support health in a variety of ways.

Antioxidants, for example, protect the body from free radicals, the unstable molecules that are produced through metabolism of and exposure to pollution, and which cause disease by damaging vital tissues and organs.

Antioxidants by color

COLOR	PHYTONUTRIENT	BENEFITS	FOUND IN
	Green		
	Lutein	Protects eyes; boosts immunity; and supports healthy tissues, skin, and blood	Kale, collard greens, cucumber, zucchini, peas, avocado, asparagus, green beans
	Chlorophyll	Detoxifying; helps build red blood cells and collagen; boosts energy and well-being	All leafy green vegetables, sprouted grasses, and microalgae
	Indoles	Has anticancer properties; supports healthy hormone balance	Brussels sprouts, broccoli, bok choy, cabbage, and turnips
	Orange/yellow		
	Carotenes (incl. alpha-, beta-, and delta-carotene)	Source of vitamin A; has anticancer and heart-protective properties; protects mucous membranes	Orange and yellow fruits and vegetables (peppers, squashes, carrots, apricots, mangoes, oranges, grapefruit)
	Xanthophylls (incl. zeaxanthin and astaxanthin)	Source of vitamin A; has anticancer properties; protects eyes and brain; strengthens the immune system	Red fish (e.g. salmon), eggs, most orange and yellow fruits and vegetables
	Red		
	Lycopene	Protects against heart disease, cancer (especially prostate), and vision loss	Fresh and cooked tomatoes, watermelon, goji berries, papaya, and rosehips
	Anthocyanins	Can help reduce the risk of heart disease, cancer, and neurodegenerative diseases	Cranberries, strawberries, raspberries, cherries, and red cabbage
	Blue/purple		
	Anthocyanins	Fights free radicals; has anticancer properties; supports healthy aging	Blueberries, eggplant, grapes, grape juice, raisins, and red wine
	Resveratrol	Has anticancer properties; helps balance hormone levels	Grapes, grape juice, red wine, mulberries, and cocoa
	White		
	Allyl sulfides	Boosts immunity; has anticancer and anti-inflammatory properties	Onions, garlic, scallions, and chives
	Anthoxanthins	Helps lower cholesterol and blood pressure; helps reduce the risk of certain cancers and heart disease	Bananas, cauliflower, mushrooms, onions, parsnips, potatoes, garlic, ginger, and turnips

DIFFERENT DIETARY PATTERNS

While we would not advocate a rigid approach to a particular diet, there are things that can be gained and adopted from traditional diets. Humans are very adaptable and it is interesting to see the ways in which different cultures have adjusted their diets to remain healthy in widely different environments.

TRADITIONAL DIETS

INUIT

The Inuit people of the Arctic have traditionally had very little access to cereals or fresh fruit and vegetables, but the manner in which they hunt and eat their mostly fish- and meat-based diet meets their nutritional needs. For example, vitamins and minerals that are derived from plant sources in other areas of the world are also present in most Inuit diets: vitamins A and D are present in the oils and livers of coldwater fishes and mammals, for instance, while vitamin C is obtained through sources such as caribou liver, kelp, whale skin, and seal offal. Because these foods are typically eaten raw or frozen, the vitamin C they contain—which would be destroyed by cooking—is instead preserved.

MEDITERRANEAN

Another traditional diet that has received publicity in recent years is the Mediterranean diet. This diet is based mainly on fresh vegetables and fruit with some whole grains, healthier oils like olive oil and those from fresh fish, red wine, and smaller quantities of meat. Studies throughout the world have shown that following a strict Mediterranean diet offers substantial protection against heart disease, cancer, and Parkinson's and Alzheimer's diseases. The biggest study into this diet has shown that it can reduce the number of deaths from these diseases; it also found that people who follow this diet show significant improvements in health, and are nine percent less likely to die young.

JAPANESE

Traditional Japanese cuisine is rich in fat-soluble vitamins from seafood and organ meats and minerals from fish broth, and contains plenty of beneficial lactofermented foods, such as tempeh and miso. Although portions tend to be relatively small, they are both filling and very nutrient-dense. In fact, Japanese people who follow this traditional diet tend to be some of the healthiest, least obese, and longest-lived people in the world.

ANCESTRAL/PALEOLITHIC

Also referred to as the caveman or hunter-gatherer diet, this modern nutritional plan is based on an ancient diet of wild plants and meat that early humans were likely to have habitually eaten during the Paleolithic era—a period of about 2.5 million years that ended around 10,000 years ago with the development of agriculture. Early humans were foragers who would have grazed opportunistically on seasonally available plants and not made the, often arbitrary, distinctions we do between weeds and crops and medicinal and culinary herbs. Although the hunter-gatherer diet comprises commonly available modern foods—mainly fish, grass-fed, pasture-raised meats, vegetables, fruit, fungi, roots, and nuts—it largely excludes dried beans, dairy products, grains, salt, refined sugar, and processed oils, which define the Western diet (overleaf). Studies of the Paleolithic diet in humans have shown improved health and fewer incidences of diseases, such as diabetes, cancer, obesity, dementia, and heart disease.

WHAT MANY OF THESE DIETS have in common is that they are plant-based, with meat reserved for feast days and occasional treats. They include plenty of oily fish so are rich in the omega-3 fatty acid DHA. Their overall balance of essential fatty acids is healthier (i.e. higher in omega 3 than 6, unlike modern diets), and they are high in antioxidants. People who follow these diets rely on seasonal fresh food produced without industrial chemicals, which means they eat a wide variety of nutrient-dense foods necessary for optimal heath throughout the year. They tend to eat sensible portions and rarely "snack" between meals.

THE WESTERN DIET

By contrast, the modern Western diet, also called the Western pattern diet, is characterized by high intakes of red meat, sugar and artificial sweeteners, high-fat foods, salt, and refined grains. It also typically contains hydrogenated and transfats, high-sugar drinks, and higher intakes of processed meat. This diet, based on studies of western populations, is associated with an elevated incidence of obesity, death from heart disease, cancer (especially colon cancer), and other western-pattern diet-related diseases. The high consumption of grains—as breakfast cereals, breads, cakes, cookies, pasta, and so on—means that grain has become a significant source of carbohydrate-energy, minerals, and, in the case of whole grains, of fiber and B vitamins. However, it is now thought that this reliance on cereals may come at a high cost to our health. Modern strains of high-gluten cereals, combined with an over-reliance on wheat-based products and an industrial approach to the processing of grain-based foods, can place a strain on our digestive systems and nutrient balance. For example, an increasing number of people have developed gluten intolerance, or gluten sensitivity, which can vary from celiac disease to feeling bloated if they eat too many cereal-based foods in

> ## "IT IS NOW THOUGHT THAT RELIANCE ON CEREALS MAY COME AT A HIGH COST TO OUR HEALTH."

a day. Cereals contain what have been termed "antinutrients," which may prevent the digestive system from absorbing several essential nutrients. The most researched antinutrients are the phytates found in the bran or outer hull of most grains, and which is part of a seed's system of preservation—it prevents the seed from sprouting until conditions are right. The phytate known as phytic acid can block the absorption of essential minerals such as calcium, magnesium, copper, iron, and especially zinc, in the gut. This may be why a diet high in improperly prepared whole grains may lead to serious mineral deficiencies and bone loss, and why consuming large amounts of unprocessed bran often initially improves bowel regularity, but may lead to irritable bowel syndrome and, in the long term, other adverse effects.

So although cereals can be a useful part of a diet, they do require careful preparation because of their antinutrient properties. Many cultures throughout the world have developed ways of preparing types of grain for human consumption. Soaking, sprouting, and souring are very common aids for grain preparation, and ensure the neutralization of phytates, enzyme-inhibitors, and other antinutrients with which seeds are naturally endowed. Some traditional preparation methods involve complex, comparatively labor-intensive steps that produce what are now considered unusual foods from common grains, but which were once part of common dietary practices. The traditional sourdough method of preparing rye bread, for example, once widespread throughout eastern Europe, helps to make rye flour far more digestible.

Modern diets in general also tend to include a larger number of dried beans, and, more recently, soy derivatives. Although including beans in your diet can be a useful source of fiber and protein, these foods also contain phytates. The phytate in soybeans, for example, means they are low in calcium and one reason why they are less healthy than you might think, though fermenting helps to make soy a more nutritious food. It is interesting to note that the traditional Japanese diet includes a lot of soy, but it is usually fermented in the form of tempeh or miso. In addition, Japanese preparation techniques eliminate most of the antinutrients in other dried beans and in grains. Soymilk is not fermented and so can be a cause of digestive problems and calcium depletion, as well as being a fairly potent phytoestrogen—potentially useful for reducing hot flashes in menopausal women, but not so suitable for children or everyone else.

CARBOHYDRATES
Including refined grains and starch

FATS
Including polyunsaturated and animal fats

35%

45%

20%

PROTEINS
Including high levels of red and processed meats

WESTERN DIET FIGURES
In a Western diet, the main nutritional building blocks of fats, carbohydrates, and protein are often processed, nutrient-poor foods high in sugar, refined grains, and saturated fats.

VARIETY IS THE SPICE OF LIFE

The good news is that if you currently eat a modern Western diet, you can easily adapt your eating habits to dramatically improve your health. Including a variety of nutrient-rich, low-energy foods, such as vegetables and fruit, in your diet both helps with weight control and can have a positive effect on your health. Eating a varied diet ensures we get a steady supply of highly bioavailable nutrients that help reduce the likelihood of conditions such as Alzheimer's disease, dementia, anxiety, depression, arthritis, some types of cancer (including breast and bowel cancer), and heart and circulatory disease.

DIETARY DIVERSITY

No single food or food group can supply all the nutrients we need, which is why a diverse diet is so important. Research consistently shows that dietary diversity protects against the onset of type 2 diabetes, for example, by balancing out blood sugar levels and protecting against blood vessel damage. A varied, seasonal diet rich in plant foods can also lower your total risk of cancer and has been shown to protect against some very specific cancers of the digestive tract. To improve the balance and variety of your diet, choose foods like multigrain breads and granola that have variety "built in," and eat side dishes and condiments, such as fruit and vegetable salads, sprouted seeds, fresh salsas, pickles, and chutneys. Stir-fries, casseroles, and soups with many ingredients are another easy way to increase diversity in your diet. Or, when grocery shopping, regularly buy a fruit or vegetable that is not familiar to you to prepare and eat. Following a varied diet also tends to be more satisfying and so reduces your sugar, salt, and saturated fat consumption—all risk factors for heart disease. Including more spices and herbs in your food can also boost its flavor and nutritional density: adding a handful of chopped fresh herbs to lettuce in a salad, for example, can add up to 75 percent extra antioxidants to the food.

Vary your diet

TYPICAL DIET	DIVERSE DIET
BREAKFAST Wheat bran cereal with milk, sugar and banana; orange juice; tea with milk	**BREAKFAST** Oatmeal made with milk, sprinkled with dried fruit, sunflower and pumpkin seeds, and seasoned with cinnamon and maple syrup; rosehip and hibiscus tea
LUNCH Wheat bread, ham, cheese, and lettuce sandwich with mayonnaise for spread; a piece of fruit	**LUNCH** Lentil soup (p212) made with ginger, turmeric, shallots, garlic and chile; served with slice of rye bread (p328) spread with butter; a piece of fruit
DINNER Chicken (or other meat) served with a vegetable and rice	**DINNER** Salmon with dill and tamari sauce (p268) served with an adzuki and mung bean salad (p226) with tomatoes and a mixed citrus and herb dressing
SNACK Potato chips	**SNACK** Multiseed crackers (e.g. wheat, pumpkin seed, flaxseed, poppy seed) spread with Hummus (p196) made with chickpeas, tahini, coriander seeds, paprika
TOTAL OF 13 FOODS	**TOTAL OF 35 FOODS**

Soughdough rye bread p328

Hummus with coriander p196

As Nature Intended

The success of traditional diets, such as the Mediterranean and Inuit diets, in sustaining good health and well-being (p11) lies in the fact that they each contain a carefully balanced range of seasonal nutrient-rich foods that are available from local sources. To get the very best from locally grown fresh produce, however, it is worth considering buying organic, because foods that are produced this way contain more of the nutrients that make these seasonal foods so beneficial to our health.

LOCAL AND SEASONAL

Adjusting your diet with the seasons can mean that, as well as being beneficial for your body's "energies," you will eat more fresh foods that can be locally sourced. Choosing local and seasonal should also encourage you to make healthier choices, and can increase your general feeling of well-being as you become more in tune with the cycles of nature. This doesn't mean that you need to become rigid or obsessive about what you eat and when; some foods, such as avocados or bananas, may simply not grow where you live. It is the principles you base your dietary habits on that is key. The 80:20 rule—eating 80 percent of local, seasonal, unprocessed foods and 20 percent of more exotic foods, or "treats"—is probably a good guideline. When people switch to more local, seasonal food, many find they become more adventurous in their cooking and eating habits. If you unpack a CSA (Community Supported Agriculture) box, for example, you may find an unrecognized vegetable or fruit that you have to discover the best way to prepare, and hopefully you will look forward to preparing and eating it again next time it is in season. Or, you may become interested in learning how to preserve them—a more traditional and low-impact way of extending the natural season of foods throughout the year.

ORGANIC BENEFITS

Organic food is produced using environmentally and animal-friendly farming methods on organic farms. These methods are now legally defined in most countries of the world and any food that is sold as organic must be strictly regulated. Organic farming recognizes the direct connection between our health and how the food we eat is produced. Artificial fertilizers are banned and farmers develop fertile soil by rotating crops and using compost, manure, and clover in order. In contrast, modern intensive agricultural practices have led to the reduction of many minerals and vitamins in the food we eat; official food composition tables in the USA and UK have shown that fruits, vegetables, meat, and dairy products all contain fewer minerals than they did in the past. As soils become depleted of minerals, such as magnesium and zinc, for example, there is less for plants grown in this soil to draw up, and therefore less for us to absorb. Minerals that are particularly affected by these intensive farming methods are iron, zinc, copper, magnesium, and selenium, and their levels of depletion can be very significant. An early study in the Journal of Applied Nutrition in 1993 reported that organically and conventionally grown apples, potatoes, pears, wheat, and corn in a suburban area of the USA were analyzed and compared for mineral content. On a per-weight basis, average levels of essential minerals were much higher in the organically grown produce than in the conventionally grown foods. The organic produce was, on average, 63 percent higher in calcium, 78 percent higher in chromium, 73 percent higher in iron, 118 percent higher in magnesium, 178 percent higher in molybdenum, 91 percent higher in phosphorus, 125 percent higher in potassium, and 60 percent higher in zinc. More recent studies have confirmed this finding and interestingly, according to population studies, many people in the western world are becoming increasingly deficient in these same minerals, leading to problems such as anemia, fatigue, subfertility, and poor immunity. Organic farming can help to halt this decline in mineral content. Levels of vitamin C, phenolic acids, and antioxidants also tend to be 60–80 percent higher in organic produce. Just as important from a health point of view is the markedly more benign balance of omega-6 and -3 fatty acids in organic meat and dairy produce as compared to conventionally produced foods.

It is not just what organic food contains, it is what it does not contain that is important. Some synthetic chemicals commonly used in nonorganic agriculture are now known to potentially disrupt the nervous, circulatory, endocrine, and reproductive systems of humans. This may be even more of a problem in babies and children,

> "IT IS NOT JUST WHAT ORGANIC FOOD CONTAINS, IT IS ALSO WHAT IT DOES NOT CONTAIN THAT IS IMPORTANT."

whose organs are developing fast. Although most countries now set safety levels for pesticide residues in food, these are based on individual chemicals, and don't take into account the cocktail effect of several pesticides, which are known to be more damaging in combination. Many food additives common in processed foods are also banned from organic food products; monosodium glutamate (MSG), Brilliant Blue, aspartame, and tartrazine, for example, are now being linked to health issues and behavioral problems in children. Organic standards also insist that animals are given plenty of space and fresh air to thrive and grow, guaranteeing that they are reared humanely and not routinely fed antibiotics to suppress disease or promote growth.

Organic is kinder to the environment, too. Organic farming works with nature, not against it, and research shows that it's better for birds, butterflies, and other wildlife. Organic farms are havens for wildlife and provide homes for bees, birds, and butterflies. In fact, plant, insect, and bird life is up to 50 percent greater on organic farms. Biodiversity is something to encourage both in our environment and on our plate.

HOW ABOUT GM FOOD?

Genetically modified (GM) crops provide another potential health hazard. GM foods, which have had their genetic material (DNA) altered to achieve desired changes in their characteristics, have been developed by seed and chemical companies as one means of responding to climate change and a growing global population, although GM technologies have consistently underperformed. There is legitimate concern about how carelessly GM foods have been assessed for safety, and evidence that they may have risks to human health and wildlife. In a recent French study in 2012, rats fed a lifelong diet of a bestselling strain of genetically modified corn developed more and bigger breast tumors, and experienced kidney and liver dysfunction. In the USA, GM foods don't have to be labeled, in spite of overwhelming public support for such a requirement in a country where GM-adulterated food is so prevalent. In most countries in Europe, farm animals are fed GM foodstuff, but actual GM foods for human consumption are not yet accepted. Examples of GM foods include soybeans, corn, white rice, tomatoes, and Brazil nuts.

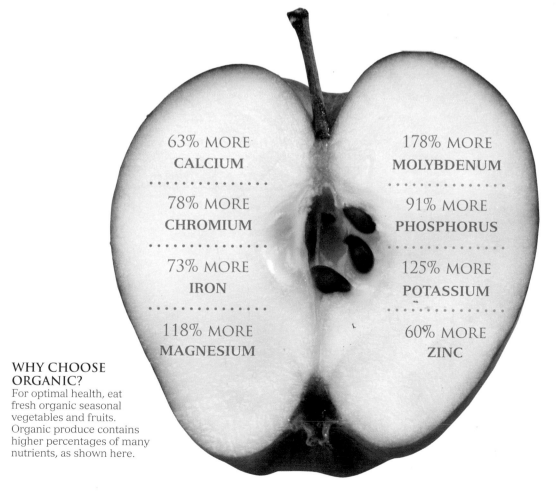

63% MORE
CALCIUM

78% MORE
CHROMIUM

73% MORE
IRON

118% MORE
MAGNESIUM

178% MORE
MOLYBDENUM

91% MORE
PHOSPHORUS

125% MORE
POTASSIUM

60% MORE
ZINC

WHY CHOOSE ORGANIC?
For optimal health, eat fresh organic seasonal vegetables and fruits. Organic produce contains higher percentages of many nutrients, as shown here.

LET FOOD BE YOUR MEDICINE

Food is the bedrock upon which a healthy life is based, and is the body's buffer against the stresses, strains, and the onslaughts of an increasingly toxic environment. Science has consistently shown that food can be used to support long-term heath as well as treat acute conditions. Ginger, for example, is a traditional remedy for nausea, honey can be as effective as conventional medicines at soothing nighttime coughs, saffron contains antioxidants that protect against age-related vision loss, garlic helps thin the blood, thus lowering the risk of stroke, and a diet rich in tree nuts can support heart health and even men's fertility. As the cost, and acknowledged side effects, of conventional medical treatments rise exponentially, we owe it to ourselves to eat the most nutritionally dense, best-quality foods. Good food is everybody's right, and in our view the best way to democratize good food is through the widespread use of organic farming and a greater attention to the concepts of local and seasonal. In reestablishing the fundamental link between food and health and exploring the benefits of traditional diets we are not looking backward, rather we are taking the best of our inherited knowledge about food and farming and applying it to a modern future.

For example, Chinese and Ayurvedic traditions have for thousands of years followed the concept that different foods have specific, healthy properties. Some foods, such as quail eggs, are considered energizing and full of concentrated life force while others, such as barley, are more soothing to the energies of the body. Traditional approaches to food also acknowledge the seasons: of recommending warming foods like oats and spices like cinnamon in winter; cleansing foods such as nettle or dandelion in spring; cooling foods like lettuce and cucumber in summer; and sustaining foods such as pumpkin and carrots in fall.

The first half of this book will help you to identify foods that have both stood the test of time as healing foods and are shown by modern research as being particularly relevant for helping to improve a health issue. The second half contains recipes, inspired by traditional cultural practices, that benefit various parts of the body or internal systems. We hope that this information will both encourage and help you affirm the connection between food and health and make food choices for yourself and your family that lead to lifelong optimal health.

Food as medicine

NAUSEA

GINGER
has a recognized ability to quell feelings of nausea.

COUGHS

HONEY
is an ancient remedy for soothing coughs and other throat complaints.

HEART

GARLIC
can help your body to fight free radicals and lower blood pressure.

LIVER

BRUSSELS SPROUTS
are a good source of sulfur, which enhances liver function.

MEMORY

BERRIES
contain antioxidants, which can help to stave off mental decline

CHOLESTEROL

NUTS & SEEDS
contain unsaturated fats, which can lower cholesterol.

SUPPLEMENTS

A balanced diet is where health begins, but there are times when your diet may not provide all the nutrients you need. A Western diet and lifestyle can also leave us vulnerable to nutritional deficiencies including iron, calcium, magnesium, folic acid, vitamins B_6, B_{12}, C, and D. Most governments produce scientifically developed recommended dietary allowances (RDAs) to cover broadly healthy people of any age or gender. These are the basis for the Reference Daily Intake (RDI) values, which regulators use to create Daily Value (DV) packaging labels. RDAs are based on the lowest levels of nutrients required to prevent deficiency diseases, such as scurvy and rickets, and do not, as our tables on pages 338–41 illustrate, reflect the higher levels required for optimum health. This is why supplement nutrient levels are often much higher than RDA levels.

Who will benefit most from supplements?

Even in healthy people, multivitamins and other supplements may help to prevent vitamin and mineral deficiencies. They also provide more nutrients than diet can alone, so they may help to protect against, or manage, certain diseases. However, the following categories highlight those people who can most benefit from taking daily supplements:

• People who have lost weight, who may be deficient in a wide range of vitamins and minerals.

• Vegetarians, who are more likely to be deficient in vitamin B_{12}, iron, vitamin D, zinc, iodine, riboflavin, calcium, and selenium.

• Vegans, who are even more likely than vegetarians to be low in protein, selenium, and B_{12}.

• People living a typical "student lifestyle" and anyone not eating a balanced diet is likely to benefit from a multivitamin supplement.

• Elderly people living in their own homes, who are often deficient in vitamin D, vitamin A, vitamin E, calcium, and zinc, and occasionally vitamin B_1 and vitamin B_2.

• Smokers, who are most likely to be deficient in vitamin C and zinc.

• Premenopausal women, who have often been found to consume low amounts of calcium, iron, vitamin A, and vitamin C.

• Pregnant women are often advised to take a folic acid supplement, and studies have shown that taking a multivitamin supplement before and during pregnancy leads to a healthier pregnancy and a healthier baby.

• Anyone living in a colder climate who does not get regular sun exposure is likely to be deficient in vitamin D, which can lead to, among other problems, an increased incidence of breast cancer, bowel cancer, depression, osteoporosis, Parkinson's and heart disease.

• Anyone who is under stress is likely to benefit from taking additional B vitamins.

• Many men and women experiencing problems with low fertility are deficient in zinc.

Are supplements safe?

Generally speaking, taking nutritional supplements from reputable companies is extremely safe, but this doesn't mean all supplements are appropriate for everyone. It is worth doing some research to find out about the potential benefits and risks of taking a supplement. There are many sources of information available to help you become well informed. If you are suffering from a specific disease, it is advisable to talk to a knowledgeable healthcare professional before taking a supplement. If you are pregnant or breastfeeding, only take those supplements specifically recommended for you to take during this time.

While many vitamins, minerals, and herbs are known to safely prevent or treat a variety of diseases, they work by altering your body chemistry—just like any medicine. So before you take a supplement, make sure you know about how it might interact with any medications you may be already taking.

Before you turn to supplements, bear in mind that using the information in this book may help you to replace depleted nutrients by eating more of a certain food. For example, if you need to replace lost potassium, you may choose to eat more bananas or drink coconut water, or eat more fresh berries to increase your vitamin C intake.

FOODS THAT HEAL

TAKE ADVANTAGE OF THE ENORMOUS **VARIETY** OF FOODS THAT HAVE INCREDIBLE **HEALTH BENEFITS** AND STAND AS A TESTIMONY TO "LET FOOD BE THY **MEDICINE**."

APPLES

 HELPS BALANCE BLOOD SUGAR LEVELS

 TACKLES DIARRHEA AND CONSTIPATION

 HELPS STRENGTHEN BONES

 HELPS LOWER CHOLESTEROL

Available in many varieties, juicy, crunchy apples have been celebrated since antiquity for their health benefits. They are **high in pectin**, a fiber, and **slow-release sugars** that help to improve **heart health** and regulate the body's **blood sugar levels**. They also contain many important vitamins and minerals, and substances that promote, among other things, strong, healthy bones.

GREEN APPLES
Like other apples, green apples contain malic acid, a useful digestive aid.

RED APPLES
Antioxidants, which can protect against neurological damage associated with conditions, such as Alzheimer's disease, are higher in red apples than in some other varieties.

YELLOW APPLES
The pectin in yellow and all other apples helps lower the body's absorption of excess dietary fats.

WHAT IS IT GOOD FOR?

BLOOD SUGAR REGULATION Fructose and antioxidant polyphenols in apples improve the metabolic balance and slow the rate at which sugar is absorbed into the bloodstream.

CONSTIPATION AND DIARRHEA Pectin has an amphoteric action. Paradoxically, it can provide relief from both constipation and diarrhea, depending on the body's needs.

PROTECTING BONES The flavonoid phlorizin, found in apple skin, may help prevent bone loss associated with menopause, because it fights the inflammation and free-radical production that lead to bone loss.

REDUCES CHOLESTEROL Pectin and other constituents, such as antioxidant polyphenols, reduce levels of "unhealthy" (LDL) cholesterol, and slow down its oxidation—a risk factor for atherosclerosis (hardening of the arteries). Polyphenols also prevent free radicals from damaging heart muscles and blood vessels.

HOW DO I GET THE BEST FROM IT?

THE WHOLE FRUIT Every part is edible. Supermarkets coat apples with wax to give a shine and keep them fresh over long periods, so always wash these apples before eating.

GO ORGANIC AND LOCAL Buy organic, and from sources as local as possible, for the freshest fruit without chemical contamination.

KEEP THE SKIN ON Peeling can remove more than half an apple's fiber, vitamin C, and iron.

HOW DO I USE IT?

A SIMPLE FOOD FOR RECUPERATION Grate 1 apple and allow to brown slightly to release the juices, making it easier to digest. Take 1–2 large spoonfuls every hour or as needed.

BAKED APPLES Core large apples, stuff with nuts, dried fruit, and spices, such as cinnamon, and bake at 350°F (180°C) until soft.

APRICOTS

 PROMOTES CLEAR SKIN   **HELPS PROTECT EYE HEALTH**   **PROMOTES BOWEL REGULARITY**   **PROTECTS AGAINST FREE-RADICAL DAMAGE**

Native to eastern Asia, apricots were cultivated by the Chinese for thousands of years before they reached the rest of the world. Low in calories yet **high in fiber** and many key vitamins, apricots can be eaten fresh or dried, and the leaves and kernels can all be used. Medicinally, they can help **improve digestion**, promote **clear skin**, and protect **vision**.

WHAT IS IT GOOD FOR?

EYE AND SKIN HEALTH Its high beta-carotene content is beneficial for aging eyes. Studies also show a regular high intake of nutrients such as vitamins C and E, zinc, and copper—all found in apricots—can reduce the risk of macular degeneration by 25 percent. They are also good for maintaining healthy skin.

DIGESTIVE HEALTH Its high fiber content aids bowel regularity, which can help prevent constipation and even bowel cancer.

ANTICANCER EFFECTS Its antioxidants can protect against free-radical damage linked to cancer and other diseases. The kernels also contain vitamin B_{17} (laetrile), shown in laboratory studies to kill cancer cells.

HOW DO I GET THE BEST FROM IT?

EAT FRESH AND DRIED Both are rich in fiber, vitamins A, C, and E, and other key nutrients. Buy dried apricots without added sulfites.

APRICOT KERNEL The seed inside the stone is edible. As well as its anticancer properties, it helps remove toxins and strengthens the body's defenses against disease.

KERNEL OIL Use the oil, which is rich in monounsaturated fats and vitamins A, C, and E, for cooking and salad dressings.

HOW DO I USE IT?

TO COUNTERBALANCE FATTY MEATS Pair with rich duck or goose meat, or include the dried fruits in stuffings or chopped into lamb stews.

LIGHTLY POACHED Poach fresh apricots in a light syrup of 1 part honey and 3 parts water. Add 6 crushed cardamom pods and ½ vanilla bean, and simmer until just tender.

PICKLED APRICOTS Japanese umeboshi, or pickled plums, are actually apricots. Eaten with rice, they stimulate digestion and prevent nausea, including nausea from hangovers.

Flesh
The very high levels of vitamin A in apricot promote healthy eyes and skin

Kernel
The kernel inside the stone is a source of a healthy oil rich in vitamin B_{17} (laetrile), known for its cancer-fighting properties

PEACHES AND NECTARINES

HELPS PREVENT
METABOLIC SYNDROME

FIGHTS FREE-RADICAL
DAMAGE TO SKIN

HELPS EXPEL
EXCESS WATER

Peaches originate from China, where they are considered an **uplifting**, **rejuvenating** fruit. Like other stone fruits, peaches and nectarines (a close relative) contain a balance of phenolic compounds—anthocyanins, chlorogenic acids, quercetin derivatives, and catechins—that work synergistically to **combat metabolic syndrome** (a group of risk factors that can lead to diabetes and heart disease).

PEACHES
These contain beta-carotene, lycopene, and lutein, which protect the heart and eyes.

NECTARINES
They have red, yellow, or white flesh and are a source of vitamins A and C and beta-carotene.

WHAT IS IT GOOD FOR?

WEIGHT MANAGEMENT Their phenolic compounds are known to have antiobesity, anti-inflammatory, and antidiabetic properties, and regular consumption of both can help prevent metabolic syndrome.

SKIN HEALTH Both are good sources of vitamin C, an essential component in the body's production of collagen. They are also a good source of the antioxidant lutein, which helps fight free-radical damage and supports healthy skin (and eyes).

DIURETIC Rich in potassium, phosphorus, and magnesium, peaches and nectarines are an antidote to a high-sodium diet and can help remove excess water from the body. They are also mildly laxative.

ANTICANCER Laboratory tests show that breast-cancer cells—even the most aggressive type—died after exposure to peach extract.

HOW DO I GET THE BEST FROM IT?

EAT IN SEASON Eat ripe stone fruits as soon as possible after buying; they can quickly become overripe and lose their nutritional benefits, and tend to bruise easily.

PRESERVE FOR LATER Both peaches and nectarines make delicious jams and preserves.

HOW DO I USE IT?

ANTIOXIDANT ICED TEA Slice 2 ripe peaches into a pan, add 2 cups water, and bring to a boil. Remove from the heat, add 8 green tea bags, and steep for 5 minutes. Gently squeeze the teabags as you remove them. Add a further 1 cup water and a little honey to sweeten, if you like. When cool, serve over ice with a mint garnish.

BREAKFAST BAGEL Top a toasted bagel with soft goat or kefir cheese and nectarine slices. A little freshly ground black pepper on top will bring out the sweetness of the fruit.

PEARS

 LOW-ALLERGY FOOD

 HAS A MILD LAXATIVE ACTION

 HELPS CALM THE NERVES

 HELPS KEEP JOINTS SUPPLE

Dozens of different varieties of pear are now available; most have paper-thin skins and a similar shape, although some, such as the Asian pear, look a little different. A cooling, uplifting, low-allergy fruit and an excellent source of **water-soluble fiber**, pears also contain useful amounts of **beta-carotene** and B vitamins, as well as traces of copper, phosphorus, potassium, and other essential elements.

WHAT IS IT GOOD FOR?

ALLERGY RELIEF Low in salicylates and benzoates, pears are less allergenic than many other fruits, and are often recommended in exclusion diets for allergy sufferers. Pear juice is often introduced as a first juice to infants. Also good for recuperation after illness.

CONSTIPATION Most of its fiber is insoluble, making it a good bulking laxative.

NERVOUS EXHAUSTION Considered to be a cooling and soothing food. Vitamin C also triggers the production of norepinephrine and serotonin, neurotransmitters that can help lift mood.

RHEUMATIC CONDITIONS Contains a combination of potassium, pectin, and tannins that help dissolve uric acid, making it ideal for those with rheumatic conditions, such as gout and arthritis.

HOW DO I GET THE BEST FROM IT?

KEEP THE SKIN ON Most of its vitamin C and dietary fiber is contained within its thin skin.

RIPEN AT HOME Pears bruise easily when ripe. Buy them slightly underripe and let them ripen at home.

DRIED Like most dried fruits, pears are high in sugar but are a good source of natural fiber. Eat just a few for a sustained energy lift.

JUICE THEM Fresh pear juice is cooling and uplifting if you are feeling hot and anxious.

HOW DO I USE IT?

UPLIFTING DRINK Boil dried pears in water for 15 minutes. Strain and reserve the hot liquid, allow to cool, then drink to relieve nervous exhaustion and symptoms of PMS.

POACH THEM Cook fresh pears gently in a light sugar syrup or wine; add a little grated ginger or cinnamon, if you like. Serve while warm, sprinkled with toasted almonds.

CONFERENCE PEAR
Fresh pears like these have higher levels of fructose, glucose, and levulose—the sweetest of all natural sugars—in them than any other fruit.

RED ANJOU PEAR
Red-hued pears, such as Red Anjou and Red Bartlett, have more antioxidant anthocyanins than green, yellow, and brown varieties.

ASIAN PEAR
These pears may sound exotic but there is no nutritional difference between these and regular varieties.

PLUMS

 HELPS PROTECT EYE HEALTH

 HAS A LAXATIVE ACTION

 HELPS BALANCE BLOOD SUGAR LEVELS

 SUPPORTS HEALTHY LIVER FUNCTION

Plums, or gages, are members of the rose family and there are more than 2,000 varieties, including the greengage, Mirabelle, and damson. Plums have good **antioxidant** and **detoxifying** properties, are a **metabolic stimulant**, and contain chromium, potassium, selenium, and other minerals, as well as **vitamin C** and **beta-carotene**. Dried plums, or prunes, are a traditional treatment for constipation.

PURPLE PLUMS
Dark-skinned varieties with a red flesh are richer in beneficial antioxidants called anthocyanins than other varieties.

GREENGAGES
Like all plums, greengages are rich in potassium, beta-carotene, and fiber.

VICTORIA PLUMS
The antioxidants in these and other plums aid skin health.

PRUNES
Dried plums can help ease constipation.

WHAT IS IT GOOD FOR?

PROTECTS EYESIGHT Its antioxidants can help prevent age-related macular degeneration (a major cause of loss of vision).

CONSTIPATION Rich in stool-bulking fibers, especially pectin, fructose, and sulfur, which help food to move effectively through the colon. Together with substances, such as sorbitol and isatin, these fibers are responsible for the fruit's well-known laxative effect.

METABOLIC STIMULANT Contains useful amounts of calcium, potassium, magnesium, and the antioxidant beta-carotene. These nutrients help regulate heart rate, blood pressure, blood sugar levels, and water balance. Damsons in particular, are noted for their ability to stimulate appetite and digestion if eaten before a meal.

DETOX Can initiate detoxification and help improve liver function. As well as improving internal health, its detoxifying properties can help promote healthy skin.

HOW DO I GET THE BEST FROM IT?

DRIED FRUIT Prunes are a good way to reap the benefits of plums all year round. They contain both soluble and insoluble fiber, which help promote bowel regularity and balance blood sugar levels.

KEEP THE SKIN ON The skin is where most of its beneficial antioxidants concentrate.

HOW DO I USE IT?

BAKE THEM Slice some plums in half, remove the pits, and bake in an oven preheated to 350°F (180°C) until they are wrinkled. Eat them plain, or drizzle with a little yogurt sweetened with honey before serving.

SWEETEN A RICE SALAD Add chopped plums and pistachio nuts to a cold brown-rice salad. Dress with extra virgin olive oil and a fruit vinegar, such as blackberry or raspberry.

KIWI FRUIT

PROMOTES COLLAGEN SYNTHESIS

HAS A MILD LAXATIVE ACTION

REDUCES TRIGYLCERIDES IN THE BLOOD

PROTECTS AGAINST COLDS AND FLU

Native to China, and sometimes called a Chinese gooseberry, this unusual-looking fruit is now grown all over the world in sunny climates. There are some nutritional differences between the two varieties, green and gold, but both are good for **digestion** and **heart health**. Their high vitamin C content also promotes **skin health** and boosts the **immune system**, fighting off any inflammation.

What Is It Good For?

GREAT SKIN Vitamin C contributes to the formation of collagen and hastening the repair from sun and wind damage.

HEALTHY DIGESTION Its mild laxative effect is linked to its fiber content. Two kiwis provide 20 percent of the daily recommended amount of fiber, and can aid digestion and maintain colon health. Also contains actinidin, an enzyme that aids the digestion of protein.

HEART DISEASE Studies show that the high levels of flavonoids and vitamins C and E in kiwis can reduce triglycerides (a type of fat) in the blood and the buildup of plaque in the arteries (atherosclerosis). The tiny black seeds contain vitamin E and omega-3 fatty acids, which act as natural blood thinners.

IMMUNITY Vitamin C boosts immunity, fights off colds and flu, and combats inflammation.

How Do I Get The Best From It?

EAT RAW ON ITS OWN Eat with a spoon, as you would a hard-cooked egg. The actinidin in green, but not gold, kiwis makes them incompatible with some foods, such as dairy produce, which they cause to curdle.

GET COLORFUL Green kiwis contain larger amounts of fiber, while gold kiwis contain higher levels of vitamin C and potassium.

How Do I Use It?

A SUMMERY SMOOTHIE Blend the flesh (seeds removed) of ¼ watermelon, 2 peeled kiwi fruit, and a peeled banana in a blender.

DETOX SOUP For a cold soup for 2, blend until smooth the flesh of 1 galia or honeydew melon, halved, (reserve the shells to serve the soup in), 1 kiwi fruit, and 1 ripe pear (seeded), a handful of green grapes, grated fresh ginger (optional), and ¾ cup aloe vera juice. Chill, pour into the melon shells, and garnish with chopped kiwi and fresh mint to serve.

GREEN KIWI
Contains significantly more fiber than gold kiwi fruit.

GOLD KIWI
Gold kiwi contains large amounts of vitamin C, vital for boosting immunity.

FIGS

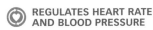 **REGULATES HEART RATE AND BLOOD PRESSURE**

 HELPS STRENGTHEN BONES

 PROMOTES BOWEL REGULARITY

Figs are a lovely, sweet, seasonal fruit, generally available from July to September, and can be enjoyed fresh or dried. Although each has its own benefits, both fresh and dried figs are beneficial foods for **blood pressure** thanks to their high potassium levels, and are also beneficial for maintaining a good **digestive system** and improving **bone health**.

PURPLE FIGS
These figs are a good source of fiber, helping promote bowel regularity and reducing the risk of bowel cancer.

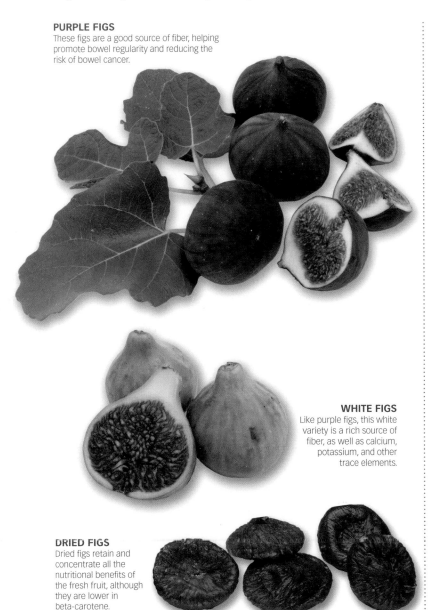

WHITE FIGS
Like purple figs, this white variety is a rich source of fiber, as well as calcium, potassium, and other trace elements.

DRIED FIGS
Dried figs retain and concentrate all the nutritional benefits of the fresh fruit, although they are lower in beta-carotene.

WHAT IS IT GOOD FOR?

BLOOD PRESSURE Fresh and dried figs contain large amounts of potassium, which is crucial for the smooth functioning of muscles and nerves, balancing fluid levels in the body, and regulating the heart rate and water balance. Figs are an ideal healthy food to eat if you have high blood pressure.

BONE HEALTH A good source of calcium, with one serving providing 10 percent of the daily recommended amount. Calcium is important in promoting the health and growth of bones. The potassium content of figs also helps reduce calcium lost through urine, meaning the body is able to absorb more calcium.

DIGESTION AND CONSTIPATION A fantastic source of fiber. Regularly including fiber in your diet is vital for maintaining a healthy digestive system, which in turn reduces the chances of constipation.

HOW DO I GET THE BEST FROM IT?

FRESH Compared to their dried counterparts, fresh figs are lower in calories and sugar. They are also higher in beta-carotene, which converts to vitamin A in the body.

DRIED Dried figs are available all year round. Compared to fresh figs, they contain more fiber, protein, calcium, potassium, magnesium, and phosphorus. They are also a great source of pectin, a form of soluble fiber, which is good for reducing blood sugar levels. They are, however, higher in calories and sugar.

HOW DO I USE IT?

AS THEY ARE Dried figs make a great sweet snack. Eat them instead of candy or chocolate, especially if you are trying to lose weight.

WITH CEREAL The health benefits of figs make them a fantastic addition to your breakfast. Adding chopped figs to granola or oatmeal is a tasty way to include them in your diet.

QUINCE

 SOOTHES STOMACH UPSETS

 CONTAINS ANTICANCER SUBSTANCES

 FIGHTS INFLAMMATION AND INFECTION

 HELPS MAINTAIN HEALTHY ARTERIES

Quince is an ancient fruit native to the Middle East that is slowly finding its place again in the modern world. It boosts the **immune system** and benefits **heart health**, while its juice is used to treat diarrhea and as a mouthwash and gargle to maintain **gum health** and treat **mouth ulcers**. This deeply fragrant fruit is too sour to be eaten raw, but cooking helps bring out its flavor and nutritional benefits.

WHAT IS IT GOOD FOR?

STOMACH SOOTHER Has an astringent quality that makes it a good general tonic for the digestive system. It is also mildly diuretic.

ANTICANCER Laboratory studies have shown the leaf and fruit contain substances that inhibit the growth of colon and kidney cancer cells.

FIGHTS FREE RADICALS Rich in antioxidant vitamins A, C, and E and unique phytonutrients, shown to have strong free-radical scavenging properties (free radicals are implicated in heart disease, diabetes, inflammatory conditions, and cancer).

HEART HEALTH Rich in potassium, which promotes a regular heartbeat and helps remove excess water from the body. Its fiber and antioxidants can contribute to healthy arteries and the regeneration of arterial walls.

HOW DO I GET THE BEST FROM IT?

BUY IN SEASON From September to November look for large firm fruits with a yellow skin. Paradoxically, for such a hard fruit, quinces can bruise easily so avoid any fruits with signs of damage or decay. Don't store for long periods, and enjoy the fragrance they impart while it lasts.

MIX WITH WATER Several laboratory studies have shown that quince steeped in hot water has an immunity-boosting effect, and may help ease symptoms of allergic dermatitis.

HOW DO I USE IT?

GOES WELL WITH APPLES Add chunks of tart quince to apple crisp, apple sauce, or apple pies to lift their texture, flavor, and aroma.

SWEETEN YOUR TEA Add a spoonful of quince jelly or preserve to green tea to sweeten, add scent, and further boost its antioxidant effect.

A VERSATILE PRESERVE Quinces are high in pectin so they make wonderful preserves.

Seeds
An extraction of the seeds produces a viscous substance, which is a traditional Middle Eastern remedy for sore throats and coughs

Leaves
Studies have shown that the leaves and fruit contain properties that can inhibit the growth of certain cancer cells

Fruit
An astringent fruit that has a general tonic effects, quince juice can be used to treat diarrhea and even as a mouthwash and gargle to maintain gum health and treat mouth ulcers

CHERRIES

 HELPS PROMOTE SLEEP

 HELPS INCREASE INSULIN PRODUCTION

 REDUCES POST-EXERCISE INFLAMMATION

 CAN HELP PREVENT GOUT

Cherries—if you pick the correct kind—can rightly be called one of today's superfoods. Montmorency cherries have the highest medicinal value because they are rich in **antioxidants**, are a good **anti-inflammatory**, and are useful in the prevention and **treatment of gout**. They are also one of very few fruits to contain melatonin, which can help treat insomnia and jetlag and can **encourage good sleep**.

DARK RED CHERRIES
Sweet cherries contain a significant amount of perillyl alcohol (POH), a chemical that may help slow or halt certain cancers.

MONTMORENCY CHERRIES
Studies show this sour, bright red variety is around 10 times more active at relieving pain than aspirin.

YELLOW AND RED CHERRIES
A very sweet variety with useful levels of vitamin C and the antioxidant beta-carotene.

WHAT IS IT GOOD FOR?

A GOOD NIGHT'S SLEEP Sour cherries are one of the few foods to contain significant amounts of melatonin, a hormone produced naturally by the body as part of our sleep–wake cycle. Studies show that a glass of sour cherry juice before bedtime can promote sound sleep.

ANTIDIABETIC Tart cherries may be useful in treating diabetes. Their abundant antioxidant anthocyanins can increase insulin production, helping regulate blood sugar levels.

ANTI-INFLAMMATORY Rich in potent antioxidants that can help fight inflammation. Drinking tart cherry juice has been shown to reduce post-exercise pain and inflammation in athletes and long-distance runners.

ARTHRITIC CONDITIONS Gout, an inflammatory condition related to arthritis, is caused by an excess accumulation of uric acid in the blood. Both sour and sweet cherries have been found to lower levels of urates in the blood, and to reduce the risk of contracting gout.

HOW DO I GET THE BEST FROM IT?

CHOOSE FRESH IN SEASON Buy organic, in season, and as local as possible for the highest nutrient content. Alternatively, pit and freeze the fresh fruits to use through the year, or choose cherry concentrates and extracts.

PICK SOUR OVER SWEET Sour cherries have higher antioxidant levels than other cherries.

HOW DO I USE IT?

DRIED CHERRIES Dried cherries can be added to cereals and yogurts.

MAKE A CHERRY PIE Cherries don't lose their medicinal value when cooked. This makes them an ideal ingredient for preserves and pies, strudels, and other desserts.

ADD TO SMOOTHIES Sweet, pitted cherries are a great addition to a fruit smoothie.

GRAPES

 HELPS REDUCE THE RISK OF CANCER

 HELPS PREVENT HARDENED ARTERIES

 HAS A MILD DIURETIC ACTION

 HELPS BALANCE BLOOD SUGAR LEVELS

For thousands of years every part of the grape plant, including the sap in the vines, has been used as medicine. Grapes, a **natural diuretic**, contain a variety of **antioxidants**, especially oligomeric proanthocyanidin complexes (OPCs), which contribute to everything from **glowing skin** to protection from **heart disease** and **free-radical damage**. OPCs are especially concentrated in grape seeds.

WHAT IS IT GOOD FOR?

ANTICANCER The high levels of flavonoids, anthocyanins, stilbenes, and many other antioxidants, especially in dark-skinned grapes, have been found to reduce the risk of cancers of the breast and prostate caused by free-radical damage. Grape antioxidant dietary fiber (GADF) also helps lower the risk of colon cancer. The seeds, in particular, are high in the antioxidant resveratrol, which has anticancer and antiaging properties.

CARDIOVASCULAR HEALTH Contains a wealth of antioxidants shown to prevent and reverse the effects of atherosclerosis (hardening of arteries). Red wine and grape juice are also high in resveratrol, which protects the heart.

DETOX AND WATER BALANCE Contains high levels of potassium and very little sodium, which encourages the body to flush out excess water and toxins.

STEADYING BLOOD SUGAR LEVELS Contains slow-release carbohydrates that assist with blood glucose control. Its antioxidant and fiber mix can also help reduce the threat of metabolic syndrome (a group of risk factors that can lead to diabetes and heart disease).

HOW DO I GET THE BEST FROM IT?

CRUNCH THE SEEDS Choose seeded varieties and eat the seeds—where OPCs, vitamin E, and linolenic acid all concentrate.

DRIED FRUIT When dried, fructose converts into a soluble fiber, fructan, which absorbs and removes cholesterol from the blood, and helps feed good bacteria in the gut.

HOW DO I USE IT?

IN A RICE DISH OR SALAD Raisins add flavor and nutrition to a rice dish, while grapes add a touch of sweetness to a green salad.

FREEZE THEM A cooling snack, frozen grapes have the same nutritional benefits as fresh.

RED GRAPES
Anthocyanins are the most abundant antioxidant in red and black grapes. They protect the heart and have anticancer properties.

Leaves
The leaves are rich in antioxidant polyphenols, beta-carotene, and vitamin K, and are a traditional remedy for pain and inflammation .

WHITE GRAPES
Flavonoid antioxidants known as catechins, which also give cocoa its medicinal power, are most abundant in white varieties.

RAISINS
Dried white grapes are an effective prebiotic, feeding good bacteria in the gut.

BLACKBERRIES

 HELPS REPAIR SUN-DAMAGED SKIN

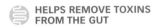 **HELPS REMOVE TOXINS FROM THE GUT**

 HELPS LOWER BLOOD PRESSURE

 CONTAINS ANTICANCER SUBSTANCES

Blackberries are high in antioxidants, of which anthocyanins are responsible for their deep purple color. Anthocyanins also fight **free-radical damage** in the body and address a range of modern conditions including **hypertension**, diabetes, cancer, vision loss, poor liver function, and **declining mental faculties**. The berries also have detoxifying properties and promote gut health.

Fruit
These berries are a source of salicylic acid, which helps lower blood pressure .....

Leaves
Reserve the leaves and brew as a tea to treat an upset stomach and boost mouth health

WHAT IS IT GOOD FOR?

SKIN HEALTH The berries are a great source of the antioxidant ellagic acid, which can help reduce damage done to skin from over-exposure to sun. Ellagic acid also prevents the breakdown of collagen, the "scaffolding" that supports firm skin and prevents inflammation.

HEALTHY GUT Contains both insoluble and soluble fiber, helpful for bowel regularity and removing toxins from the gut.

HEART PROTECTIVE Blackberries contain salicylic acid, a compound with properties similar to aspirin (also known as acetylsalicylic acid), which could help protect against heart disease and lower blood pressure.

ANTICANCER PROPERTIES Ellagic acid has been shown to stop the growth of cancer cells in laboratory tests.

HOW DO I GET THE BEST FROM IT?

FRESH IS BEST The nutrients deteriorate quickly so eat freshly picked or within a few days of purchase. Eat at room temperature.

LEAVES The leaves contain tannin and gallic acid, a natural antibiotic. Brewed in a tea, they are a traditional remedy for acute diarrhea, mouth ulcers, and bleeding gums.

HOW DO I USE IT?

ADD TO A CRISP Add to an apple crisp for added flavor and antioxidant benefits.

MAKE A VINEGAR Blackberry vinegar adds a real lift to salad dressings and marinades. Mixed with a little water, the vinegar is also a useful remedy for sore throats and a fever. Cover fresh blackberries in white wine or apple cider vinegar. Store in a cool dark place for 3 weeks. Strain the vinegar into a pan, add 2 cups superfine sugar for every 2 cups strained liquid, and boil gently for 5 minutes. Decant into sterilized, tightly sealed bottles and use within a year.

BLACKCURRANTS

HELPS REGULATE BLOOD PRESSURE

PROTECTS AGAINST NEURODEGENERATION

HELPS PROTECT AGAINST CATARACTS

FIGHTS URINARY TRACT INFECTIONS

High in vitamin C, with useful levels of **potassium** and phosphorus, blackcurrants also contain a range of different anthocyanins, **antioxidants** that protect against **heart disease**, cancer, and neurological disorders, such as **Alzheimer's disease**. The fruits also have antibacterial properties and promote **better vision**. Too sour to eat fresh on their own, they make good cordials, syrups, and jams.

WHAT IS IT GOOD FOR?

HEART HEALTH Its potassium content helps maintain a regular heartbeat, and acts as a diuretic and blood-pressure regulator. Its antioxidants also help prevent damage to blood vessel walls, which can lead to atherosclerosis (hardening of the arteries).

BRAIN FOOD Anthocyanins, which give the berries their color, help protect the brain from the free-radical damage associated with dementia and Alzheimer's disease.

BETTER NIGHT VISION Antioxidants in the fruit have been shown to improve night vision, relieve eyestrain, and help prevent cataracts.

URINARY TRACT INFECTIONS Has a similar antibacterial action to cranberries: regular consumption of the juice can help fight urinary tract infections (UTIs).

IMMUNITY-BOOSTING TONIC Its mixture of vitamin C and antioxidants is good as a general tonic to help protect and boost immunity, and heal wounds more quickly.

HOW DO I GET THE BEST FROM IT?

ADD SUGAR Turn into preserves or add the fresh fruits to other sweeter fruits in desserts.

A HEALTHY SEED OIL The oil is rich in vitamin E and several unsaturated fatty acids, such as alpha-linolenic acid and gamma-linolenic acid. Regular consumption may help skin conditions, such as eczema and dermatitis.

USE THE LEAVES A tea made from the leaves can be used to treat coughs and sore throats.

HOW DO I USE IT?

SYRUP Turn the fruit into a sweet syrup or cordial, which retains its antioxidants and other immunity-boosting phytochemicals.

TEA Add a small handful of leaves to a teapot, cover with boiling water, leave to infuse for a few minutes, strain, and drink as required.

Fruit
Weight-for-weight, blackcurrants contain three times as much vitamin C as oranges. Too sour to eat raw, make them into sweetened cordials to enjoy their benefits ......

Leaves
Add the leaves to boiling water to make a tea that can help treat coughs and sore throats

BLUEBERRIES

 SLOWS THE GROWTH OF PROSTATE CANCER

 HELPS PREVENT COGNITIVE DECLINE

 EFFECTIVE AGAINST GASTROENTERITIS

 HELPS PROTECT EYE HEALTH

Native to North America, blueberries have long been valued for their nutritional and medicinal properties. They contain **antibacterial** compounds that fight off stomach bugs and **antioxidants** to **prevent eye damage** and improve both **eyesight** and **memory**. They also promote **prostate health**. Much sweeter than many small berries, they can be eaten fresh on their own to reap all the benefits.

Berries
Studies show that blueberries have some of the highest levels of active antioxidants per serving of any food

Leaves
Tea made from the leaves can be used to prevent urinary tract infections and regulate blood sugar levels

WHAT IS IT GOOD FOR?

PROSTATE HEALTH A rich source of concentrated proanthocyanidin compounds, which can slow the growth and spread of various cancers. Recent laboratory studies show that blueberry extract also significantly slows the growth of prostate-cancer cells.

IMPROVED MEMORY It may have a positive effect on the nervous system. Also studies show it can increase levels of dopamine—a vital neurotransmitter—thus improving memory. May also alleviate cognitive decline.

HEALTHY GUT Contains anthocyanins, antibacterial antioxidants effective against causes of gastroenteritis, such as *E. coli*. Also combats the bacteria that cause diarrhea.

SUPPORTING VISION Anthocyanins can help improve eye health by protecting against retinal degeneration. They may also help prevent the eye condition glaucoma because of their collagen-enhancing properties.

URINARY TRACT INFECTIONS Recent studies confirm its usefulness in treating urinary tract infections (UTIs).

HOW DO I GET THE BEST FROM IT?

BUY ORGANIC Blueberries belong to a "dirty dozen" list of fruits that generally have the most pesticide residues. Eating organic is the only way to avoid chemical contamination.

LEAVES The leaves contain similar levels of antioxidants to that of the fruit. Use to prevent UTIs and regulate blood sugar levels.

HOW DO I USE IT?

FOR BREAKFAST Add to cereal or yogurt, or freeze to preserve them for longer and include them in a breakfast shake or smoothie.

LEAF TEA Pour boiling water on the leaves, infuse, strain, and drink as a tea that contains antibacterial and hypoglycemic properties.

To *freeze blueberries,* spread them in a single layer on a large baking pan, and place in the freezer overnight. When completely frozen, transfer the berries to a freezer bag; force as much air out of the bag as possible. Return to the freezer for storage.

CRANBERRIES

 FIGHTS URINARY TRACT INFECTIONS

 HELPS FIGHT GUM DISEASE

HELPS ALLEVIATE HEAVY PERIODS

HELPS PREVENT STOMACH ULCERS

Native to North America, these rather sour red berries are packed with **antioxidants** and have a number of health benefits. They are both **astringent** and **antibacterial**, helping, among other things, to promote good **gum health**. Beyond that they contain a unique substance that helps prevent infections from taking hold in the urinary tract, kidney, and bladder.

Fruit
Cranberries were used by Native American People to treat bladder and kidney infections

Juice
To get the best from cranberry juice, look for brands low in sugar

Dried cranberries
Adding the dried fruit to cereals and granola is a simple way to include more antioxidants in your diet

WHAT IS IT GOOD FOR?

URINARY TRACT INFECTIONS Contains nondialyzable material (NDM) that prevents infections of the urinary tract (UTIs), bladder, and even kidneys.

PROTECTING TEETH The antioxidant proanthocyanidin, which gives the berries their bright red color, can inhibit enzymes associated with the buildup of plaque, acid formation in teeth, and receding gums.

TONING AND ASTRINGENT Its astringent and slightly antiseptic nature helps alleviate heavy periods, diarrhea, upset stomachs, sore throats, and laryngitis.

DIGESTION Preliminary research suggests that NDM may also prevent *Helicobacter pylori* bacteria from attaching to stomach walls, giving it a useful role in preventing ulcers.

HEALTHY HEART Its high vitamin C and anti-inflammatory antioxidant content can protect against inflammation and heart disease by reducing oxidative stress caused by free radicals in the body.

HOW DO I GET THE BEST FROM IT?

JUICE Fresh cranberry juice gives you the overall benefits of the fruit. Sugar feeds bacteria that can cause urinary tract infections in the first place, so look for unsweetened, varieties. Better yet, juice the berries yourself.

DRIED Eat the dried berries to enjoy most of the fruit's benefits throughout the year. Only the vitamin C content is heavily diminished.

HOW DO I USE IT?

MAKE A TEA Add 1 heaped tsp dried berries to 2 cups water in a pan. Simmer over low heat for 10–15 minutes, strain, and drink.

IN BETWEEN BRUSHING Chew dried berries thoroughly to release their gum-protecting properties and to give gums a gentle massage.

ELDERBERRIES

 HELPS FIGHT COLDS AND THE FLU

 HAS A MILD DIURETIC ACTION

Elderberries are the fruit of a woodland tree common throughout Europe, North America, and Asia. It was once regarded as a **complete medicine chest** because all parts of the plant can be used medicinally. The fruits and flowers, most commonly consumed today, have **immunity-boosting** and **diuretic effects**. The raw berries are an acquired taste, but cooking makes them more palatable.

WHAT IS IT GOOD FOR?

STRENGTHENING IMMUNITY The flowers are a traditional remedy for relieving lung congestion. They promote sweating and can cool fevers, and are also anti-inflammatory. Syrup made from the berries is a well-proven way to boost immunity at any time, but especially in winter against colds and flu.

DETOX The fruits are known to have a mild diuretic and laxative action.

HOW DO I GET THE BEST FROM IT?

PRESERVE THE FRUITS Raw elderberries are too sour for some tastes. Turning them into jams, preserves, compotes, and syrups is the best way to get the most benefit from them.

FLOWERS The flowers can be used to make everything from a lightly sparkling elderflower "champagne" to a useful gargle to soothe sore throats. Chemicals in the flowers may also help to reduce swelling in mucous membranes in the sinuses.

HOW DO I USE IT?

A HEALING SYRUP Add 2 cups strained juice from the berries to 1 cup honey and mix together well. For colds and flu, take 2 tsp as needed.

ELDERFLOWER TEA Add 2–4 fresh flower heads (or 2 tsp dried herb per cup) to a teapot, add boiling water, leave to infuse for a few minutes, strain, and drink as a tea to fight coughs and congestion.

MAKE A CORDIAL Place 2lb (900g) berries in a pan with 1 cup water. Simmer over low heat until the berries release their juice. Crush and strain, reserve the juice, and return to the pan with 1 cup superfine sugar and a 1in (2.5cm) piece of fresh ginger, grated (optional). Simmer for 1 hour. Strain and store in a tightly sealed sterilized bottle and chill. Use within 3 months. To drink, dilute to taste.

BERRIES
Elderberries get their color from antioxidant flavonoids that help prevent damage to the body's cells.

FLOWERS
The flowers (and berries) may help relieve nasal congestion.

GOJI BERRIES

 HELPS MAINTAIN MUSCLE STRENGTH

 SUPPLIES OXYGEN TO CELLS

 HELPS PROMOTE PEACEFUL SLEEP

 PROTECTS EYES FROM FREE-RADICAL DAMAGE

These berries belong to the broader nightshade family that includes chile peppers and tomatoes. Also called wolfberries, they are rich in a combination of **antioxidant** nutrients that benefit **cardiovascular health**, muscle health, and vision. They also contain a variety of **carotenoids**, including beta-carotene, known to boost **metabolic processes** and promote **good sleep** and **memory**.

FRESH WOLFBERRIES
Wolfberries don't store or travel well, which is why they are eaten dried as goji berries.

DRIED GOJI BERRIES
The antiaging effects attributed to goji berries are due to their high antioxidant capacity.

WHAT IS IT GOOD FOR?

MUSCLE HEALTH Contains betaine, a nutrient that helps build muscle, and beta-sitosterol, which helps prevent the inflammation that causes sore muscles.

METABOLIC SUPPORT Pyridoxine (vitamin B_6) is involved in numerous metabolic processes, aids the production of energy, and boosts the oxygen-carrying capacity of red blood cells. One serving of the berries contains nearly half the daily requirement of pyridoxine.

NEUROLOGICAL SUPPORT Betaine, used by the liver to produce choline, helps to soothe nerves, promote restful sleep, and has a role to play in enhancing memory.

VISION Abundant in lutein and zeaxanthin, antioxidants that have a proven ability to protect and maintain eye health.

ANTIOXIDANT BOOST Contains around 10 times the antioxidant capacity of blueberries, contributing to cardiovascular- and immune-system health. It may also protect against degenerative and inflammatory diseases, such as diabetes and arthritis. Its high antioxidant levels also mean it is a healthy skin food.

HOW DO I GET THE BEST FROM IT?

DRIED Wolfberries deteriorate quickly once harvested. Dehydrating them preserves their nutritional benefits. Choose sulfite-free organic varieties to ensure a low toxic load.

JUICE Choose goji berry juice if you don't enjoy the dried fruit: it contains all the health benefits of the dried fruit except the fiber.

HOW DO I USE IT?

AS THEY ARE Eat as a snack during the day to boost energy or satisfy cravings.

BREAKFAST FRUIT Soak in water and add to granola, oatmeal, fruit, yogurt, and smoothies, or add to home-baked breakfast bars.

MULBERRIES

⚡ **HELPS RESTORE VITALITY**

◉ **RELIEVES TIRED EYES**

◯ **SOOTHES NERVES, PROMOTES SLEEP**

☰ **HELPS EASE BLOATING AND CONSTIPATION**

Mulberries are an ancient fruit with a long tradition of use as a medicine, including as a **tonic** for the whole body. All parts of the plant, from root to tip, can be used medicinally, though these days we tend to concentrate only on the fruit and leaves, which are high in **antioxidant** anthocyanins and **cancer-fighting** resveratrol and vitamin C. They also protect against **eye damage** and act as a **sedative**.

WHAT IS IT GOOD FOR?

STRENGTHENING TONIC Can be used as a general tonic to restore vitality. The berries contain a useful amount of iron to benefit the kidneys, liver, and blood, and also resveratrol (also found in grape seeds), which has anticancer properties. Their high antioxidant content helps prevent heart disease and diseases associated with chronic inflammation.

EYE HEALTH The fruit and leaves contain zeaxanthin, which helps protect eyesight. Traditionally, mulberry was used to combat "dry conditions," such as dry skin and eczema, and a dry mouth and throat; its moistening properties can ease dry, strained eyes.

SEDATIVE A tea made from the fresh fruit or a teaspoon of the fruit preserve steeped in water is a traditional remedy for insomnia.

DIGESTIVE HEALTH Strengthens the digestive tract and can ease bloating and constipation.

LOWERS FEVERS A cooling food, it can be useful for treating fevers and heatstroke.

HOW DO I GET THE BEST FROM IT?

EAT DRIED Fresh mulberries don't store well, so enjoy their benefits in dried form—a good substitute for raisins.

MAKE A TEA FROM THE LEAVES The leaves, harvested after the first frosts of the fall season, have antibacterial properties.

BE GENTLE Picked fresh from the tree, the berries are a healthful treat, but they are more fragile than other berries so pick carefully.

HOW DO I USE IT?

ADD THE LEAVES TO A SALAD The young, tender leaves can be eaten raw in salads.

MAKE A JAM The berries are high in pectin and so make an excellent jam.

A NATURAL SWEETENER Add dried berries to regular or green tea to gain extra nutrients.

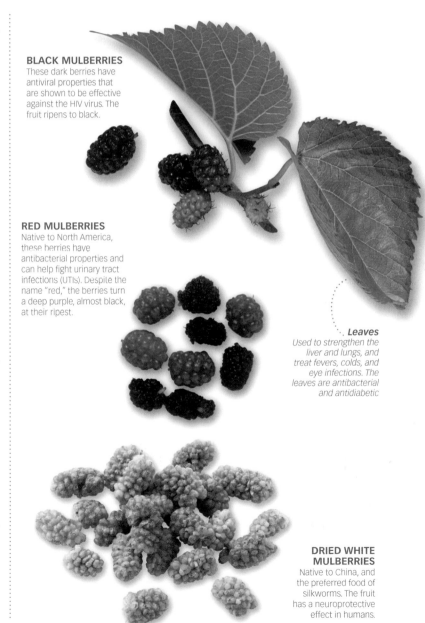

BLACK MULBERRIES
These dark berries have antiviral properties that are shown to be effective against the HIV virus. The fruit ripens to black.

RED MULBERRIES
Native to North America, these berries have antibacterial properties and can help fight urinary tract infections (UTIs). Despite the name "red," the berries turn a deep purple, almost black, at their ripest.

Leaves
Used to strengthen the liver and lungs, and treat fevers, colds, and eye infections. The leaves are antibacterial and antidiabetic

DRIED WHITE MULBERRIES
Native to China, and the preferred food of silkworms. The fruit has a neuroprotective effect in humans.

RASPBERRIES

 MINIMIZES THE ABSORPTION OF FAT

 HELPS TONE THE UTERUS

 CONTAINS CANCER-FIGHTING SUBSTANCES

Recent studies confirm that raspberries contain a vast array of **antioxidants** with a host of potential benefits in **regulating metabolism** and **fighting diseases**. One of these antioxidants is the anti-inflammatory compound, ellagic acid, which is **cancer-protective**. The leaves can be used medicinally as a **tonic in pregnancy**, and in particular, preparing the uterus for a birth.

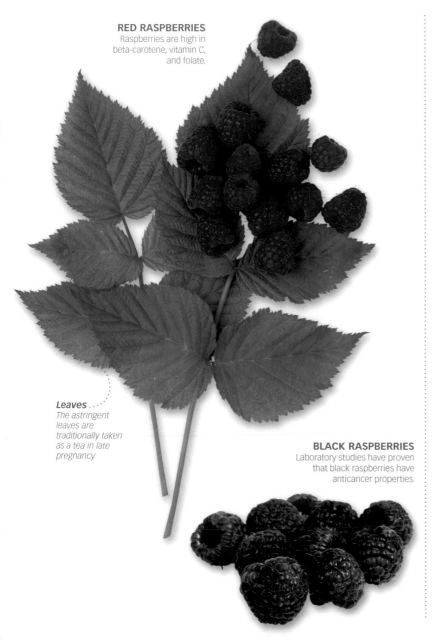

RED RASPBERRIES
Raspberries are high in beta-carotene, vitamin C, and folate.

Leaves
The astringent leaves are traditionally taken as a tea in late pregnancy

BLACK RASPBERRIES
Laboratory studies have proven that black raspberries have anticancer properties.

WHAT IS IT GOOD FOR?

METABOLIC AID Preliminary research suggests rheosmin, a phenolic compound, can suppress the digestion and absorption of fat, and stimulate the metabolism. Another compound, tiliroside, has a similar action, and may also help regulate blood sugar levels.

PREGNANCY AID The leaves are rich in tannins that may help tone and strengthen the uterus. However, only drink raspberry leaf tea during the last two months of pregnancy.

CANCER FIGHTER Phytonutrients in red and black berries may inhibit the development of certain cancers. Particular studies have focused on the potential of black raspberries to protect against DNA mutations and inhibit the growth of tumors. In laboratory tests, black raspberries have halted the development of esophageal and colon cancer. The anti-inflammatory compound, ellagic acid, which is cancer-protective, may also help with bowel conditions.

HOW DO I GET THE BEST FROM IT?

EAT ORGANIC Recent research on organic raspberries has shown the organic fruits to be significantly higher in their total antioxidant capacity than nonorganic berries.

MAKE SURE THEY ARE RIPE Studies show that fully ripe raspberries contain significantly more antioxidants than unripe fruits.

HOW DO I USE IT?

MAKE A JAM Extend the short season of raspberries by preserving them as jam.

MAKE A LEAF TEA Put 1 tsp dried leaves (or 2 tsp fresh) per ⅔ cup water in a teapot, cover with boiling water, leave to infuse for 10 minutes, strain, and drink as required. Raspberry leaf tea should only be drunk in the last 2 months of pregnancy; avoid it completely in the first 2 trimesters.

STRAWBERRIES

 HELPS PREVENT BLOOD VESSEL DAMAGE

 SOOTHES UPSET STOMACHS

 CONTAINS ANTICANCER SUBSTANCES

Fresh strawberries are a high **antioxidant** food. As well as being a rich source of **vitamin C**, they contain manganese, folate, potassium, B vitamins, and the beneficial **flavonoids**, quercetin and kaempferol. In addition, they have **heart-healthy** properties, benefit the **digestive system**, and are the only fruit to have seeds—a source of small amounts of omega-3 fatty acids—on their exterior.

WHAT IS IT GOOD FOR?

HEART HEALTH Apart from vitamin C, the berries are rich in quercetin and kaempferol, both of which can prevent "unhealthy" (LDL) cholesterol in the blood from oxidizing and damaging artery walls (atherosclerosis).

DIGESTION A tea made from the leaves is a traditional remedy to soothe acid indigestion. Fiber in the fruit can aid a sluggish bowel.

ANTICANCER Contains the antioxidant compound ellagic acid that scavenges for, binds to, and helps neutralize cancer-causing chemicals in the body.

HOW DO I GET THE BEST FROM IT?

EAT SEASONALLY Strawberries are grown all over the world and are available through the year, but they do not store well and quickly lose their nutrients once picked. They are most delicious and nutritious when eaten fresh in season.

GO ORGANIC Most strawberries are treated with high amounts of pesticides and fungicides. Eating organic is the only way to avoid this chemical contamination.

HOW DO I USE IT?

STRAWBERRY AND CUCUMBER SALAD Try this unusual and detoxifying combination: hull and halve 1lb (450g) strawberries and cut 1 cucumber into thin slices. Toss in a bowl and season with freshly ground black pepper (which brings out the flavor of the strawberries). Blueberries make a nice additional ingredient so add a few, if you like.

MAKE A TEA Stomach-soothing strawberry tea is best made from just-picked young strawberry leaves. Place a handful of fresh leaves in a teapot. Cover with boiling water and allow to steep for 5 minutes. Add honey, if you like, strain, and serve. If fresh leaves aren't available, use dried.

Leaves
Fresh or dried strawberry leaves can be used to make a tea that can soothe upset stomachs

Berries
Nutrients in strawberries help prevent cholesterol from damaging artery walls

CITRUS FRUITS

🫁 **HELPS PREVENT KIDNEY STONES**   ❤ **HELPS LOWER CHOLESTEROL**   ⬚ **AIDS HEALTHY DIGESTION**   ✺ **HELPS REMOVE ACCUMULATED TOXINS**

This family of juicy fruits not only includes lemons, limes, oranges, and grapefruit, but also tangerines, mandarins, and less widely eaten fruits, such as pomellos and kumquats. Their **vitamin C** content is legendary, and regular consumption can help reduce the risk of **heart disease**, **kidney stones**, and **infections** of all kinds. They also boost **good digestion** and have alkalizing and **detoxifying** properties.

LEMONS
Lemons have antibacterial properties proven to fight the Vibrio species of bacteria, responsible for cholera.

LIMES
The vitamin K in limes is essential for healthy blood clotting.

ORANGES
Orange juice may help prevent kidney stones (calcium oxalate stone formation).

GRAPEFRUITS
High in vitamin C, these fruits can help reduce the severity of inflammatory conditions, such as asthma.

WHAT IS IT GOOD FOR?

KIDNEY STONES Lemons have the highest concentration of citrate; consuming dilute lemon juice or unsweetened lemonade daily has been shown to decrease the rate of stone formation. Orange juice may also help.

HEART HEALTH Contain hesperidin, which can reduce symptoms of hypertension, and pectin (fiber) and limonoid compounds, which can slow atherosclerosis (hardening of the arteries) and reduce "unhealthy" (LDL) cholesterol in the blood. Antioxidant flavones can also lower the risk of strokes in women.

RELIEVES INDIGESTION Mixed with hot water, lemon juice can relieve heartburn, nausea, acid indigestion, and stomach aches. It may also have an antiparasitic effect.

ALKALIZING AND DETOXIFYING Lemons are a natural diuretic and can help reduce swelling, inflammation, and edema (water retention). Also antibacterial, they flush out the bacteria that cause urinary tract infections (UTIs).

HOW DO I GET THE BEST FROM IT?

USE THE PEEL Citrus peel is full of beneficial antioxidants and has a high concentration of the fruit's limonoids. Modern science shows citrus peel fights free radicals, balances blood sugar levels, and supports thyroid health.

FOOD SYNERGY The vitamin C in citrus fruits helps the body absorb non-heme iron, a form of iron from plant sources, such as vegetables.

HOW DO I USE IT?

A JEWELED SALAD Chop the fruit of 5 large peeled oranges and place in a bowl. Add the seeds of 1 pomegranate and its juice. Add the juice of 1 orange, 3 tbsp olive oil, chopped fresh mint, and pepper, and mix gently.

MIX WITH WATER Start the day with a glass of warm water and lemon juice to alkalize and cleanse your system.

BANANAS

 HELPS STRENGTHEN BONES

 PROTECTS AGAINST ULCERS

 CONTAINS SLOW-RELEASE SUGARS

LOWERS RISK OF HEART DISEASE AND STROKE

Bananas are an extremely versatile and healthy fruit. They are **rich in potassium**, which is essential for **maintaining blood pressure** at healthy levels, and are **natural antacids**, which makes them a soothing and healing choice for **upset stomachs** and **ulcers**. The ripe fruit consists of nearly 90 percent natural **slow-release sugars**—ideal for athletes and busy people alike.

WHAT IS IT GOOD FOR?

BONE HEALTH Its potassium content slows the urinary calcium loss associated with a modern diet that is high in salt. Also contains prebiotic compounds that feed good bacteria in the gut. A healthy gut increases the body's ability to absorb key nutrients such as calcium, which is crucial for bone health.

SOOTHING THE STOMACH Has antacid effects that protect the stomach from ulcers. Also helps activate cells that build the stomach lining, and eliminates the bacteria that cause stomach ulcers. These antacid effects are also good for easing heartburn.

ENERGY BOOSTER The fruit contains both quick-release glucose and slow-release fructose, so it supplies energy in 2 ways.

CARDIOVASCULAR HEALTH An extremely good source of potassium and fiber. Studies show that potassium- and fiber-rich diets reduce the risk of stroke and heart disease. Potassium is also essential for the maintenance of a healthy level of blood pressure.

FOR CONSTIPATION Its high fiber content helps bowel regularity and eases constipation.

HOW DO I GET THE BEST FROM IT?

EAT RIPE FRUIT To get the most antioxidants, eat when the skin is yellow with a few brown or black spots, and the flesh is ripe, almost to the point of spoilage.

HOW DO I USE IT?

IN THE BLENDER Banana works well with many flavors and helps to thicken the texture, so it is a good base for a fruit smoothie.

TO SWEETEN CEREALS Add to your cereal or oatmeal as a natural sweetener and as an extra source of fiber.

A FROZEN TREAT Bananas can be frozen and eaten as an alternative to ice pops, or puréed and served as an alternative to ice cream.

FRUIT
The potassium in bananas lowers blood pressure and insures against brittle bones.

Heart
Like an artichoke, the outer bracts (leaves) and flowers are removed to reveal a pale, edible heart.

FLOWER
In some Asian cuisines, the flower (or inflorescence) is eaten both cooked and raw. It is high in vitamin C and beta-carotene and is a traditional remedy for menstrual cramps.

DATES

 PROMOTES BOWEL REGULARITY

 CONTAINS SLOW-RELEASE SUGARS

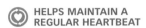 **HELPS MAINTAIN A REGULAR HEARTBEAT**

 SOOTHES COUGHS AND SORE THROATS

The date palm, one of the oldest trees cultivated by man, has its origins in the desert around the Persian Gulf. **Immunity-boosting** dates are high in **potassium**, supply **slow-release sugars**, and provide a range of other **essential nutrients**, for example, they are a **good source of fiber**, protein, **minerals** including magnesium, manganese, selenium, and zinc, and trace elements, such as boron.

FRESH DATES
When ripe, the berries of the date palm tree are sweet and have the texture of a firm pear.

SEMIDRIED DATES
Semidried dates are not as sweet as dried dates, but retain all the gut-friendly fiber and nutrients.

DRIED DATES
These dates provide all the benefits of the fresh berries in a concentrated form.

WHAT IS IT GOOD FOR?

SUPPORTING DIGESTION A great source of soluble and insoluble fiber, aiding digestion and promoting bowel regularity. Also contains tannins, which have an astringent quality that is useful for treating stomach upsets and intestinal troubles.

BALANCING BLOOD SUGAR High in sugar, dates still defy the dogma that all sugar is bad. Their sugar is released slowly, so they benefit blood sugar control. Their soluble fiber content also aids blood glucose regulation.

HEART HEALTHY A very good source of potassium, an essential mineral that maintains proper muscle contractions, including those of the heart. Potassium also promotes a healthy nervous system and efficient metabolism by the body. The soluble fiber in dates also helps to lower "unhealthy" (LDL) cholesterol levels in blood.

COLDS AND FLU As an infusion, extract, syrup, or paste, dates are a traditional remedy for sore throats, colds, and bronchial catarrh.

HOW DO I GET THE BEST FROM IT?

DRIED The drying process concentrates all the nutrients so just a few dates will supply good amounts of nutrients and fiber. Look for dates that have not been treated with sulfites.

FRESH Fresh dates are usually only available for a few weeks in late summer, often from specialty supermarkets. They contain much more vitamin C than the dried fruit.

HOW DO I USE IT?

IN CEREALS AND BREADS Adding chopped dates to granola makes a great healthy breakfast. Dates are also a staple ingredient of sweet loaves, such as date and nut bread.

A SWEET SUBSTITUTE Dates are a delicious, sweet yet healthy snack, and can be eaten as a replacement for candy or chocolate.

MANGOES

 FEEDS GOOD BACTERIA IN THE GUT

 CONTAINS ANTICANCER SUBSTANCES

 HELPS PROTECT EYE HEALTH

 PROTECTS AGAINST COLDS AND FLU

Throughout Asia, the mango has both spiritual and medicinal significance. It is the national fruit of India, Pakistan, and the Philippines, and the national tree of Bangladesh. Mangoes are high in the antioxidants **beta-carotene** and **vitamin C**, and so are good for boosting the **immune system**, protecting **eyesight**, and aiding **digestion**. They also help neutralize **free-radical damage** in the body.

WHAT IS IT GOOD FOR?

DIGESTION Contains enzymes that aid the breakdown and digestion of protein, and also fiber, which keeps the digestive tract working efficiently. Dietary fiber has more long-term benefits as well, lowering the risk of developing colon cancer, heart disease, type-2 diabetes, and diverticular disease.

ANTICANCER EFFECTS Laboratory tests show the triterpene compound, lupeol, a kind of plant hormone found in mangoes, is effective against both prostate and skin cancers.

EYE HEALTH Rich in beta-carotene, a powerful antioxidant that helps reduce the effects of free-radical damage in the body, including the skin and eyes. It also helps prevent age-related macular degeneration (loss of vision).

IMMUNITY An average-sized mango contains up to two-thirds of the daily recommended intake of vitamin C, which plays a key role in boosting the immune system and so helps reduce the incidence of colds and flu.

HOW DO I GET THE BEST FROM IT?

KEEP IT FRESH Eat as fresh as possible. Mangoes bruise easily, so unless you are using them immediately, buy hard fruits and let them ripen at home. When you can't find fresh, dried mango is a good substitute.

ADD DAIRY Studies suggest the bioavailability of beta-carotene in the fruit improves by 19–38 percent if combined with a little dairy.

HOW DO I USE IT?

QUICK MANGO SMOOTHIE Blend 2 peeled, chopped mangoes, 1 cup cold milk or yogurt, and 1½ tbsp honey, until smooth.

MANGO SALSA Dice and mix 1 ripe mango, ½ red onion, ½ sweet red bell pepper, 1 small cucumber, 1 small finely chopped jalapeño chile, and 3 tbsp each lime juice and chopped fresh cilantro. Season and serve with fish.

Mango flesh
Contains prebiotic dietary fiber, which helps feed good bacteria in the gut

Green mango
In Southeast Asia, green mango is used shredded in salads. Green mangoes have more vitamin C and more pectin than ripe mangoes, but have a very sour taste

MELONS

 HELPS PROTECT EYE HEALTH

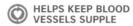 **HELPS KEEP BLOOD VESSELS SUPPLE**

 HELPS SPEED WOUND HEALING

Aromatic melons are, perhaps surprisingly, members of the gourd family, which includes cucumber and squash. They were first cultivated in Persia and northern Africa nearly 4,000 years ago, and later by ancient Greeks and Romans. Rich in **beta-carotene**, **vitamin C**, and assorted **antioxidants**, they are good for **immune support**. They also contain potassium, which normalizes **blood pressure**.

HONEYDEW
It has the highest sugar content of any melon, but also contains vitamin C, folate, and potassium.

WATERMELON
Red-fleshed watermelon is a rich source of the plant pigment lycopene, which helps lower the risk of heart disease.

CANTALOUPE
This is the most nutrient-dense melon: a single serving provides around half your daily vitamin C and A needs.

WHAT IS IT GOOD FOR?

EYESIGHT Melons derive their bright color from the antioxidant beta-carotene, important for skin and bone health and for preventing age-related macular degeneration (loss of vision). Cantaloupes also contain lutein and zeaxanthin, which are good for eye health.

BLOOD FLOW Citrulline, an amino acid in the rind and flesh of watermelon, can stimulate the production of nitric oxide, which relaxes and expands blood vessels, lowering blood pressure and enhancing blood flow.

BLOOD PRESSURE Contains a useful amount of potassium, a natural diuretic that helps to normalize blood pressure. Watermelons are rich in lycopene, which helps lower the risk of heart disease.

WOUND HEALING The citrulline in watermelon plays a role in the production of the amino acid arginine, which boosts immune function and speeds wound healing.

HOW DO I GET THE BEST FROM IT?

DETOX Melons are an excellent food for light detox days. Their water content (around 95 percent) is highly mineralized, and has an alkalizing and diuretic effect.

GENTLE ON YOUR TUMMY Easy to digest, it also provides useful carbohydrates for energy.

EAT THE SEEDS The dried seeds contain healthy unsaturated fats and fiber, and make a nutritious addition to savory dishes.

HOW DO I USE IT?

SPICE UP YOUR CANTALOUPE Sprinkle a little freshly ground black pepper onto cantaloupe slices to enhance their flavor.

RAINBOW SALAD Slice watermelon, kiwi, and soft goat cheese into cubes, serve on bed of arugula or watercress, dress with balsamic vinegar, and scatter with sesame seeds.

PAPAYA

CONTAINS NATURAL DIGESTIVE ENZYMES

HELPS FIGHT INFECTIONS

HELPS LOWER CHOLESTEROL

REDUCES CATARACT AND GLAUCOMA RISK

Also called paw paw or tree melon, papaya has become a commercial crop that is now widely available. It is known to have **antibacterial** properties and promotes good **digestion**, and almost every part of the plant can be used. In the West, we tend to focus only on its brightly colored orange flesh, which is a good source of **antioxidant** carotenoids, such as **beta-carotene**, that protect **eyesight**.

WHAT IS IT GOOD FOR?

DIGESTION Contains the enzymes papain and chymonpapain. Both have been shown to aid digestion, prevent constipation, and, in combination with the fruit's natural fiber, cleanse the colon. Papain is also helpful in healing and preventing stomach ulcers.

FIGHTS "BUGS" The seeds are effective against salmonella, *E. coli*, and staphylococcus infections. They can be used to support liver function and have an antiparasitic function, which helps rid the body of intestinal parasites.

HEALTHY FIBER Its natural fiber helps control blood pressure and regulate levels of "unhealthy" (LDL) cholesterol in the blood. Its dietary fiber is also important in preventing diseases, such as bowel cancer.

EYE HEALTH The beta-carotene and vitamins C and E in papaya help reduce the risk of cataracts, glaucoma, and age-related macular degeneration (loss of vision).

HOW DO I GET THE BEST FROM IT?

DON'T THROW THE SEEDS AWAY The seeds are edible either fresh or dried. They have a peppery flavor and can be used in cooking.

JUICE IT Papaya juice helps restore the good bacteria in the stomach, which is especially important after an illness or taking antibiotics.

GO GREEN Papain, a beneficial digestive enzyme, is found in greatest abundance in green, unripe papayas.

HOW DO I USE IT?

MAKE A CHUTNEY To benefit from the high concentration of papain in unripe papaya, make a spicy chutney for meats and cheeses.

SHRIMP AND PAPAYA Arrange cooked large shrimp and papaya slices on a bed of lettuce. Drizzle with a dressing of walnut oil, lime juice, Dijon mustard, honey, salt, and pepper.

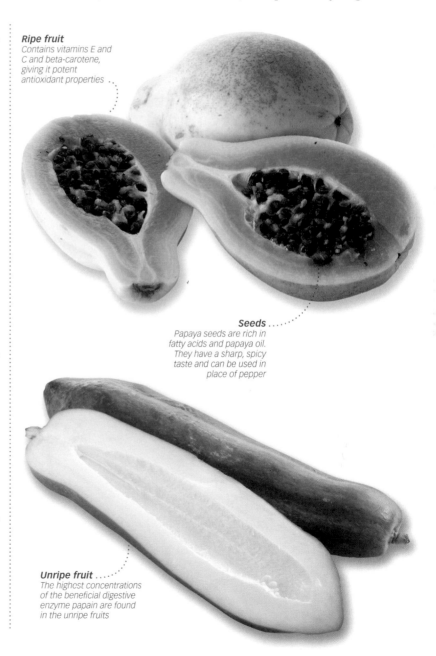

Ripe fruit
Contains vitamins E and C and beta-carotene, giving it potent antioxidant properties

Seeds
Papaya seeds are rich in fatty acids and papaya oil. They have a sharp, spicy taste and can be used in place of pepper

Unripe fruit
The highest concentrations of the beneficial digestive enzyme papain are found in the unripe fruits

POMEGRANATE

 REDUCES THE RISK OF PROSTATE CANCER

 HELPS KEEP BLOOD VESSELS SUPPLE

BLOCKS ENZYMES THAT DESTROY CARTILAGE

 PROVIDES ANTIVIRAL PROTECTION

Native to modern-day Iran and Iraq, pomegranate has been used as a folk medicine for thousands of years. The juice contains substances that support a **healthy prostate** and **antioxidants** to maintain the elasticity of the **arteries**. All parts of the plant are used as medicine in the Ayurvedic traditions; in the West, the arils (seeds) and their juice are most valued for their **antiviral** and **antibacterial** properties.

Seeds
Oil from the seeds contains isoflavones similar to those found in soy

Rind
Pomegranate rind is used in many medicinal traditions for making teas and gargles. Recent studies show it contains chemicals that are antibiotic and have cancer-fighting properties

WHAT IS IT GOOD FOR?

MEN'S HEALTH Drinking a glass of the juice every day has been shown to lower levels of prostate-specific antigen (PSA) in men. (The higher a man's PSA level is, the greater his risk of death from prostate cancer.)

HEART PROTECTIVE Its polyphenol compounds keep arteries elastic and so help lower blood pressure and the risk of heart disease and stroke. It also stops free radicals from oxidizing "unhealthy" (LDL) cholesterol in the blood and causing plaque to build up on artery walls (atherosclerosis).

JOINT HEALTH Antioxidant flavonols have been shown to significantly reduce the activity of proteins that cause inflammatory conditions, such as arthritis. Preliminary studies show that pomegranate extract (equivalent to one glass of juice) can block the production of an enzyme that destroys cartilage in the body.

FIGHTS INFECTION The juice has antiviral properties, and studies show that extracts of the fruit are effective against dental plaque.

HOW DO I GET THE BEST FROM IT?

EAT THE SEEDS The fruit is a high-fiber food, but only if you eat the seeds, which also contain unsaturated fats, beneficial isoflavones (plant hormones similar to those found in soy), and other micronutrients.

POMEGRANATE MOLASSES This concentrated form of the syrup contains all the nutritional values of pomegranate.

HOW DO I USE IT?

AS A "VINEGAR" Pomegranate molasses is a delicious substitute for balsamic vinegar in dressings, marinades, and glazes.

SUPERFRUIT SALAD Combine pomegranate seeds with pear, pineapple, and orange segments, chopped fresh mint, and lettuce. Drizzle with a honey-sweetened dressing.

A **drizzle of** pomegranate molasses brings a tangy, sweet-sour flavor and an antioxidant boost to a simple salad dressing of olive oil, lemon, and black pepper.

PINEAPPLE

 EASES SYMPTOMS OF INFLAMMATORY BOWEL

 ENHANCES SPERM QUALITY

 SPEEDS RECOVERY FROM SPORTS INJURIES

Thirst-quenching and cooling, pineapple is a good source of **manganese**, which can boost men's fertility, and contains significant amounts of **vitamin C**. The core contains the proteolytic enzyme bromelain, a powerful **anti-inflammatory** used to treat bowel and joint problems. Its anti-inflammatory and **astringent** quality makes it a good choice for **treating sore throats**.

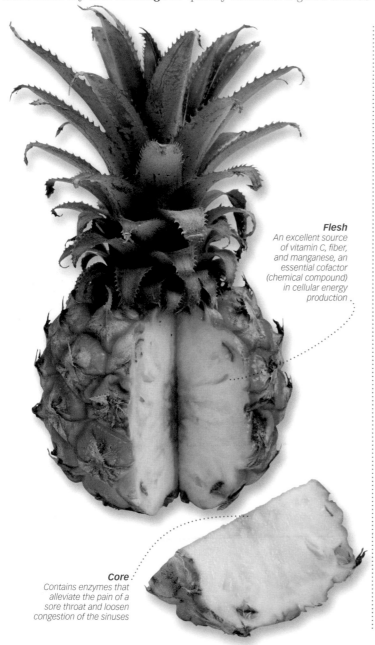

Flesh
An excellent source of vitamin C, fiber, and manganese, an essential cofactor (chemical compound) in cellular energy production

Core
Contains enzymes that alleviate the pain of a sore throat and loosen congestion of the sinuses

WHAT IS IT GOOD FOR?

INFLAMMATORY BOWEL The juice can ease the symptoms of colitis, an inflammatory bowel condition marked by abdominal pain and bloating, diarrhea, wind, and dehydration. Most bromelain is concentrated in the core and stem. However, researchers have found that the juice provides enough of the enzyme to have a medicinal effect.

MEN'S FERTILITY Its high manganese content helps restore vitality and can help boost fertility by improving sperm motility.

STAYING FLEXIBLE Bromelain has shown promise in treating and preventing inflammatory conditions, such as arthritis, and may facilitate recovery after sports injuries.

DIGESTION Bromelain extract is an effective digestive aid, while using the juice as a marinade for meat dishes helps tenderize them, making them more easily digestible.

HOW DO I GET THE BEST FROM IT?

FRESH IS BEST The nutrients and enzymes disappear quickly once cut or cooked. When ripe, almost to the point of spoilage, the fruit's antioxidant levels are at their highest.

EAT THE CORE Bromelain concentrates in the fibrous core of the fruit.

JUICE IT The juice can help lower fever, ease sore throats, and acts as a natural expectorant.

HOW DO I USE IT?

A TANGY SORBET Juice 1 large pineapple, pour 1 cup into a large pan, and add ⅔ cup superfine sugar. Boil to a syrup. Allow to cool. Add the pineapple pulp from the juicer and the juice of 3 large oranges. Pour into a plastic container. Freeze, removing it occasionally to give the sorbet a stir.

SALSA Dice and combine pineapple, chile, red onion, garlic, fresh cilantro, and lime juice.

Coconut

 FIGHTS BACTERIA, VIRUSES, AND FUNGI

 ENHANCES METABOLISM

 PROVIDES ENERGY FOR THE BRAIN

 INCREASES "HEALTHY" (HDL) CHOLESTEROL

We may think of coconut as a nut, but it is a fruit, or drupe, similar to peaches and plums. It is native to the Indo-Pacific region, where it is called the "tree of life." Its medicinal properties, which benefit, among others, the heart, brain, and stomach, stem from its unique **healthy fat content**, antibacterial effects, and **balance of sugar**, **dietary fiber**, proteins, antioxidants, **vitamins**, and minerals.

What Is It Good For?

A NATURAL ANTIBIOTIC Lauric acid—a fatty acid in coconuts—helps the body combat a wide spectrum of bacteria and viruses that cause colds, flu, herpes, gum disease, ulcers, and urinary tract infections, among others. The fruit also contains caprylic acid, found to be a potent antifungal that can fight disorders, such as candidiasis, thrush, and athlete's foot.

METABOLIC BALANCE The oil is high in medium-chain triglycerides (MCTs), healthy fats that help lower the risk of heart disease. MCTs can help with weight management by reducing appetite, boosting metabolism, and increasing the activity of fat-burning cells.

FEEDING THE BRAIN Studies show that the brains of Alzheimer's sufferers can utilize the ketones produced when MCTs are metabolized as an alternative energy source. This may help ameliorate some symptoms of the disease.

IMPROVING CHOLESTEROL RATIOS MCTs increase "healthy" (HDL) cholesterol without raising "unhealthy" (LDL) cholesterol levels.

How Do I Get The Best From It?

CHOOSE THE RIGHT OIL Virgin coconut oil is not chemically treated (refined, bleached, and deodorized), so MCT content remains intact.

IN YOUR COOKING Coconut oil is very heat stable so use for roasts and in savory dishes.

How Do I Use It?

AN ALTERNATIVE TO SPORTS DRINKS Hydrating coconut water from the immature fruit is a superior drink for restoring electrolyte balance during and after sports.

NOURISHING SALAD DRESSING Coconut oil, which is solid at room temperature, enhances the absorption of fat-soluble nutrients, such as carotenoids. Blend with other more "liquid" ingredients, such as vinegar, honey, or thinner oils, to make an excellent dressing.

COCONUT FRUIT
Contains less fat than many seeds and nuts, such as almonds, and less sugar and more protein than popular fruits, such as bananas, apples, and oranges.

Coconut water
A pure and perfect balance of electrolytes, it was given intravenously to soldiers during the Second World War when regular IV saline solution ran out

COCONUT OIL
Coconut oil is high in healthy fats that help lower the risk of heart disease.

COCONUT MILK
Coconut milk, obtained primarily by extracting the juice from the white kernel, is rich in beneficial fats.

AVOCADO

 HELPS KEEP JOINTS SUPPLE

 HELPS LOWER BLOOD PRESSURE

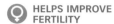 **HELPS IMPROVE FERTILITY**

The avocado has the distinction of being the fruit with the highest fat content. This may sound unhealthy, but its **beneficial monounsaturated oils**, which can lower blood pressure and lubricate joints, have earned it the title "the olive oil of the Americas." The flesh and oil contain **antioxidants** and are **anti-inflammatory**, helping to lower the risk of diseases, such as **arthritis,** and boost women's fertility.

AVOCADO
The flesh contains a favorable balance of potassium and sodium that can help lower blood pressure.

AVOCADO OIL
The oil is pressed from the flesh of the avocado, not the seed, and is known for its ability to protect the heart and fight free-radical damage.

WHAT IS IT GOOD FOR?

ANTI-INFLAMMATORY The fats of this fruit are unique. They include phytosterols, plant hormones, such as campesterol, beta-sitosterol, and stigmasterol, that help to keep inflammation under control. It also contains polyhydroxylated fatty alcohols (PFAs), which are anti-inflammatory. Also a source of omega-3 fatty acids, which help lubricate joints and reduce arthritic symptoms.

LOWERING BLOOD PRESSURE A good source of potassium and low in sodium. As a result, it can reduce the risk of high blood pressure and stroke. Also very rich in antioxidants and monounsaturated fats, which offer protection from heart disease and stroke.

FERTILITY BOOST The healthy fats have been shown to dramatically boost fertility and increase the success of IVF treatment.

HOW DO I GET THE BEST FROM IT?

PEEL WITH CARE The majority of the avocado's nutrients concentrate in the dark green flesh near the skin. Quick or careless peeling means you lose these benefits. Cut the fruit lengthwise into quarters and peel off the skin in sections as you would a banana.

A RICH OIL The oil makes an excellent base for salad dressings and marinades, and can be used in sautés and as a dipping oil.

HOW DO I USE IT?

A COLORFUL SALAD Add avocado to a salad to increase the absorption of key fat-soluble antioxidants, such as lycopene and beta-carotene, in the other vegetables.

GUACAMOLE This classic Mexican dip is quick and easy to make, and is also great as a healthy accompaniment to fish dishes. Mash 1 avocado, a couple of diced tomatoes, and a squeeze of lime juice into a paste, and add chopped fresh cilantro to taste.

BROCCOLI

 PROMOTES PROSTATE HEALTH

 PROMOTES COLLAGEN SYNTHESIS

 HELPS STRENGTHEN THE IMMUNE SYSTEM

 HELPS PROTECT EYE HEALTH

This cruciferous vegetable has been widely studied for its medicinal properties, which include antibacterial and **immunity-boosting** activities. It is rich in **vitamin C** and **fiber** and has the highest level of **carotenoids**—particularly eye-healthy lutein—of all brassicas. It is also an excellent source of indole-3-carbinol, a chemical that boosts **DNA repair** in cells and appears to block the growth of cancer cells.

WHAT IS IT GOOD FOR?

PROSTATE HEALTH Diets high in broccoli are associated with a lower risk of aggressive prostate cancer.

SKIN FOOD Contains abundant pantothenic acid, beta-carotene, and sulfur compounds, all of which encourage great skin. It is also rich in vitamin C, which aids the formation of collagen and helps to repair damaged tissue.

IMMUNITY BOOST Higher in vitamin C than many citrus fruits, and rich in beta-carotene antioxidants, broccoli is an ideal food to eat to maintain a healthy immune system.

EYE HEALTH Has a useful amount of lutein, an antioxidant that promotes eye health and may also benefit the heart and circulation.

HOW DO I GET THE BEST FROM IT?

STEAM IT Eat raw or steam lightly to retain its vitamin C, iron, and chlorophyll content.

TRY A CHANGE OF COLOR Purple sprouting broccoli generally contains more antioxidants and more of the phytochemical sulforaphane, which gives broccoli its detoxifying and anticancer reputation.

SPROUT THE SEEDS The sprouts are lower in nutrients than the vegetable, but higher in sulforaphane, thought to help prevent cancer.

HOW DO I USE IT?

HEART-HEALTHY MEAL Stir-fry with soba (buckwheat) noodles. The rutin content of buckwheat, the vitamin C in broccoli, and the healthy fats in olive oil together can lower cholesterol levels.

SALAD BOOSTER The raw leaves and sprouts can add a serious nutritional boost to salads.

ADD TOMATOES Eating broccoli together with tomatoes can slow the growth of prostate cancer more effectively than eating either vegetable on its own.

PURPLE BROCCOLI RABE
Contains more antioxidants than green varieties, but is more prone to nutrient loss when cooked.

GREEN BROCCOLI
Higher in vitamin C than many citrus fruits.

BROCCOLI SPROUTS
Higher than mature broccoli in the anticancer antioxidant sulforaphane.

Leaves
These contain more beta-carotene than the flower or stalks

CABBAGE

 HELPS HEAL ULCERS

 SUPPORTS HEALTHY LIVER FUNCTION

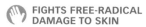 **FIGHTS FREE-RADICAL DAMAGE TO SKIN**

Many people don't consider cabbage a "love to eat" vegetable nowadays, but before we lost the habit of eating bitter foods it was revered as a warming, calming, **balancing**, and grounding food. It is now known to **clear the blood**, boost **skin health**, and is a remarkable remedy for **ulcers**. Its bitterness stimulates gastric juices to digest food more effectively, and it is also a mild **diuretic**.

GREEN CABBAGE
Contains a broad spectrum of nutrients including vitamin U—a potent ulcer remedy.

RED CABBAGE
Contains 2–8 times more vitamin C than other cabbages, and is rich in additional antioxidant anthocyanins.

BRUSSELS SPROUTS
These sprouts are higher in anticancer glucosinolates than other cabbages.

BOK CHOY
A good source of beta-carotene and vitamins C and B_6.

WHAT IS IT GOOD FOR?

HEALS ULCERS Contains ample amounts of vitamin U, or S-methylmethionine. Vitamin U heals stomach and duodenal ulcers quickly.

SUPPORTS LIVER FUNCTION It stimulates the production of glutathione, the body's most important internally produced antioxidant, which plays a role in liver detoxification.

HEALTHY SKIN Contains vitamins C and K, and antioxidants that protect skin from free-radical damage. Its sulfur content may be useful in healing acne and eczema.

ANTIPARASITIC Its high sulfur content helps maintain a gut free from parasites. It is also fiber-rich and promotes bowel regularity.

HOW DO I GET THE BEST FROM IT?

COOK IT LIGHTLY Cabbage retains more of its nutritional and medicinal benefits if lightly cooked or eaten raw.

TRY BOK CHOY Lighter in texture and taste, bok choy is also rich in vitamins A, B_6, and C, beta-carotene, calcium, potassium, and fiber.

GET COLORFUL Purple cabbage has more vitamin C and antioxidant anthocyanins, which help lower the risk of heart disease, diabetes, and certain types of cancer.

USE THE OUTER LEAVES The outer leaves have more vitamin E and contain about 30 percent more calcium than the inner leaves.

HOW DO I USE IT?

WRAPS The large leaves make ideal wraps. Use like tortillas and fill with ingredients, such as rice, beans, and different vegetables.

JUICE IT The juice is especially good for skin and ulcers. If you find the taste too strong, try mixing it with celery juice.

FERMENT IT Eating sauerkraut is a great way to cleanse the digestive tract and encourage healthy gut flora.

KALE

 HELPS STRENGTHEN BONES

 HELPS FIGHT INFLAMMATION

 HELPS LOWER CHOLESTEROL

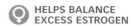 **HELPS BALANCE EXCESS ESTROGEN**

Science has revealed kale to be rich in beta-carotene, **vitamins C and K**, and **folate**, causing its popularity to grow in recent years. It is an exceptional source of **chlorophyll**, and its calcium and iron content are highly bioavailable (easily absorbed). It helps balance **hormones** and lower **cholesterol**, and its **antioxidants** and omega-3 fatty acids give kale strong **anti-inflammatory** properties.

WHAT IS IT GOOD FOR?

BONE BUILDING Its high calcium, magnesium, and vitamin K content helps strengthen bones, benefitting those with osteoporosis.

ANTIOXIDANT BOOST Contains multiple antioxidants, including kaempferol and quercetin, which are responsible for anti-inflammatory benefits in diseases, such as diabetes, arthritis, stroke, and heart disease.

LOWERS CHOLESTEROL Its fiber binds with cholesterol to remove it from the blood, lowering the risk of heart disease and stroke.

HORMONE BALANCING Contains indoles, natural substances that boost DNA repair and have an antiestrogen effect that can protect against and arrest the spread of estrogen-dependent cancers, such as breast cancer.

HEALING ULCERS The juice is rich in sulfur, which can aid the healing of stomach and duodenal ulcers.

DIGESTIVE STIMULANT Its bitter flavor aids digestion and eases lung congestion.

HOW DO I GET THE BEST FROM IT?

ADD LEMON Serving kale with a lemon dressing or another acidic citrus fruit as part of a meal boosts the absorption of its iron and calcium content.

COOK BRIEFLY The less you cook kale, the more nutrients you retain. Cooking lightly also leaves the plant's cholesterol-lowering properties intact.

HOW DO I USE IT?

ADD TO JUICES Blend kale juice with spicy ginger and apple juice, or try a cleansing mixture of celery, kale, and coconut water.

KALE PESTO Replace the basil and pine nuts in a pesto recipe with 1lb (450g) kale leaves, ribs removed, and 2½ cups toasted walnuts. Add to soups, stews, hot pasta, or dressings.

CURLY KALE
The antioxidants kaempferol and quercetin, which help fight inflammation, top the list of kale's beneficial properties.

CAVOLO NERO
This deep blue-green variety is rich in chlorophyll and folate.

PURPLE KALE
Purple varieties contain more anthocyanins—antioxidant red pigments—than green.

HORSERADISH

 ANTIBIOTIC AND ANTIBACTERIAL

 HELPS REMOVE TOXINS FROM THE BODY

HAS A DIURETIC ACTION

 HELPS CLEAR CONGESTION

This pungent root contains an array of nutrients in small amounts, but its volatile oils are responsible for the **medicinal** effects of horseradish. Its potent oil, allyl isothiocyanate, boosts **metabolism** and gives it **antibiotic** and **antibacterial** properties against food-borne pathogens. This is why, in the days before refrigeration, horseradish was eaten with fish or meats as a kind of insurance policy.

HORSERADISH ROOT
Its volatile oils can fight food-borne pathogens, such as *listeria* and *E. coli*.

HORSERADISH LEAVES
The young leaves, which can be eaten raw, contain oils that aid digestion.

WASABI
Sometimes called Japanese horseradish, wasabi is not true horseradish but a root with similar properties.

WHAT IS IT GOOD FOR?

ANTIBIOTIC AND INSECTICIDAL Laboratory tests have shown horseradish to be active against a variety of harmful bacteria, such as *listeria*, *E. coli*, and *staphylococcus*. Allyl isothiocyanate is also effective against intestinal worms.

DETOX As a stimulating food it can aid digestion, boost circulation, and help lower fevers by promoting perspiration.

BENEFITS THE URINARY SYSTEM Traditionally, it has been used to help treat water retention, urinary infections, and kidney stones.

COMBATS SINUS INFECTIONS Stimulates the flow of mucus, and opens and cleanses the sinuses in much the same way as chile peppers. Try taking horseradish at the first signs of cold, flu, or coughs.

HOW DO I GET THE BEST FROM IT?

FRESH AND RAW If grated and left to stand too long, or cooked for long periods, it loses its potency, so eat horseradish fresh and raw.

EAT THE LEAVES The small tender leaves have a pleasant flavor with just enough "bite" to lift an everyday salad. The older leaves can be cooked and used as you would spinach or kale.

SERVE WITH VEGETABLES Studies show that serving vegetables, such as broccoli, with a little horseradish or wasabi can increase the amount of nutrients absorbed by the body.

HOW DO I USE IT?

ADD TO CONDIMENTS Freshly grated, it mixes well with mayonnaise, sour cream, yogurt, or cream cheese with fresh herbs and seasoning.

FOR HOARSENESS Infuse 2 tbsp grated horseradish root and 1 tbsp apple cider vinegar in ⅓ cup boiling water for 1 hour. Strain and add 1¼ cups honey. Take 1 tbsp hourly until the condition eases.

Sweet Peppers

 PROMOTES COLLAGEN SYNTHESIS   **HELPS PROTECT AGAINST CATARACTS**   **MAINTAINS HEALTHY BLOOD VESSELS**   **CONTAINS ANTICANCER SUBSTANCES**

Part of the nightshade family, which includes tomatoes, potatoes, and eggplant, peppers are rich in **antioxidants** to benefit **heart** and **eye health**. Their vitamin C content boosts **collagen** levels and they may also help to prevent **lung cancer**. They don't contain the beneficial compound capsaicin found in chiles, but weight-for-weight they contain more essential nutrients, because you can eat more of them.

What Is It Good For?

SKIN AND BONES Contains vitamin C, necessary for the synthesis of collagen, the main structural protein in the body that maintains the integrity of blood vessels, skin, and bones.

EYE HEALTH Possibly due to a combination of beta-carotene, vitamin C, lutein, and zeaxanthin, peppers have been shown to be protective against cataracts and age-related macular degeneration (loss of vision).

HEART HEALTH Antioxidant levels, including beta-carotene, capsanthin, quercetin, and luteolin, may vary between varieties, but all have been shown to prevent the oxidization of cholesterol, the cause of free-radical damage to the heart and blood vessels. Diets high in antioxidants can also help prevent blood clot formation and reduce the risk of stroke.

LUNG CANCER Beta-cryptoxanthin, found mostly in red peppers, may help prevent lung cancer in those at risk.

How Do I Get The Best From It?

RED BENEFITS Red peppers have significantly higher nutrient levels than green, including lycopene, which helps to protect against cancer of the prostate, cervix, bladder, and pancreas, and lowers the risk of heart disease.

COOK THE RIGHT COLOR Cooking lowers vitamin C levels in green peppers, but increases their beta-carotene content; in red peppers it increases vitamin C levels and lowers its beta-carotene. Yellow peppers are high in vitamin C, so may be the best choice if you want more of this vitamin, but overall, cooked red peppers are more nutritious.

How Do I Use It?

EAT RAW Slice and use as crudités with dips or salsas, or simply add to fresh salads.

STUFFED PEPPERS Fill with rice, mushrooms, other vegetables, and fresh herbs.

GREEN PEPPERS
This immature fruit eventually ripens to a bright red color. Even at this stage, it contains twice as much vitamin C as an orange.

RED PEPPERS
Red peppers, including romano peppers, offer superior quantities of nutrients and antioxidants to other colored peppers.

YELLOW PEPPERS
Yellow and red peppers contain 3 times as much vitamin C as an orange.

CHILES

 HELPS REMOVE TOXINS FROM THE BODY

 HELPS LOWER CHOLESTEROL

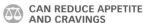 **CAN REDUCE APPETITE AND CRAVINGS**

 HELPS CLEAR CONGESTION

The chile pepper, the hottest member of the capsicum family, is a fruit pod from the plant belonging to the nightshade family. Its volatile oils, particularly capsaicin, account for its strong, spicy, pungent character and **antioxidant** and **anti-inflammatory** effects, which give chile its **cholesterol-lowering**, **blood-sugar balancing**, and **appetite-suppressing** properties. Capsaicin can also aid **detoxification**.

Piri piri
Hot

FRESH CHILES
Some varieties are hotter than others, but the heat can vary enormously even between peppers of the same variety.

Jalapeño
Mild

Scotch bonnet
Super hot

WHAT IS IT GOOD FOR?

DETOX The heat in capsaicin can help remove toxins by promoting increased sweating.

KEEPS ARTERIES CLEAR Studies show that capsaicin can help reduce "unhealthy" (LDL) cholesterol levels in obese individuals.

WEIGHT MANAGEMENT Hot chiles in quantities normally used for seasoning can stimulate digestion, reduce hunger and cravings, and boost metabolism.

CLEARS CONGESTION Hot chiles increase mucus secretion in the lungs and nose.

ANTIDIABETIC There is evidence that hot chiles can help regulate blood sugar levels.

HOW DO I GET THE BEST FROM IT?

AS HOT AS YOU DARE For an occasional spicy meal, use the hottest chiles you can tolerate to get the most from their capsaicin content.

DRIED SEEDS Most of us throw the seeds away, yet they contain the most capsaicin. Dry the seeds, combine with seasonings, such as salt and garlic, and grind to a coarse powder to add a quick zing to any savory dish.

CONTROL THE HEAT The heat of fresh chiles can vary. If you want to control how much heat you include in a dish, try using dried hot cayenne or milder chili powder blends instead, which are still rich in capsaicin.

HOW DO I USE IT?

AS A THERAPY FOR COLDS Add chile pepper and garlic to chicken soup as a therapeutic meal for colds, sinusitis, and bronchitis.

AS A MEDICINAL KICK IN DISHES Add chili and cayenne powders to salsas, chutneys, marinades, and rubs for an additional kick.

PICK THE FRESHEST PRODUCE Choose fresh chiles with bright, deep colors and glossy, firm, taut skins. Buy only as many as you need and use them up quickly.

DRIED CHILES
The dried seeds and flakes make a useful seasoning. The seeds contain the highest amounts of capsaicin.

CAYENNE POWDER
Unlike standard chili powder, which can be a mixture of spices, ground cayenne comprises pure hot chiles.

Whichever jewel-colored chile variety you select, the heat and beneficial capsaicin is concentrated in the seeds and white membrane inside.

CUCUMBERS

 DETERS ESTROGEN-BASED CANCERS

 HAS A DIURETIC ACTION

 PROMOTES A HEALTHY DIGESTIVE TRACT

 HELPS LOWER CHOLESTEROL

The watery composition of this member of the gourd family is packed with bioavailable (easily absorbed) **minerals**, **vitamins**, and **electrolytes**, making it an ideal way to increase your daily nutrients. Cucumber also contains **phytoestrogens** and digestive enzymes that **benefit the gut**. It is known for being a classic cooling food, helping to maintain the body's **water balance** on hot days.

CUCUMBERS
Keep the skin on to retain all the beneficial nutrients.

ENGLISH CUCUMBERS
Although 98 percent water, cucumber contains a highly available mix of vitamins and minerals.

WHAT IS IT GOOD FOR?

HELPFUL PHYTOESTROGENS Contains lariciresinol, secoisolariciresinol, and pinoresinol—three lignans (plant hormones) that help reduce the risk of cardiovascular disease and several types of cancer including breast, uterine, ovarian, and prostate.

MAINTAINS WATER BALANCE Its ability to balance water in the body makes cucumber important for heart and kidney problems. It also has a mild diuretic action and can help prevent constipation.

SUPPORTS URINARY FUNCTION The caffeic acid in cucumber helps prevent water retention. Other nutrients it contains help dissolve uric acid accumulations and can aid in the treatment of kidney and bladder stones.

PROMOTES A HEALTHY GUT Contains erepsin, a digestive enzyme that helps break down protein. It also acts as an antiparasitic and helps cleanse and tone the intestines.

LOWERS CHOLESTEROL Contains beneficial plant sterols that can help lower "unhealthy" (LDL) cholesterol levels.

HOW DO I GET THE BEST FROM IT?

EAT THE SEEDS The seeds have diuretic properties and so are worth consuming.

EAT THE SKIN The skin is a good source of silicon, chlorophyll, and bitter chemicals that aid digestion. It also contains the highest concentration of cholesterol-lowering sterols.

HOW DO I USE IT?

MAKE A COOLING DIP Grate a cucumber and mix with Greek yogurt, minced garlic, lemon juice, olive oil, and fresh mint for a tzatziki, or spices and natural yogurt for an Indian raita.

DRINK IT Juice with other vegetables, add slices to a cold pitcher of water, or brew the skin as a tea to ease swollen hands and feet.

WINTER SQUASHES

 HELPS FIGHT INFLAMMATION

 LOWERS RISK OF HEART DISEASE AND STROKE

PROMOTES BOWEL REGULARITY

 SUPPORTS A HEALTHY PREGNANCY

Their bright orange flesh signals that all squashes have similar nutritional and medicinal benefits. They are good sources of healthy **carbohydrate**, **magnesium**, and antioxidant **carotenoids**, and are known to improve **cardiovascular health**, **digestion**, and benefit **pregnant women**. Unlike watery summer squashes, these squashes (which store well through winter) usually have tough rinds.

WHAT IS IT GOOD FOR?

HEALTHY CARBOHYDRATE About half its carbohydrate content is in the form of complex carbohydrates, or polysaccharides (including pectin). This makes it anti-inflammatory and antioxidant. It also has insulin-regulating properties.

CARDIOVASCULAR HEALTH Its wide range of nutrients, such as alpha- and beta-carotene, vitamin C, manganese, and magnesium, are all heart-healthy, helping protect against stroke and normalize blood pressure. Its folate content reduces homocysteine levels which, when too high, are a risk factor for heart disease.

BOWEL HEALTH Squashes are high in fiber, which promotes bowel regularity.

PREGNANCY Contains large amounts of folate, so it is a good food choice during pregnancy. While folate deficiency isn't the sole cause of birth defects, adequate levels of this B vitamin can help protect against neural tube defects.

HOW DO I GET THE BEST FROM IT?

SEEDS All squash seeds are edible and contain healthy fats, protein, and fiber. The seeds have long been used in traditional medicine for prostate and urinary problems, and their high-fat, low-carbohydrate content is useful for heart health.

EAT THE RIND Choose varieties with a thin rind, such as butternut. Cook with the rind on to make the most of the nutrients it contains.

BUY ORGANIC Squashes absorb heavy metals and other toxins from the soil, so buy organic.

HOW DO I USE IT?

ROASTED SEEDS Place rinsed seeds on a baking sheet. Bake for 15 minutes at 300°F (150°C) to preserve their beneficial fatty acids.

BAKED SQUASH Cube, toss in olive oil, season, and bake at 350°F (180°C) for 35–40 minutes.

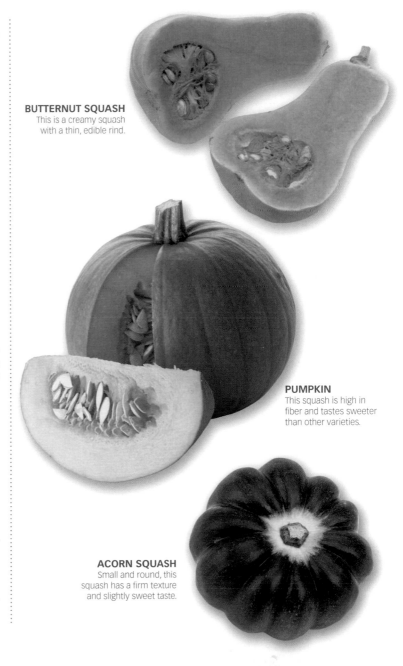

BUTTERNUT SQUASH
This is a creamy squash with a thin, edible rind.

PUMPKIN
This squash is high in fiber and tastes sweeter than other varieties.

ACORN SQUASH
Small and round, this squash has a firm texture and slightly sweet taste.

ZUCCHINI

 HELPS MAINTAIN WATER BALANCE

 HELPS REDUCE AN ENLARGED PROSTATE

 LOWERS RISK OF HEART DISEASE AND STROKE

 HELPS BALANCE BLOOD SUGAR LEVELS

Related to melons, cucumbers, and other squash, zucchini are a light, cleansing food. They contain a high volume of **water**, are **low in calories**, and can **ease prostate conditions** in men. Their **vitamin C** and potassium levels are higher than in other squash, and they also contain **beta-carotene**, phosphorus, and folate.

GREEN ZUCCHINI
Nutrients, such as folate and vitamin C, are concentrated in the skin.

Squash blossoms
The edible flower is high in folate and potassium

YELLOW SUMMER SQUASH
Particularly rich in antioxidant carotenes, such as lutein and zeaxanthin.

WHAT IS IT GOOD FOR?

DIURETIC AND LAXATIVE Phytonutrients in zucchini promote bowel regularity and aid water balance.

PROSTATE HEALTH Helps ease the symptoms of enlarged prostate, including frequent and painful urination, and increased risk of urinary tract infections (UTIs).

HEART HEALTH Contains magnesium, a mineral proven to reduce the risk of heart attack and stroke. Also contains folate, which breaks down homocysteine, a substance that raises the risk of heart attacks and stroke.

METABOLIC BALANCE Fiber, vitamin C, and beta-carotene help regulate blood sugar levels. Amounts of manganese can help the body metabolize protein and carbohydrates, digest fat, contribute to sex hormone production, and lower blood pressure.

HOW DO I GET THE BEST FROM IT?

EAT THE WHOLE PLANT From their skins to their seeds, zucchini and other summer squash are almost entirely edible. As cooling, sedative foods, they are useful for treating tired adrenals and frayed nerves. They can't be stored for long, so eat quickly while fresh.

EAT THE SKIN Important nutrients—including lutein and zeaxanthin, which promote healthy eyes—are concentrated in their skins.

JUICE THEM Their water content is highly mineralized and bioavailable (easily absorbed). Juice for a quick mineral boost.

HOW DO I USE IT?

TRY IT RAW Try adding julienne strips to your regular salad, or eat as crudités with dips.

STUFFED SQUASH Slice the squash in half lengthwise, remove the seeds, and fill with grains, lentils, and/or vegetables. Bake in the oven at 400°F (200°C), or until tender.

CORN

 FIGHTS AGE-RELATED VISION LOSS

 HELPS REDUCE AN ENLARGED PROSTATE

 PROMOTES A HEALTHY DIGESTIVE TRACT

Much corn is now genetically modified, and modern yellow varieties are bred for their high sugar content. However, heirloom varieties, particularly blue corn, have a **high nutritional value** that can balance **blood sugars**, boost **eye health**, soothe the **urinary tract**, and are available as organic and GM-free. Yellow corns contain more **beta-carotene**, while red and blue contain more **anthocyanins**.

WHAT IS IT GOOD FOR?

EYE HEALTH Carotenoids, such as zeaxanthin and lutein support eye health and prevent age-related macular degeneration.

PROSTATE HEALTH Partly due to its significant potassium content, corn silk can soothe urinary tract irritation, is a useful diuretic, and can treat an enlarged prostate.

DIGESTIVE HEALTH Corn contains soluble dietary fiber that regulates the flow of waste material through the digestive tract. Soluble fiber also helps to control blood sugar levels.

HOW DO I GET THE BEST FROM IT?

POPCORN Without added butter, sugar, and salt, popcorn is a great high-fiber, low-calorie food. Try using organic blue and multi-colored heirloom corn for extra benefits.

CORNMEAL Ground from dried corn, cornmeal is available in fine to coarse grades. Drying the corn improves the availability of B vitamins such as niacin, thiamine, pantothenic acid, and folate. Stoneground varieties are higher in nutrients and flavor.

EAT RAW OR LIGHTLY COOKED Add baby corn or raw kernels to salads or stir-fries.

HOW DO I USE IT?

MAKE A TEA Make a medicinal tea by steeping ¼ cup fresh corn silk in boiling water for 5 minutes. Strain and drink as a mild diuretic.

POLENTA Boil ground cornmeal in water or stock until thick. Let cool and firm up, and then bake in the oven at 350°F (180°C) or slice and broil it.

MAKE A CORN CHOWDER Strip the kernels from 6 cobs and simmer in boiling water until tender. Sauté some onions and garlic, put them in a blender with the kernels and some of the broth, and purée until smooth. Serve topped with fresh corn kernels and cilantro leaves.

Corn silk
The silky threads inside the husk are a useful diuretic and can relieve prostate enlargement

Fresh corn on the cob
Good source of skin- and eye-healthy beta-carotene and lutein

BLUE CORN
Contains 30 percent more protein than yellow corn. Beneficial antioxidants include protocatechuic acid (which gives green tea its healthy properties).

BABY CORN
Harvesting corn while young means the cob, with its beneficial soluble fiber, can be eaten.

ARTICHOKE

 HELPS BALANCE BLOOD SUGAR LEVELS

 HELPS LOWER CHOLESTEROL

 AIDS THE DIGESTION OF FAT

 A MILD LAXATIVE AND DIURETIC

This edible member of the thistle family is among the top 10 highest **antioxidant-rich** foods. It is high in **dietary fiber**, and was traditionally eaten by the Greeks and Romans to maintain a **healthy gut**, promote **bowel regularity**, and **alleviate upset stomachs**. It also has a reputation for "cleaning the blood" by **detoxifying** the liver and gallbladder, reducing **cholesterol**, and balancing **blood sugars**.

Leaf
Stimulates the flow of bile and can ease constipation, diarrhea, and bloating

Heart
Contains inulin to keep blood sugar levels in balance

WHAT IS IT GOOD FOR?

BALANCES BLOOD SUGAR LEVELS The leaves and heart contain plant fibers including inulin (a prebiotic that feeds healthy gut flora), which helps maintain steady blood sugar levels.

REDUCES CHOLESTEROL The antioxidant flavonoid silymarin helps reduce "unhealthy" (LDL) cholesterol and raise "healthy" (HDL) cholesterol levels. It also protects the liver.

EASES INDIGESTION The leaves and hearts contain cynarine, a phytochemical that stimulates bile, helps digest fat, and prevents indigestion. May be particularly useful in cases of irritable bowel syndrome.

AIDS DETOXIFICATION A mild laxative and diuretic that supports kidney and liver health.

ENCOURAGES HEALTHY GUT Acts as a prebiotic food that encourages the growth of bifidobacteria in the gut.

HOW DO I GET THE BEST FROM IT?

LEAVES AND HEARTS Easy to digest, both leaves and hearts have similar nutritional and medicinal properties that benefit the liver.

MAKE A TEA Boil the fresh or dried leaves to make an antioxidant-rich, heart-healthy tea with a clean, slightly sweet taste.

HOW DO I USE IT?

CHOOSE SMALLER PRODUCE Look for smaller globes with dark, thick, fleshy leaves. Larger vegetables can be tough and tasteless.

HOW TO COOK IT Cook by boiling until tender. Dip the leaves into melted butter (or an olive oil and lemon dressing) and pull off the flesh at the base of the leaves with your teeth. Gently clear away the prickly thistle to reach the tender edible heart at the center.

MARINATED HEARTS Artichoke hearts marinated in healthy olive oil are delicious in salads, as part of a dip, or by themselves.

Toning, strengthening artichokes are best served simply. Cut away the spiky top and tough outer leaves, and boil or steam until just tender. Marinate in olive oil, lemon slices, parsley, freshly ground black pepper, and salt.

Eggplants

 PROTECTS THE HEART AND BLOOD VESSELS

 HELPS BALANCE BLOOD SUGAR LEVELS

 HELPS REMOVE TOXINS FROM THE BODY

Eggplants, which grow on vines, are part of the same nightshade family that includes peppers and potatoes, and there are several varieties ranging in size, shape, and color. They all contain beneficial amounts of **antioxidants** as well as potassium, folate, magnesium, **beta-carotene**, and **fiber**, while their medicinal properties include balancing **blood sugar** levels and boosting **gut health**.

PURPLE EGGPLANT
Contains fiber that benefits digestion, and antioxidants that prevent cell damage.

BABY EGGPLANT
Has all the same benefits as the classic purple variety.

WHITE EGGPLANT
Lacks the protective dark pigments, but still contains heart-healthy chlorogenic acid.

What Is It Good For?

HEART HEALTH Dark purple varieties are particularly rich in the antioxidant polyphenol, chlorogenic acid, as well as caffeic acid and flavonoids, such as nasunin, which protect the heart from oxidative stress caused by free radicals in the body.

BALANCES BLOOD SUGAR LEVELS The antioxidant chlorogenic acid also helps slow the release of glucose into the bloodstream after a meal.

DETOX Beyond promoting bowel regularity and water balance, some studies have shown that eggplant can help remove harmful chemical substances from the body.

How Do I Get The Best From It?

CHOOSE CAREFULLY Eggplant spoils fairly quickly so choose firm, glossy examples. Ideally, eat within a day of purchase.

LEAVE THE SKIN ON Eggplant's antioxidants concentrate in the skin, which tenderizes as you cook it. Some white varieties have a tougher skin that may need to be peeled before cooking.

HOW TO COOK IT Bake, roast, or fry. When fried, its spongy texture will soak up large amounts of oil; to prevent this, first sprinkle eggplant slices with salt and leave in a colander to drain. Rinse well, press firmly to remove excess water, and cook.

How Do I Use It?

BABA GANOUSH This classic dish is made from eggplant fried or baked until soft, and puréed with lemon juice, garlic, and olive oil. Spread on bread or use as a vegetable dip.

STUFFED EGGPLANT For a satisfying main meal, slice an eggplant in half lengthwise, hollow out, and stuff with a mixture of healthy grains, such as quinoa, wild rice, or bulgur, and vegetables.

TOMATOES

 HELPS REMOVE TOXINS FROM THE BODY

 HELPS KEEP BLOOD VESSELS SUPPLE

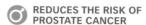 **REDUCES THE RISK OF PROSTATE CANCER**

Although strictly a fruit, tomatoes are widely used as a vegetable in savory dishes. They are rich in **beta-carotene**, vitamin C, and **lycopene**—a superstar of medicinal food substances and the source of their vibrant red color. Lycopene has been found to reduce the risk of **prostate** and **breast cancer**, lower **cholesterol**, protect **eyes and skin**, and boost **immunity**.

WHAT IS IT GOOD FOR?

DETOX Tomatoes are abundant in potassium, which reduces water retention. They are also a good source of glutathione, which helps the body remove fat-soluble toxins.

HEART HEALTH Contains large amounts of vitamins C and E and beta-carotene, all of which support heart health. However, lycopene is most important—it helps strengthen the walls of blood vessels and remove cholesterol from the blood.

PROSTATE CANCER Many cancers are linked with oxidative stress caused by free radicals in the body, and antioxidant foods, such as tomatoes, are known to be preventive. Research into prostate cancer shows that regularly eating raw or cooked tomatoes can reduce the development and spread of cancer.

HOW DO I GET THE BEST FROM IT?

JUICE One glass of tomato juice can contain 74 percent of your recommended daily vitamin C intake, other key vitamins, such as K, B_1, B_2, B_3, B_5, and B_6, and minerals, such as potassium, manganese, and iron.

COOKED When cooked, the lycopene content in tomatoes increases by 5 or 6 times.

KEEP THE SKIN ON The highest concentration of carotenoids is found in the skin.

HOW DO I USE IT?

SALSA Finely chop 2–3 medium tomatoes, 1 small onion, and 2 chiles. Add some finely chopped fresh cilantro, lime juice, 1 tsp water, and salt to taste. Mix well before serving.

HOMEMADE TOMATO JUICE Put 3¼lb (1.5kg) tomatoes, roughly chopped, in a saucepan. Add 1 chopped onion and 1 chopped celery stick, 2 tbsp sugar, and 1 tsp salt. Add some black pepper and, if you like, a few drops of chili sauce. Cook gently over low heat until souplike. Strain and chill before drinking.

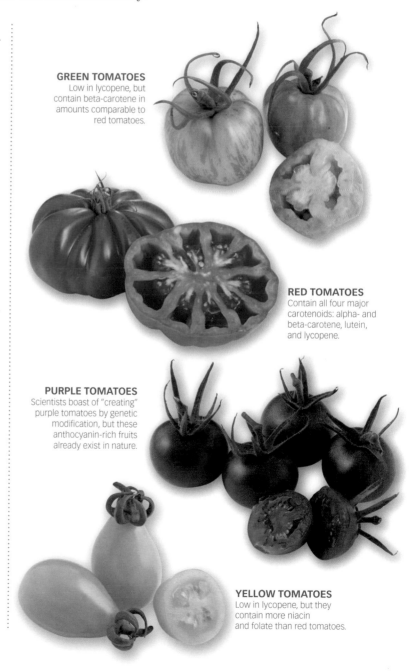

GREEN TOMATOES
Low in lycopene, but contain beta-carotene in amounts comparable to red tomatoes.

RED TOMATOES
Contain all four major carotenoids: alpha- and beta-carotene, lutein, and lycopene.

PURPLE TOMATOES
Scientists boast of "creating" purple tomatoes by genetic modification, but these anthocyanin-rich fruits already exist in nature.

YELLOW TOMATOES
Low in lycopene, but they contain more niacin and folate than red tomatoes.

LETTUCE

 HAS NATURAL SEDATIVE PROPERTIES

 HELPS EASE BLOATING AND DISCOMFORT

 STRENGTHENS HEART AND BLOOD VESSELS

We may think of lettuce as simply a base for more flavorful foods, but it is a useful source of **folate** and **soluble fiber** in the form of pectin. How rich it is in other nutrients depends on the variety—deeply colored lettuces have greater stores of **beta-carotene**. It is also considered to be **cooling**, **diuretic**, and **calming** for the nerves. The milky juice in darker, bitter varieties contains a **sedative**, lactucarium.

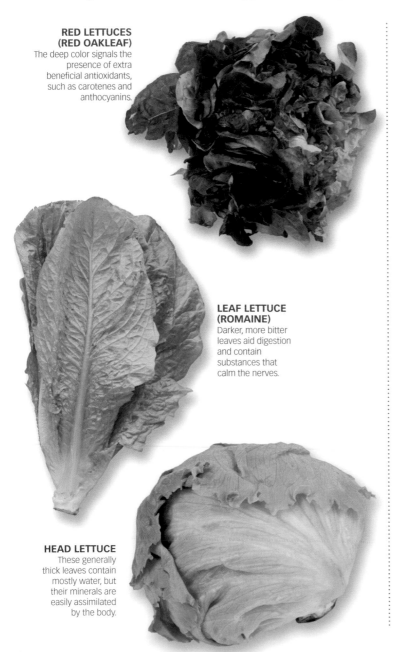

RED LETTUCES (RED OAKLEAF)
The deep color signals the presence of extra beneficial antioxidants, such as carotenes and anthocyanins.

LEAF LETTUCE (ROMAINE)
Darker, more bitter leaves aid digestion and contain substances that calm the nerves.

HEAD LETTUCE
These generally thick leaves contain mostly water, but their minerals are easily assimilated by the body.

WHAT IS IT GOOD FOR?

SEDATIVE Wild lettuce is a traditional herbal sedative. The dark, bitter lettuces contain lactucarium, which can relax nerves, reduce palpitations, and induce sleep.

DIGESTIVE AID AND DIURETIC Contains useful amounts of fiber and can help soothe gassy or griping pains. The watery nature of lettuce also helps to flush toxins from the body.

HEALING HEMORRHOIDS The astringent nature of lettuce can help strengthen blood vessels and may help treat hemorrhoids.

HOW DO I GET THE BEST FROM IT?

CHOOSE LARGE LEAVES Large, loose lettuce leaves are richer in essential nutrients, especially chlorophyll, iron, beta-carotene, and vitamin C, than paler, tightly packed head lettuces, such as iceberg (mostly water).

BEYOND GREEN Ancient lettuce varieties were a rich array of colors. Red lettuces contain extra antioxidant pigments that enhance your daily intake of nutrients.

FRESH AND CRISP Its nutritional value depends on the variety, time of year, and how long it has been stored. To get the best out of lettuce and other salad leaves, buy what is in season and always choose fresh heads, leaves, or "living salad" leaves and not prewashed, bagged varieties of lettuce.

HOW DO I USE IT?

MIX IT UP Its watery texture and neutral, refreshing taste makes lettuce a good partner for fresh fruit.

MAKE A CALMING TEA Tea brewed from lettuce leaves is a useful nighttime sedative. Simmer 3–4 large, deeply colored lettuce leaves with 1 or 2 mint leaves in 1¼ cups water for 15 minutes. Remove from the heat, strain, and drink.

SPINACH

  HELPS STRENGTHEN BONES

 CONTAINS ANTICANCER PROPERTIES

HELPS FIGHT INFLAMMATION

HELPS PREVENT ATHEROSCLEROSIS

Packed with **vitamins** and **minerals**, spinach contains more than a dozen different **antioxidant** flavonoid compounds that have **anti-inflammation properties** that protect against **heart disease** and help to **neutralize the free radicals** that compromise the immune system and are linked to cancer. Its considerable vitamin K content also helps to **protect bones**.

WHAT IS IT GOOD FOR?

BONE HEALTH A single serving provides more than twice the daily recommended intake of vitamin K, which is important for maintaining healthy bones. It is especially good at protecting the elderly from bone fractures.

REDUCED CANCER RISK Studies have shown it can help to reduce the risk of certain cancers. Specifically, the antioxidant kaempferol appears to be protective against prostate and ovarian cancer risk.

ANTI-INFLAMMATORY Its high levels of antioxidants, particularly neoxanthin and violaxanthin, have anti-inflammatory effects.

HEART HEALTH Its vitamin C and beta-carotene work together to prevent the oxidization of "unhealthy" (LDL) cholesterol, which can lead to hardening of the arteries.

HOW DO I GET THE BEST FROM IT?

COOKED VS. RAW While raw spinach is nutritious, cooked spinach is even more so. Its iron content is more available and it provides considerably larger amounts of beta-carotene, lutein, vitamins, and minerals.

SERVE WITH CITRUS FRUITS Contains oxalic acid, which prevents us from absorbing all its iron and calcium. If eating raw, serve with a lemon dressing or a glass of orange juice to increase absorption of these vital minerals.

HOW DO I USE IT?

CITRUS SPINACH SALAD Toss 2 generous handfuls of spinach leaves, ½ finely chopped red onion, 1 orange, peeled and separated into segments, and 2 tbsp toasted pine nuts in a bowl. For the dressing, mix 2 tbsp each of orange juice, white vinegar, olive oil, honey, and Dijon mustard with 1 tbsp chopped fresh cilantro. Season and serve.

SPINACH PESTO Substitute basil leaves with spinach in any pesto recipe.

SPINACH
Among the many nutrients in spinach, the carotenoids lutein and zeaxanthin can help to protect the eyes.

MICROGREENS
These contain more antioxidants and other nutrients than the mature leaves.

WATERCRESS

 CONTAINS ANTICANCER SUBSTANCES

 PROMOTES CLEAR SKIN

 AIDS OPTIMAL DIGESTION

HAS A DIURETIC ACTION

This salad leaf is a member of the cruciferous vegetable family, which includes cabbage and broccoli. Its numerous health benefits include reducing the risk of certain **cancers**, aiding **digestion**, maintaining the body's **water balance**, and acting as a **natural antibiotic** to **boost immunity**. It doesn't have a particular growing season and so can be grown and harvested all year round.

Leaves
Contain digestive enzymes and are rich in vitamins C and K, iron, beta-carotene, and B vitamins

WHAT IS IT GOOD FOR?

REDUCED CANCER RISK A great source of the antioxidants vitamin C and beta-carotene, which help fight free radicals. Studies have found that regularly eating cruciferous vegetables can help reduce the risk of cancers of the colon, rectum, and bladder.

SKIN DETOX Rich in sulfur, which aids protein absorption, blood purification, and cell building, and promotes healthy skin and hair.

DIGESTIVE AID The chlorophyll that gives watercress its green color is rich in digestive enzymes that help the body fully utilize the nutrients in any meal.

MAINTAINS WATER BALANCE It is rich in potassium, so is natural diuretic and diet aid.

FIGHTS COLDS AND FLU The volatile oils that give it its peppery taste are a good remedy for coughs, colds, flu, and bronchial ailments.

HOW DO I GET THE BEST FROM IT?

JUICE A natural antibiotic. Add to freshly prepared juices to detox and boost clear skin.

BUY ORGANIC If watercress is not grown in controlled conditions, it runs the risk of being contaminated with harmful bacteria. Buying organic means it will contain neither the bacteria nor any pesticides.

EAT FRESH Watercress quickly loses its nutrients. Consume within 5 days of buying.

HOW DO I USE IT?

WATERCRESS SOUP A traditional remedy for inflammatory conditions including achy joints, swollen gums, and mouth ulcers. Simmer ½lb (225g) each of watercress and sliced carrots in water or vegetable stock until the watercress reduces to one-third in volume. Blend and season to taste before serving.

SALAD INGREDIENT The perfect base to any salad; use instead of, or with, lettuce.

MUSTARD GREENS

 HELPS REMOVE TOXINS FROM THE BODY   **CONTAINS ANTICANCER SUBSTANCES**   **HELPS LOWER CHOLESTEROL**   **HELPS FIGHT INFLAMMATION**

Pungent, peppery mustard greens are the leaves of a mustard plant. They range from bright green to deep purple and are high in **antioxidants** and **anti-inflammatory** properties, and can help **detoxify** the body and lower "unhealthy" (LDL) **cholesterol**. The plant also produces hot, bitter-tasting brown seeds that are used to make Dijon mustard, and which are frequently used in Indian cooking.

WHAT IS IT GOOD FOR?

DETOX The antioxidant beta-carotene and vitamins C and K help neutralize toxins and remove them from the body, providing effective detox support.

CANCER PREVENTION A combination of antioxidant, detoxification, and anti-inflammatory properties contribute to cancer prevention. Mustard greens are also rich in sulfurous chemicals, called glucosinolates, which break down into cancer-fighting isothiocyanates. Studies have linked the leaves to the prevention of bladder, colon, breast, lung, prostate, and ovarian cancers.

LOWERS CHOLESTEROL Rich in natural substances called sulforaphanes. These help remove the "unhealthy" (LDL) cholesterol that increases the risk of heart disease.

BROAD SPECTRUM ANTIOXIDANT Contains key antioxidants including hydroxycinnamic acid, quercetin, isorhamnetin, and kaempferol, which help lower the risk of inflammation and oxidative stress caused by free radicals in the body.

HOW DO I GET THE BEST FROM IT?

HOW TO COOK IT Cooking decreases the availability of its anticancer properties so add raw to salads. However, light steaming boosts its cholesterol-lowering properties.

SPROUT THE SEEDS The seeds, rich in volatile oils, can be sprouted. Add to salads or soups.

HOW DO I USE IT?

HEALTHY SAUTÉ Sauté chopped onions and garlic until tender in a few tablespoons of broth or stock. Add roughly chopped mustard greens and cook until just wilted. Toss with sesame oil and season to taste before serving.

PASTA SAUCE Chop tomatoes and mustard greens and mix with pine nuts, goat cheese, and a little olive oil. Stir through hot pasta.

DEEP GREEN
Sulfurous chemicals support the heart and tissues, and aid detoxification.

PURPLE LEAF
Has the same nutritional value as green leaves, but also contains extra antioxidant pigments.

MIZUNA
These spidery leaves can be grown in the garden or bought at farmers' markets.

ARUGULA

 SUPPORTS HEALTHY LIVER FUNCTION

 HELPS PROTECT AGAINST INFECTIONS

 HELPS PROTECT EYE HEALTH

 HAS ANTI-ULCER PROPERTIES

Once used mainly for its **energizing** medicinal qualities in stimulating **digestion** and protecting against **stomach ulcers**, arugula is now prized as a unique, peppery, **low-calorie**, **detoxifying** salad ingredient. The arugula plant is a relative of broccoli and cabbage and has many of the same benefits, including boosting the **immune system** and maintaining **eye and skin health**.

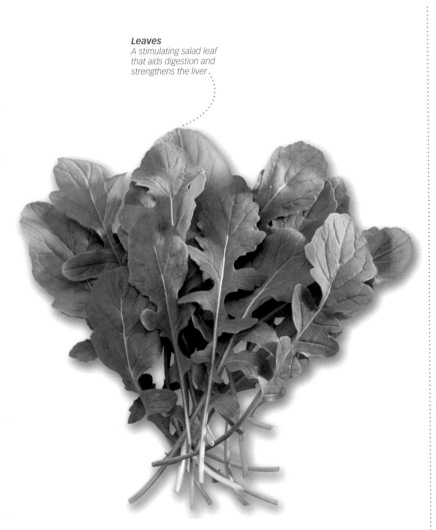

Leaves
A stimulating salad leaf that aids digestion and strengthens the liver.

WHAT IS IT GOOD FOR?

DETOX Sulfurous chemicals in arugula stimulate circulation, strengthen the liver, and have mild diuretic and laxative properties.

IMMUNE HEALTH Arugula contains very high levels of vitamin C and beta-carotene. These nutrients have proven immunity-boosting properties and help the body defend itself against infections. During digestion arugula releases isothiocyanates, which are protective against cancer.

HEALTHY EYES Arugula contains large quantities of eye-healthy lutein and zeaxanthin. Including these nutrients in your diet can reduce the risk of age-related macular degeneration (loss of vision).

DIGESTIVE HEALTH Studies show arugula can stimulate digestion and also help protect against stomach ulcers.

HOW DO I GET THE BEST FROM IT?

REPLACE OTHER SALAD LEAVES Unlike spinach, its iron and calcium levels are highly available because of its low levels of oxalate.

EAT RAW AND FRESH Arugula begins to lose its nutrients soon after picking. Heat can further degrade its nutritional value. For this reason it is best to buy it fresh and use it as quickly as possible after purchase.

HOW DO I USE IT?

ARUGULA PESTO Blend 4 generous handfuls of arugula, 3 crushed cloves of garlic, 3 tbsp pine nuts, and ¼ cup olive oil in a blender. Gradually add 1½oz (45g) pecorino cheese. Blend until smooth, then stir through hot pasta or mix with hot new potatoes.

SUPER SIMPLE SALAD Arugula is best eaten fresh and raw, so use it as the base of a salad. Combine with lycopene-rich tomatoes and dress the salad with a simple olive oil dressing for an antioxidant-rich meal.

DANDELION

 SUPPORTS HEALTHY LIVER FUNCTION

 HAS A MILD DIURETIC ACTION

HELPS BOOST IMMUNITY

PROMOTES HEALTHY SKIN

Think of the dandelion as a superfood rather than a weed: it is a **nutritional powerhouse**, and can be used as a **diuretic** and **liver cleanser**. Every part can be used. Collect the leaves before the familiar yellow flowers emerge to ensure the least bitter taste, and gather the flowers once they turn yellow. Never collect wild plants from chemically treated lawns or gardens.

WHAT IS IT GOOD FOR?

LIVER CLEANSER Helps clear inflammation and congestion of the liver and gallbladder.

DIURETIC A natural source of potassium, making it a safe, gentle diuretic.

IMMUNE SUPPORT Rich in antioxidants that help fight infection and speed wound healing.

HEALTHY SKIN A good source of vitamin C, which supports collagen formation—the foundation of youthful skin and healthy gums.

HOW DO I GET THE BEST FROM IT?

LEAVES These supply all the major antioxidant vitamins, including vitamins C and E.

FLOWERS Dandelion flowers contain useful amounts of beta-carotene, vitamin C, iron, and other nutrients. The colorful petals contain antioxidant flavonoids, which help lower blood pressure and boost immunity.

ROOTS The root, which can be dried and used as a caffeine-free coffee substitute, has a mild laxative and diuretic effect. It also has antiviral properties and contains inulin, a prebiotic that encourages healthy gut flora.

HOW DO I USE IT?

MAKE A PESTO Use the leaves on their own, or combine with nettles, and blend to a paste in a food processor with pine nuts, garlic, Parmesan cheese, and olive oil to make a springtime alternative to classic pesto.

DANDELION TEA Fresh or dried, all parts of the plant can be brewed into a refreshing tea that has diuretic properties.

ADD TO SALADS AND STIR-FRIES Add the yellow flower petals to salads and stir-fries, or pickle the flower heads in vinegar to preserve their nutritional benefits beyond the period they are in season.

ROAST THE ROOTS Cook like parsnips. They taste sweetest from fall to early spring.

Flower
Contains flavonoids and coumaric acid derivatives that can help lower blood pressure

Leaf
Traditionally used to help remove excess water and toxins from the body

Root
Rich in choline, a B vitamin that supports heart health and is also antidiabetic

NETTLES

 HAS A POWERFUL DIURETIC ACTION

 HELPS REDUCE AN ENLARGED PROSTATE

 BOOSTS IRON STORES TO COMBAT FATIGUE

HELPS BALANCE BLOOD SUGAR LEVELS

Many gardeners consider stinging nettles to be a weed, but they have long been used to **treat painful muscles** and joints, eczema, **arthritis**, gout, and **anemia**. Today, they are used to benefit the blood, treat **urinary tract infections**, urinary problems during the early stages of an **enlarged prostate**, hay fever, or in compresses or creams to treat joint pain, sprains and strains, tendonitis, and **insect bites**.

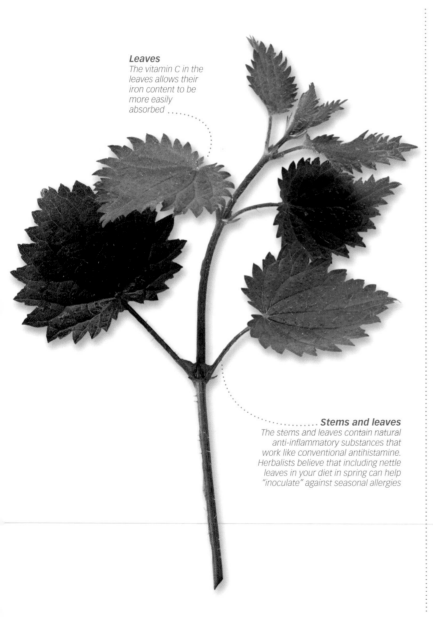

Leaves
The vitamin C in the leaves allows their iron content to be more easily absorbed

Stems and leaves
The stems and leaves contain natural anti-inflammatory substances that work like conventional antihistamine. Herbalists believe that including nettle leaves in your diet in spring can help "inoculate" against seasonal allergies

WHAT IS IT GOOD FOR?

DIURETIC It keeps water flowing through the kidneys and bladder, washing bacteria away and stopping urine crystals from developing into kidney stones.

HEALTHY PROSTATE Nettles are comparable to finasteride (a commonly prescribed medication) for reducing the symptoms of prostate enlargement. Unlike finasteride, it doesn't decrease prostate size, but does improve urinary flow, and reduce post-urination dripping and the urge to urinate.

BLOOD BUILDER Its iron content makes it a wonderful blood builder, and its vitamin C ensures better iron absorption. It is also a good source of vitamin K, which aids clotting.

DIABETIC CONDITIONS Nettle tea can help balance blood sugar levels.

RHEUMATIC CONDITIONS It can eliminate uric acid from joints. Studies suggest that nettle extract can help those with rheumatoid arthritis to lower their NSAID (nonsteroidal anti-inflammatory drug) use.

HOW DO I GET THE BEST FROM IT?

PICK FRESH PLANTS Avoid nettles treated with pesticides. Young nettle tops are full of nutrients and have a mild, pleasant flavor.

AS A TEA Steep fresh or dried nettles in hot water for 10–15 minutes for a detoxifying, diuretic tea. For prostate health, drink several cups of nettle root tea a day.

HOW DO I USE IT?

SPRING DETOX SOUP Sauté nettles, onion, leeks, and celery in butter, purée in a blender or food processor with stock and a little yogurt, and season to taste to serve.

YOUNG NETTLE PESTO Substitute basil leaves with nettles in any pesto recipe. Young spring leaves are more palatable and more potent.

CHICORY

 PROMOTES A HEALTHY DIGESTIVE TRACT

 HAS A MILD DIURETIC ACTION

 HELPS REMOVE TOXINS FROM THE BLOOD

 HAS NATURAL SEDATIVE PROPERTIES

Blanched white chicory (Belgian endive), green-leaf chicory, and red-leaf varieties (radicchios), are the most familiar types of this bitter leaf. Grown in the dark, the popular white chicory lacks the usual array of vitamins, but it retains the **volatile oils** and other substances that **aid digestion,** and acts as a **detoxifier** and a mild diuretic. Chicory contains natural sedative compounds to **ease stress and pain**.

WHAT IS IT GOOD FOR?

INTESTINAL HEALTH Rich in mucilaginous (gumlike) fiber, which helps lubricate the intestines and soften stools.

BETTER DIGESTION Its bitter constituents stimulate bile production, increase appetite, and aid digestion. Chicory can also help combat excessive wind and indigestion.

AIDS DETOXIFICATION It is a natural diuretic and mildly laxative. As a good source of dietary fiber, it helps removes toxins from the blood and tissues.

MILD SEDATIVE Both chicory and radicchio contain the substance lactucopicrin, which contributes to their bitter taste and has sedative and analgesic properties.

ANTIOXIDANT Although it lacks most other vitamins, chicory is rich in the useful antioxidant beta-carotene, which can help protect against cancer.

HOW DO I GET THE BEST FROM IT?

EAT IT RAW While it can be eaten lightly braised, you will receive more of chicory's vitamin C, folate, and beta-carotene content if you eat it raw.

EAT IT FRESH Both chicory and radicchio are relatively fragile and only keep for a few days in the refrigerator crisper before wilting.

HOW DO I USE IT?

A NATURAL SCOOP Use the leaves of the witloof chicory, also known as Belgian endive, which have a naturally curved shape, as crudités to serve with a variety of dips, or fill the leaves with different toppings or a stuffing made of rice and vegetables and serve them as a finger food or an appetizer.

ENLIVEN STIR-FRIES AND SALADS The mildly bitter flavor of chicory and radicchio gives a pleasant edge to salads and stir-fries.

WHITE CHICORY (WITLOOF OR BELGIAN ENDIVE
The thick leaves and delicate white flesh are a source of folate, beta-carotene, and vitamin K, and also contain traces of calcium and magnesium. Green-leaf chicory has similar nutrients.

RED-LEAF CHICORY (RADICCHIO)
Contains higher levels of the antioxidant anthocyanin and volatile oils that aid digestion.

GREEN BEANS

 PROVIDES CELLULAR ENERGY

 STRENGTHENS CONNECTIVE TISSUE

 HELPS BUILD STRONG BONES

 PROTECTS AGAINST FREE-RADICAL DAMAGE

Fresh green beans, which are the same species as the dried versions we use in chili con carne and baked beans, are edible pods picked early in the plant's growth cycle; as they mature, the pods become tough, fibrous, and inedible. The beans are a **good source of vitamin C** and folate, and have useful amounts of **calcium** and **protein**. This makes them **heart-protective** and **anti-inflammatory**.

GREEN BEANS
Contain a wide spectrum of carotenoids and flavonoids, which pack an antioxidant punch.

PURPLE BEANS
Purple pod beans can be eaten raw and add tremendous color to fresh salads; the pods turn green when cooked.

RUNNER BEANS
Mature plants produce a pink/deep purple edible bean similar in flavor to a lima bean. Runner beans aid water balance through their strong diuretic properties.

FAVA BEANS
Fava beans are rich in isoflavones—plant hormones with heart-protective and anticancer properties.

WHAT IS IT GOOD FOR?

ENERGY BOOSTING Contains twice the amount of iron as spinach, so it's a good way to make up iron loss during menstruation. Iron is a component of red blood cells that transport oxygen from the lungs to cells throughout the body. It is also is a key element in making energy and the body's metabolism.

SKIN, HAIR, AND NAILS Provides an easily absorbed type of silicon, important for the formation of healthy connective tissues and strengthening nails.

BONE HEALTH Abundant in vitamin K, which activates osteocalcin, the main noncollagen protein found in bones that locks calcium molecules together inside the bone.

FIGHTS FREE RADICALS Levels of the antioxidants lutein, beta-carotene, violaxanthin, and neoxanthin are comparable to those in carotenoid-rich vegetables, such as carrots.

DETOX Beans have strong diuretic properties and help to speed the elimination of toxins from the body.

HOW DO I GET THE BEST FROM IT?

DON'T CUT THEM Where you can, just trim the beans and cook them whole to preserve their nutrients.

HOW TO COOK THEM Cook until "al dente" (slightly crunchy), or steam briefly to ensure their vitamin C content is retained.

HOW DO I USE IT?

VERSATILE Add to salads, soups, and stews, or serve as a side dish. Pair tender varieties with lighter meats, such as poultry, and more robust, coarser varieties, such as runner beans, with red meats.

GET BEYOND BUTTER Serve with a dressing of olive oil, lemon, and garlic to bring out their flavor and boost their nutritional value.

OKRA

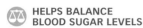 **HELPS BALANCE BLOOD SUGAR LEVELS**

 AIDS DETOXIFICATION SYSTEM

 HELPS PROTECT EYE HEALTH

 PROMOTES A HEALTHY PREGNANCY

Okra, also known as bhindi and lady's fingers, is a flowering plant that belongs to the mallow family. It has a unique, slightly peppery taste somewhere between eggplant and asparagus. Its main medicinal value lies in its extraordinary combination of **soluble and insoluble fiber**, which helps lower **blood sugar** levels, cleanse the **intestines**, and feed **good gut bacteria.**

What Is It Good For?

ANTIDIABETIC A rich source of many nutrients, including fiber, vitamin B_6, and folate. B vitamins slow the progress of diabetic neuropathy and reduce levels of homocysteine, a risk factor for this disease. The soluble fiber also helps to stabilize blood sugar levels.

BRILLIANT DETOX Abundant in both soluble and insoluble fiber. Soluble fiber absorbs water and helps bulk up stools, and helps lower "unhealthy" (LDL) cholesterol in the blood. Insoluble fiber helps keep the intestinal tract healthy, binding to toxins and aiding their removal. This decreases the risk of some forms of cancer, especially colorectal cancer.

PROTECTING VISION In addition to having good amounts of beta-carotene, it contains zeaxanthin and lutein. These compounds are essential for maintaining good vision.

FOLATE-RICH Okra is a good source of folate, a nutrient that enriches red blood cells, protects the heart, and lowers the risk of birth defects in babies.

How Do I Get The Best From It?

LEAVE IT WHOLE The more you slice okra, the more it exudes a gelatinous substance, which some people find off-putting. Avoid this by trimming just the ends without puncturing the inner pod, and don't overcook it.

HOW TO COOK IT Cook lightly and quickly by steaming, grilling, or adding to a stir-fry to preserve its essential nutrients.

How Do I Use It?

ADD TO A SALAD If you are tired of the same lettuce, tomato, and cucumber salad, try slicing whole grilled okra into a salad and drizzle with a chile and lime dressing.

ADD TO STEWS Use in soups and stews and curries as a thickener.

GREEN OKRA
Okra is high in fiber in the form of mucilaginous gums and pectins. If you find purple okra it will have the additional cancer-protective antioxidant anthocyanin.

Seeds
Oil pressed from okra seeds is rich in heart-friendly polyunsaturated fats and is often used in African cooking

Peas

 PROMOTES A HEALTHY DIGESTIVE TRACT

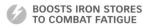 **BOOSTS IRON STORES TO COMBAT FATIGUE**

 HELPS FIGHT INFECTION

 PROMOTES HEALTHY SPERM

While neither exotic nor rare, this naturally sweet legume has a nutrient content that guarantees it a place in the medicinal food world. Peas are rich in **vitamin K**, **manganese**, and **vitamin C**, and are a good source of **folate** and **trace elements**. Their **insoluble fiber content** is good for the gut and also helps to reduce the risk of **heart disease** and **stroke**.

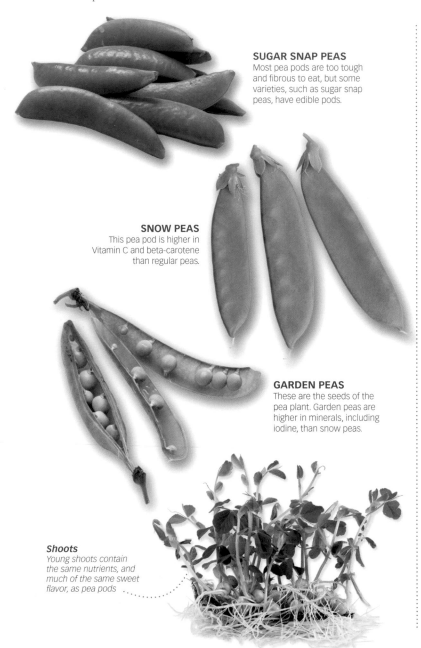

SUGAR SNAP PEAS
Most pea pods are too tough and fibrous to eat, but some varieties, such as sugar snap peas, have edible pods.

SNOW PEAS
This pea pod is higher in Vitamin C and beta-carotene than regular peas.

GARDEN PEAS
These are the seeds of the pea plant. Garden peas are higher in minerals, including iodine, than snow peas.

Shoots
Young shoots contain the same nutrients, and much of the same sweet flavor, as pea pods

What Is It Good For?

DIGESTION Its fibrous content makes it useful for maintaining a healthy digestive tract.

ENERGY BOOST A good source of iron, which helps prevent anemia and combats fatigue.

IMMUNITY Rich in vitamin C; a single serving of peas or snow peas supplies half your daily needs. Peas, especially pea shoots, also contain phytoalexins, an antioxidant that can inhibit *H. Pylori*, the bacterium that causes stomach and duodenal ulcers, and stomach cancer.

MEN'S HEALTH Glycodelin-A, a substance found in snow peas, can help strengthen sperm and improve their ability to fertilize a female egg.

EYE HEALTH The carotenoid pigment in green peas is lutein, which is well known for reducing the risk of cataracts and macular degeneration (loss of vision).

How Do I Get The Best From It?

EAT RAW Get the best flavor and nutrients by eating fresh peas straight from their pods.

FROZEN OR DRIED The sugar in fresh peas quickly turns to starch with storage. Frozen peas are processed immediately after picking, which is why they tend to taste sweeter. Dried peas are sold in green and yellow varieties (usually split), and you can also buy dried wild peas. All of them are great for enjoying the benefits of peas beyond their summer season.

How Do I Use It?

AS AN ALTERNATIVE TO LETTUCE Swap salad leaves for pea shoots in a stir-fry or salad.

SNOW PEAS WITH CASHEWS Heat 1 tsp coconut oil in a skillet. Add 3 handfuls of snow peas and the zest of ½ orange and cook on low heat for 3–4 minutes. Season and serve scattered with a handful of cashew nuts for a skin-nourishing dish.

ASPARAGUS

 HAS A MILD LAXATIVE ACTION

 REMOVES ENERGY-DRAINING TOXINS

 HELPS STRENGTHEN THE IMMUNE SYSTEM

 HELPS KEEP BLOOD VESSELS SUPPLE

Asparagus is a member of the lily family. It has been prized for millennia for its unique flavor, succulent texture, and medicinal qualities: it has **detoxifying properties** and contains **antioxidants** that strengthen the heart and blood vessels. Traditional Chinese medicine also suggests it can benefit people with **respiratory illnesses** and **ease menstrual problems**.

WHAT IS IT GOOD FOR?

SUPPORTS THE GUT Asparagus contains inulin, a prebiotic that encourages healthy gut flora. Also has mild laxative and diuretic properties.

BOOSTS ENERGY Aspartic acid neutralizes excess ammonia in the body, which could otherwise result in a sense of feeling drained and lacking in vigor.

ANTI-INFLAMMATORY Contains rutin and glutathione, which protect cells against oxidative stress by free radicals in the body, promote a healthy immune response, and can strengthen blood vessels.

PROTECTS THE HEART AND MORE A great source of B vitamins, especially folate, which may help control homocysteine, a substance that promotes heart disease, cancer, and cognitive decline. Increased folate intake during pregnancy can help fight birth defects.

SKIN HEALTH A combination of detoxifying properties and beta-carotene in asparagus has a purifying effect on the skin.

HOW DO I GET THE BEST FROM IT?

BUY IN SEASON To get the most nutrients, always buy it in season. Depending on area, asparagus season lasts from February to June.

USE IT QUICKLY Asparagus deteriorates quickly when stored. Buy and use within a couple of days to get the maximum benefit.

HOW TO COOK IT Broil or steam for 3–5 minutes (avoid boiling). Or braise quickly in a little vegetable broth to ensure the maximum flavor and retention of nutrients.

HOW DO I USE IT?

IN SALADS Add cooked cold asparagus to a colorful salad to make a delicious light meal.

AS A SPECIAL INGREDIENT Cook and serve with hot pasta, cooked fresh fish and chicken, or add to vegetable quiche.

GREEN ASPARAGUS
It contains more stress-busting B vitamins than other varieties. If you find purple asparagus, it will contain additional antioxidant pigments called anthocyanins.

WHITE ASPARAGUS
This lacks natural antioxidant pigments, but is rich in aspartic acid and cholesterol-fighting phytochemicals.

CELERY AND CELERIAC

 HELPS LOWER BLOOD PRESSURE

 HAS A DIURETIC ACTION

 PROMOTES FEELING OF FULLNESS

 PROMOTES HEALTHY JOINTS AND MUSCLES

There is more to bitter, aromatic celery than a pleasant crunch; in Eastern medicine, both the stalks and roots are used to **treat high blood pressure**. Celery and its close cousin celeriac are mildly **diuretic** and help reduce levels of the **stress hormone** cortisol. They are also rich in **B vitamins**, trace elements, **fiber**, and **circulation-supporting coumarins**. Its taste and nutritional quality are highest when in season.

SEEDS
Rich in volatile oils and essential fatty acids.

STALKS
The water and fiber content can aid weight control.

CELERIAC CORM
High in phosphorus, which benefits the nervous, lymphatic, and urinary systems.

WHAT IS IT GOOD FOR?

LOWERS BLOOD PRESSURE Contains coumarins, which help lower blood pressure and aid water balance, and phthalides, anti-coagulants that reduce the risk of blood clots and stroke and lower stress hormone levels.

A DIET AID Celery is mostly water and fiber—two things that can aid weight control. Adding celery to your meal may help you to eat more slowly and chew more thoroughly, and therefore increase a feeling of fullness.

SOURCE OF SILICON It contains good amounts of silicon as well as vitamin K, which is not only beneficial for skin and hair but also for joints, bones, muscles, arteries, and connective tissues.

HOW DO I GET THE BEST FROM IT?

STALKS Low in calories and high in fiber, the stalks (and leaves) have, in addition to their other benefits, diuretic and laxative properties.

SEEDS Rich in volatile oils, traditionally used as a diuretic and sedative, and to reduce inflammation and treat menstrual discomfort. Studies show they may help lower blood pressure and "unhealthy" (LDL) cholesterol. Use as a seasoning or brewed as a tea.

HOW DO I USE IT?

COMBINE WITH FRUIT Celery is one of the few vegetables that combine well with fruit. Slice some into a fruit salad for extra crunch.

ADDS FLAVOR The phthalides in celery and celeriac have no flavor of their own but can act as a natural flavor enhancer in meals.

AS A COLD REMEDY Combine celery juice with a little lemon juice to help treat the feverish symptoms of cold and flu.

JUICE IT Both stalk and corm yield an alkalizing, revitalizing, and detoxifying juice that helps regulate the body's water balance.

FENNEL

 EASES STOMACH CRAMPS

 CONTAINS ANTI-INFLAMMATORY OILS

 A GENTLE HORMONE REGULATOR

 HAS A DIURETIC ACTION

Aromatic fennel looks like a larger version of its relative dill, but has a distinct aniseed flavor. Since Roman times it has been valued for it ability to soothe **digestive troubles.** It also helps to relieve **water retention** and regulate **female hormones**. A low-calorie source of **vitamin C**, dietary fiber, and potassium, it also contains a range of **antioxidants** and **anti-inflammatory** volatile oils.

WHAT IS IT GOOD FOR?

STOMACH SOOTHER It encourages healthy digestion and eases stomach cramps. Can be effective against worms and parasites due to the volatile oil anethole, which gives fennel its characteristic aniseed flavor.

EASING COUGHS AND COLDS A syrup made from the juice is traditionally used to thin mucus and make coughs more productive.

HORMONE REGULATION Its estrogenic qualities may help bring hormonal balance to females of all ages—from young mothers to women in menopause.

MAINTAINING WATER BALANCE Fennel can relieve water retention and bloating.

HOW DO I GET THE BEST FROM IT?

HOW TO COOK IT The tender stems can be added to soups or roasted in oil. Fennel can also be eaten raw in salads.

MAKE USE OF THE SEEDS A mild, cooled tea made from the seeds and sweetened with a touch of honey is a time-honored way of settling the stomach and easing colic in babies.

HOW DO I USE IT?

BREW A TEA Boil 1 tsp of fennel seeds in 1 cup water or milk and drink as required.

HEALING SYRUP To make a syrup from fennel juice as a traditional remedy for coughs, juice the whole plant—or steep the seeds in a little boiling water to make a strong decoction—and mix with lemon juice and honey to taste.

LIGHTLY ROAST Slice the bulb into wedges, arrange in an ovenproof dish, season, dot with butter, add a generous handful of fresh thyme, and bake at 350°F (180°C) until tender.

MAKE A SOUP To ease menstrual symptoms, cook equal quantities of fennel, asparagus, and fresh parsley in a broth of water and milk until soft. Purée, season to taste, and serve.

SEEDS
Contain concentrated volatile oils that sooth upset stomachs.

BULB AND LEAVES
Contain anti-inflammatory and antioxidant substances including rutin, quercetin, kaempferol glycosides, and anethole.

RHUBARB

 HELPS STRENGTHEN BONES

 PROTECTS AGAINST NEURO-DEGENERATION

 HELPS LOWER CHOLESTEROL

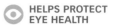 **HELPS PROTECT EYE HEALTH**

Although we think of rhubarb as a fruit, it is actually a vegetable and a member of the buckwheat family. It is too sour to eat raw, but even cooked it contains a number of beneficial properties, including helping to **strengthen bones** and protect against **neurological damage**. It is also a good source of **fiber** and is known to help reduce "unhealthy" (LDL) **cholesterol** levels in the blood.

OUTDOOR RHUBARB
Field rhubarb has bright green leaves and is less tender than the forced variety, but has a better flavor.

FORCED RHUBARB
Forced rhubarb is grown in the dark, but it has all the same healing properties.

WHAT IS IT GOOD FOR?

BONE HEALTH Contains calcium and notable amounts of vitamin K, especially important for protecting against bone fractures as we age.

PROTECTING THE BRAIN Adequate vitamin-K levels can protect against the neurological damage linked to Alzheimer's disease. Vitamin K is also a useful clotting agent for blood, so may protect against bleeding and stroke.

HEART HEALTH Studies show that including rhubarb in your diet can help reduce an overbalance of "unhealthy" (LDL) cholesterol levels in the blood. It is also a good source of fiber and has moderate levels of vitamin C.

EYE HEALTH Contains useful amounts of lutein, which can reduce the risk of age-related macular degeneration (loss of vision).

HOW DO I GET THE BEST FROM IT?

RED IS BETTER THAN GREEN Red stalks contain more beta-carotene than green varieties. They also contain small amounts of polyphenolic flavonoid compounds, such as zeaxanthin and lutein.

MAKE SURE IT'S RIPE Rhubarb contains oxalic acid, which prevents the absorption of nutrients, such as iron and calcium. Most oxalic acid concentrates in the leaves, but it can be especially high in unripe stalks too. Look for stalks that are deeply colored.

COOK IT The stalks are sour and considered inedible raw, so always cook before eating.

HOW DO I USE IT?

SPICE IT UP Sauté garlic and onions in olive oil, add chopped rhubarb, root vegetables, and presoaked lentils. Add a little stock, season with pungent curry spices, and simmer until tender. Serve over rice.

AS A FRUIT Use in preserves, jams, muffins, and fruit pies instead of cherries and berries.

ONION FAMILY

 HAS A POWERFUL ANTIBIOTIC ACTION

 HELPS LOWER CHOLESTEROL

FEEDS GOOD BACTERIA IN THE GUT

The onion family is part of the allium family, which also includes garlic. The Chinese, East Indians, Ancient Greeks, Romans, and even Egyptians all revered onions, and modern science has proved them right. Onions contain dozens of medicinal chemical compounds that have **antibacterial** and **anti-inflammatory** actions in the body and promote good **heart** and **gut health**.

WHAT IS IT GOOD FOR?

ANTIBACTERIAL ACTION The sulfur compounds in onions—including thiosulfinates, sulfides, and sulfoxides—are responsible for their powerful antibacterial and antiviral action, and unique taste.

HEART HEALTH A good source of heart-healthy quercetin. This flavonoid helps avoid heart disease by preventing blood clots and cholesterol from sticking to arterial walls. Over time, quercetin can also help raise levels of "healthy" (HDL) cholesterol in the blood.

HEALTHY GUT Contains a fiber called inulin and a range of other fructo-oligosaccharides. These compounds, known as prebiotics, provide the right food to encourage the growth of healthy bacteria in the gut. This may be why including more onions in your diet has a role to play in preventing bowel cancer.

HOW DO I GET THE BEST FROM IT?

RAW IS BEST Its benefits are mostly lost when cooked. To enjoy at its medicinal best, use raw or braise lightly in stock or broth.

USE STRONG VARIETIES Highly flavored onions contain the most healthful compounds.

HOW DO I USE IT?

A SIMPLE COLD REMEDY Mix onion juice with honey and take 2–3 tsp daily when you are fighting a cold or feel one coming on.

A VARIETY OF TASTES Onions and shallots add punch and bite to omelets, soups, and stews, while leeks lend a rich, creamy flavor. Scallions are ideal in stir-fries or with steamed fish, and can enliven mashed potato.

SPROUT THE SEEDS Add sprouting onion seeds to salads, sandwiches, and other dishes.

RAMPS These immature flowering stalks, available in late spring/early summer, are delicious in a spring detox salad.

RED ONION
Pigments known as anthocyanins give red onions an antioxidant boost.

WHITE ONION
Contains the flavonoid quercetin, which can help prevent heart disease.

SPRING ONION
Even "baby" onions such as these contain immunity-boosting sulfur compounds.

LEEK
This mild-flavored relative of the onion stimulates appetite, and is a gentle diuretic and laxative.

GARLIC

 A NATURAL ANTICOAGULANT

 HELPS STRENGTHEN THE IMMUNE SYSTEM

 REMOVES TOXINS AND POLLUTANTS

 CONTAINS ANTICANCER SUBSTANCES

The main beneficial ingredients of this member of the allium family are allicin and diallyl sulfides—sulfurous compounds that are **antibacterial** and **antifungal**. Garlic is universally recognized for its health-promoting benefits: **aiding the circulatory** and **digestive** systems, boosting the **immune system**, lowering **blood pressure**, and fighting **heart disease**. It even helps to **eliminate toxins**.

DRIED GARLIC BULB
Contains abundant antibiotic and antifungal sulfur compounds including allicin, alliin, and ajoene.

Wild garlic leaves
Use sparingly in salads, pestos, soups, and risottos for extra flavor

FRESH GARLIC
Has the same benefits as the dried bulb and with edible stems.

WILD GARLIC
Only the leaves and flowers are usually eaten, making it easier to digest than bulb garlic. The leaves contain chlorophyll in addition to adenosine.

Flowering stalks
Garlic scapes are harvested in late spring/early summer and can be added to salads

GARLIC SCAPES
These are immature flowering stalks of garlic that have the same benefits as the mature bulb, but with a mild flavor.

WHAT IS IT GOOD FOR?

HEART HEALTH The sulfur in garlic stimulates nitric oxide production in blood vessels. This relaxes and improves their elasticity, helping lower blood pressure and reducing the risk of stroke and atherosclerosis (hardening of the arteries).

IMMUNITY Its volatile oils are antibiotic and can be used to treat colds and coughs.

DETOXIFYING Contains sulfhydryl, which works by helping to remove toxic substances, such as heavy metals, from the body.

CANCER Garlic is recognized for helping to prevent numerous types of cancer, including bowel, breast, and lung cancer. It purportedly also helps treat prostate and bladder cancer.

REGULATES BLOOD SUGAR LEVELS A regular intake of garlic lowers the amino acid homocysteine, a risk factor in diabetes and heart disease.

HOW DO I GET THE BEST FROM IT?

FRESH IS BEST Choose fresh rather than bottled in water or oil, because its healthful allicin compounds degrade dramatically.

TRY BLACK GARLIC Fermented black garlic has a molasses-like balsamic flavor, twice the amount of antioxidants of white garlic, and leaves no trace of bad breath after eating it.

HOW TO COOK IT Cooked garlic doesn't have the same levels of allicin as raw, but it does retain other compounds. Let it stand for 10 minutes after crushing or slicing to allow the allicin to develop before being heated. Microwaving kills off nearly all its benefits.

HOW DO I USE IT?

FRESH GARLIC Cook the stems like leeks, or slice and use in soups and omelets or as a garnish for salads.

EAT RAW Scatter raw over cooked vegetables.

BEETS

 HAS A LIVER-CLEANSING ACTION

 LOWERS THE RISK OF HEART ATTACK

 IMPROVES BLOOD'S OXYGEN UPTAKE

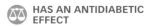 **HAS AN ANTIDIABETIC EFFECT**

They may look tough, but beets are a delicate vegetable with a unique group of **antioxidants**, known as betacyanins. These pigments give beets their strong color and are the source of their medicinal benefits: **supporting the liver**, **improving circulation**, and **purifying the blood**. Eaten raw, they have a crunchy texture; once cooked, they taste soft and buttery. Their leaves **aid digestion**.

WHAT IS IT GOOD FOR?

SUPPORTS THE LIVER Its phytochemicals stimulate the production of glutathione, a detoxifying antioxidant that combines with an array of antioxidant pigments to aid liver function and neutralize and excrete toxins.

STRENGTHENS THE HEART Its antioxidants lower cholesterol and blood pressure, while the B vitamins improve nerve function, helping maintain a strong regular heartbeat.

NOURISHES THE BLOOD A combination of iron and antioxidants helps feed and purify the blood while improving its oxygen uptake, making beets a useful remedy for anemia.

ANTI-INFLAMMATORY Contains choline, a B vitamin that supports heart health, and is also antidiabetic.

HOW DO I GET THE BEST FROM IT?

EAT FRESH Grated in a salad, it adds crunchy texture, lively color, and boosts nutrients.

USE THE LEAVES Beet greens are even more nutrient-packed than the root and are rich in bone- and blood-healthy vitamin K and beta-carotene, which is great for the skin and eyes, among other things.

HOW TO COOK IT Lightly steamed or roasted is best. The freshest beets will cook faster, helping retain essential nutrients.

HOW DO I USE IT?

JUICE IT The juice can lower blood pressure within an hour of drinking. Regular intake can lower the risk of heart disease, and is used as part of an anticancer regime in some clinics.

COMBINE IT Eat with carrots in salads (or as a juice) to boost energy, improve appetite, and aid hormone regulation during menopause.

LEAFY SALAD Use the leaves raw in salads as a slightly bitter digestive aid or lightly steam it like spinach.

RED BEETS
Liver-healthy betacyanins are the dominant antioxidant pigments in this root.

Leaves
Sometimes called chard, beet leaves of all varieties are rich in protein, fiber, vitamins, and minerals

Root
Cook with the skin and trimmed stems on to prevent the beneficial pigments from bleeding away

GOLD BEETS
Immunity-boosting betaxanthins, particularly vulgaxanthin, are the main antioxidant pigments in this variety of beet.

CARROTS

 AIDS DIGESTION AND A FEELING OF FULLNESS

 HELPS LOWER CHOLESTEROL

 POWERFUL ANTIOXIDANT

 HELPS MAINTAIN GOOD EYESIGHT

The benefits of carrots are hinted at in their name; they are rich in beta-carotene (from which the body makes vitamin A). A diet high in carotenes is associated with significant decreases in the incidence of **some cancers**. Carrots also aid **digestion**, help **weight control**, contain silicon, which benefits skin and nails, and promote **eye health** due to their beta-carotene, lycopene, and lutein content.

ORANGE CARROTS
Contain beta-carotene and the eye-healthy antioxidants lutein and lycopene.

PURPLE CARROTS
Contain extra antioxidant pigments that may benefit diseases, such as arthritis and heart disease.

WHAT IS IT GOOD FOR?

WEIGHT CONTROL High fiber promotes a feeling of fullness and aids bowel regularity.

CHOLESTEROL FIGHTING Contain a form of calcium easily assimilated by the body that may help lower "unhealthy" (LDL) cholesterol levels.

SKIN CONDITION In addition to beta-carotene, lutein, and lycopene, carrots contain silicon, which promotes healthy skin and nails.

SEEING CLEARLY Lutein and lycopene help maintain good eyesight and night vision.

HOW DO I GET THE BEST FROM IT?

EAT IT RAW A raw carrot a day can reduce the risk of cancers of the esophagus, stomach, intestines, and prostate. The essential oils in carrots protect against intestinal parasites.

FRESH IS BEST As soon as a carrot is picked, its beta-carotene content begins to decline. Buy loose carrots rather than those in plastic bags and consume as quickly as possible.

DON'T THROW THE GREENS AWAY Carrot tops are edible and rich in protein, minerals, and vitamins. Use in small amounts in salads and dressings, as a garnish instead of a fresh herb, or brew into an antiseptic, diuretic tea.

HOW DO I USE IT?

A GREAT BASE FOR JUICE Juicing gives the highest concentration of beta-carotene. It makes a good base ingredient for fruit and vegetable juice mixes.

CHILDREN'S LUNCHBOXES A few carrot sticks a day can help strengthen and clean children's teeth, and may also help encourage lower-jaw development and avoid overcrowded teeth.

PURÉE INTO A SOUP Use as a healing, strengthening dish for stomach upsets, or if you have poor digestion.

A tea made from chlorophyll-rich carrot tops makes a delicious, detoxifying drink. Choose organic carrots with leaves that haven't been treated with chemicals.

RADISHES

⚙ **SUPPORTS HEALTHY LIVER FUNCTION**

♡ **HELPS LOWER BLOOD PRESSURE**

⤷ **TREATS CONGESTION AND INFLAMMATION**

Belonging to the cruciferous family of vegetables, fiery-tasting radishes grow in a variety of sizes, shapes, and colors, and are available all year round. Both the roots and leaves are rich in **vitamin C**, potassium, magnesium, **B vitamins**, and trace elements, which help to fight **hypertension**. Its pungent essential oils help support a **healthy liver** and fight inflammation and congestion.

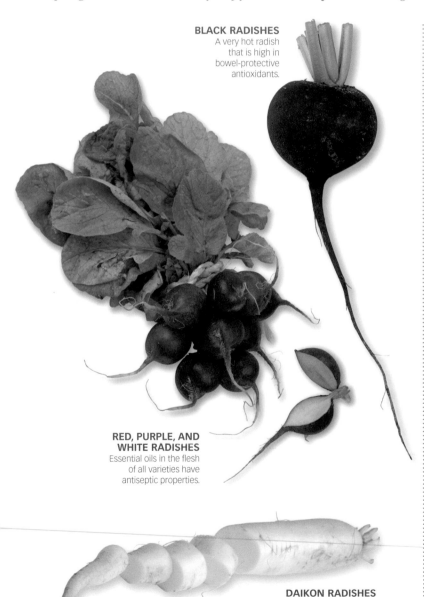

BLACK RADISHES
A very hot radish that is high in bowel-protective antioxidants.

RED, PURPLE, AND WHITE RADISHES
Essential oils in the flesh of all varieties have antiseptic properties.

DAIKON RADISHES
In Chinese medicine, the daikon radish is considered cooling and is used to soothe coughs, bronchitis, and laryngitis.

WHAT IS IT GOOD FOR?

DETOX The radish is a useful tool for fat digestion because it stimulates the flow of bile. It also has a cleansing, decongesting action on the gallbladder, liver, and blood. Traditionally, radishes have been used to help break up gallstones and kidney stones. They also have a diuretic and laxative action.

FIGHTS HYPERTENSION Radishes are high in potassium, which helps keep blood pressure low.

CLEARS CONGESTION The high vitamin C content in radishes can help treat colds and the flu. The juice pressed from grated, fresh radish root is a traditional remedy for coughs, inflamed joints, and gallbladder problems.

HOW DO I GET THE BEST FROM IT?

USE THE GREEN TOPS Radish leaves contain 6 times more vitamin C than the roots, and also supply calcium.

LOOK FOR DAIKON RADISHES The daikon radish, a staple of Eastern cooking, is high in the enzyme myrosinase: it both aids digestion and, during the digestive process, produces isothiocyanate, an antioxidant that has anticancer benefits.

HOW DO I USE IT?

JUICE IT Make a fiery detox drink by juicing apples, celery, and radishes. As a cold remedy, try mixing equal parts of radish juice and honey. Take 1 tbsp 3 times a day.

A SIMPLE SIDE DISH Gently braise radishes in butter and vegetable stock. Turn off the heat, add some fresh watercress, season, and serve.

ENERGIZING SALAD Make a salad from thinly sliced radish, a soft leaf lettuce (e.g. butter lettuce), and ruby grapefruit segments. Dress with a mustard vinaigrette containing some of the grapefruit juice.

POTATOES

 HELPS FIGHT INFLAMMATION

 HELPS LOWER BLOOD PRESSURE

 HELPS CALM THE NERVES

Potatoes are a surprisingly good source of vitamin C, potassium, fiber, B vitamins, copper, tryptophan, manganese, and even lutein. Their alkaline nature helps to **detoxify** and balance excess **acidity** in the body and relieve the **inflammation** and pain of **ulcers**. They are a **natural sedative** and encourage healthy **blood circulation**, and the skin contains chlorogenic acid, which helps prevent cell mutation.

WHAT IS IT GOOD FOR?

REDUCING INFLAMMATION Alkalizing and anti-inflammatory, potatoes soothe stomach and duodenum ulcers and reduce stomach acidity. They may also relieve the inflammation associated with arthritis.

HIGH BLOOD PRESSURE Potatoes are high in chlorogenic acid and anthocyanins, chemicals that help to lower blood pressure. The polyphenol in purple potatoes may also help.

CALMING THE NERVES Potatoes contain tryptophan, an amino acid with natural sedative properties.

HOW DO I GET THE BEST FROM IT?

USE THE JUICE Drinking the juice is a quick way to benefit from its anti-inflammatory properties. Wash and grate several red-skinned potatoes, put in cheesecloth, and squeeze to remove the juice. Drink as needed.

KEEP THE SKIN ON Potato nutrients leech into the cooking water and so lose a great deal of their nutritional value if they are peeled before boiling. When buying potatoes, avoid those that are already washed. The washing process destroys their natural protective coating, making them more vulnerable to bacteria and thus decay. Buy organic potatoes to ensure the skins are free from pesticides.

HOW DO I USE IT?

POTATO AND NETTLE RÖSTI Boil potatoes until al dente (still slightly firm). When cool, roughly grate, blend with a handful of chopped nettles, season, shape into small flat cakes, and shallow-fry. Drain and serve.

POTATO SALAD Use red-skinned potatoes in a potato salad for an extra dose of antioxidants.

CRUSHED POTATOES AND WILD GARLIC Cook new potatoes until just tender and crush rather than mash them together with a handful of wild garlic and butter or oil.

White flesh
The sedative tryptophan in potatoes makes them a good choice if you are stressed

Red skin
Contains antioxidant anthocyanins, which are good for the heart

NEW POTATOES
New potatoes are eaten with the skin on, which is rich in nutrients.

PURPLE POTATOES
In Korea, the purple potato is eaten as a way to lose weight.

SWEET POTATOES

 HELPS BALANCE BLOOD SUGAR LEVELS

 FIGHTS FREE-RADICAL DAMAGE TO SKIN

PROTECTS AGAINST INFECTION

They may look uninteresting, but sweet potatoes are a superfood. A single sweet potato contains more than a day's worth of **beta-carotene** and nearly all your daily **vitamin C** requirements. They help combat **free radicals** in the body, benefit **skin health**, and support the **immune system**. Because of their high level of slow-release carbohydrates, they can also help maintain **steady blood sugar levels.**

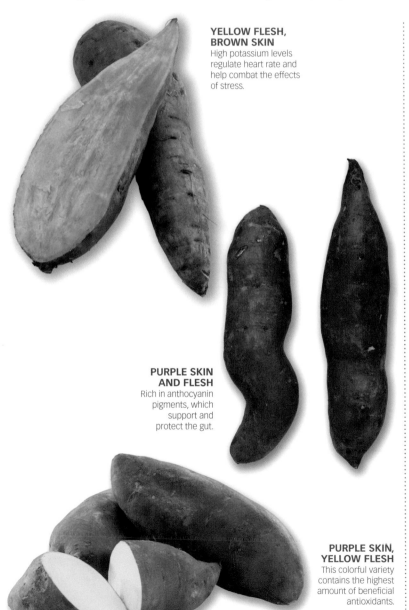

YELLOW FLESH, BROWN SKIN
High potassium levels regulate heart rate and help combat the effects of stress.

PURPLE SKIN AND FLESH
Rich in anthocyanin pigments, which support and protect the gut.

PURPLE SKIN, YELLOW FLESH
This colorful variety contains the highest amount of beneficial antioxidants.

WHAT IS IT GOOD FOR?

GLUCOSE CONTROL Sweet potatoes are a traditional treatment for diabetes. They contain slow-release carbohydrates and the hormone adiponectin, a combination that helps keep blood sugar levels steady.

BEAUTIFUL SKIN Its high levels of beta-carotene means sweet potato benefits skin by fighting the free radicals that cause skin aging.

IMMUNE BOOSTING High in beta-carotene and vitamin C, regular consumption of sweet potatoes can strengthen the immune system and help develop resistance to infection, and may also provide anticancer benefits.

HOW DO I GET THE BEST FROM IT?

KEEP THE SKIN ON The skin is healthy and contains nutrients similar to that of the flesh underneath. To get your full complement, eat sweet potatoes with their skins on.

HOW TO COOK THEM Steaming or boiling, rather than roasting, preserves their slow-release carbohydrates and essential nutrients.

ADD SOME FAT Eat with a little butter or oil to ensure all the antioxidants, such as beta-carotene, are fully absorbed.

THINK PURPLE The purple-fleshed sweet potato is rich in antioxidant and anti-inflammatory anthocyanins—primarily peonidins and cyanidins—that can protect against irritable bowel and ulcerative colitis.

HOW DO I USE IT?

MASHED Peel and cut roughly into chunks. Boil for 30 minutes or until soft, mash with butter, and serve. Add brown sugar, cinnamon, and/or nutmeg for extra flavor.

AS A SALAD Add steamed (or leftover) sweet potatoes and sliced red peppers to arugula or spinach. Dress with a balsamic vinegar dressing. Add goat cheese too, if you like.

TURMERIC

 HELPS RELIEVE ARTHRITIC PAIN

 HELPS PREVENT HARDENED ARTERIES

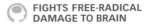 **FIGHTS FREE-RADICAL DAMAGE TO BRAIN**

 CONTAINS ANTICANCER SUBSTANCES

Known to be extremely beneficial for health, turmeric is a key ingredient in almost any curry, and can be used fresh or as a powder. Its main healthy constituent is curcumin, a well-researched **antioxidant** and powerful **anti-inflammatory** that helps to fight **free-radical damage** and prevent and treat **arthritis**, **cardiovascular problems**, **diabetes**, and even **neurological conditions**.

WHAT IS IT GOOD FOR?

ANTI-INFLAMMATORY Contains potent volatile oils with anti-inflammatory properties and, perhaps most importantly, curcumin, which gives it its vibrant color. Curcumin has a medicinal effect comparable to drugs, such as hydrocortisone and phenylbutazone, and can be used to provide relief from rheumatoid arthritis, treat inflammatory bowel disease, protect against diabetes, and avoid heart disease and stroke by preventing the build-up of plaque in the arteries.

ALZHEIMER'S PROTECTION Curcumin reduces the build-up of the protein amyloid-b in the brain. Amyloid-b causes oxidative (free radical) damage and inflammation in the brain and is one of the main causes of Alzheimer's disease. Antioxidants in turmeric help to fight this free-radical damage.

CANCER PROTECTION In laboratory studies, curcumin has been shown to stop the growth and spread of cancer cells.

HOW DO I GET THE BEST FROM IT?

FRESH OR DRIED The fresh root can be used in place of ginger in most meals. The powder is a key component in most Indian curries.

LEAVES The leaves can be used to flavor dishes, such as curries, or to wrap around food during cooking.

DON'T FORGET THE OIL Curcumin is better absorbed in the presence of oils, such as coconut, olive, ghee, and butter. Heating it slightly aids absorption.

HOW DO I USE IT?

AN ANTIOXIDANT DRINK Stir 1 tbsp turmeric powder into warm whole or low-fat milk to treat painful joints or eczema.

A SPICY RICE DISH Enliven brown rice with cashews and raisins, and season with turmeric, cumin, and toasted coriander seeds.

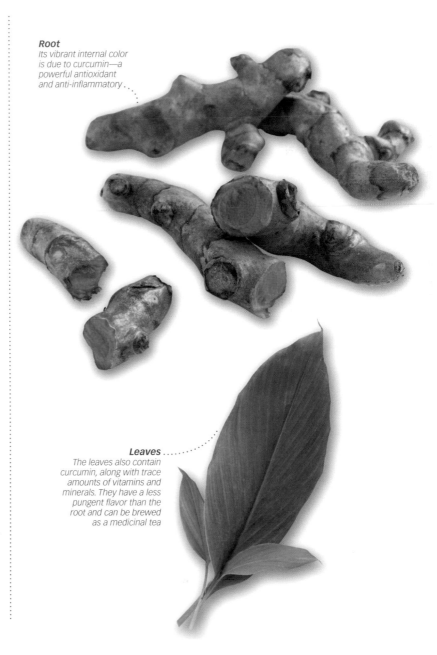

Root
Its vibrant internal color is due to curcumin—a powerful antioxidant and anti-inflammatory.

Leaves
The leaves also contain curcumin, along with trace amounts of vitamins and minerals. They have a less pungent flavor than the root and can be brewed as a medicinal tea

GINGER

 HAS POWERFUL ANTI-INFLAMMATORY OILS

 HELPS ALLEVIATE ARTHRITIC PAIN

 REDUCES SYMPTOMS OF NAUSEA

This pungent root is known for its ability to settle **upset stomachs** and **alleviate nausea**. Its active constituent, gingerol, is a relative of capsaicin and piperine, found in hot chiles. Studies show that its volatile oils have **anti-inflammatory** properties similar to those of NSAIDs (nonsteroidal anti-inflammatory drugs) so it can ease the symptoms of **colds and flu, headaches,** and **menstrual pains.**

MATURE GINGER ROOT
Gingerol has analgesic, sedative, antipyretic, and antibacterial effects; another component, zingerone, is an antioxidant.

YOUNG GINGER ROOT
Contains the same substances as the mature root, but the thinner pink/purple skin doesn't need to be peeled.

PICKLED GINGER
Made from young roots, it is naturally pink and contains beneficial anthocyanin antioxidants.

WHAT IS IT GOOD FOR?

FIGHTS INFLAMMATION Reduces inflammation, lessens pain, and can lower medication intake in cases of osteoarthritis.

NAUSEA Studies show it can ease morning sickness, motion sickness, and nausea caused by cancer chemotherapy and after surgery.

DIGESTIVE HEALTH Protects and heals the gut, hastens the movement of food through the gastrointestinal tract, and reduces wind, bloating, and cramps. It also awakens the taste buds and gets digestive juices flowing.

HOW DO I GET THE BEST FROM IT?

PEEL IT CAREFULLY The richest resins and volatile oils concentrate in and near the skin so peel carefully. The best way to peel ginger is with a teaspoon. Gently scrape the skin off rather than using a vegetable peeler.

EAT FRESH Whenever possible, choose fresh ginger. It is not only superior in flavor to dried but contains higher levels of active constituents, such as gingerol and zingibain. Store in a dry place.

LOOK FOR YOUNG ROOTS Most supermarkets sell the mature roots, though Asian supermarkets often sell the younger pale pink roots. These don't need peeling, are juicier, and have a milder taste.

HOW DO I USE IT?

SOOTHING SYRUP For sore throats or congestion, make a syrup of 2 tsp each ginger juice, turmeric, and black pepper, 1 tsp each honey and vinegar, and 3 tbsp water. Use as needed. An easy way to collect the juice is to grate the root and squeeze the juice from the shreds.

MAKE A TEA Mix 1 tsp freshly grated ginger, the juice of ½ lemon, and 1 tsp honey in a mug. Add boiling water. Take at the first signs of a cold or chill, or for indigestion or nausea.

MUSHROOMS

 CLEANSING AND ANTI-INFLAMMATORY

 FEEDS GOOD BACTERIA IN THE GUT

 GOOD SOURCE OF VITAMIN D

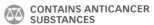 **CONTAINS ANTICANCER SUBSTANCES**

Most commercial mushroom varieties are actually the same mushroom at different stages of growth, and share common medicinal traits. Others, such as shiitake, rei-shi, and wild wood ear, are "super" mushrooms with extraordinary **healing powers**. All types contain varying degrees of **fiber**, protein, **B vitamins**, and **vitamin D**. They are also known to have **anti-inflammatory** and **antibacterial** effects.

WHAT IS IT GOOD FOR?

ANTIOXIDANT All mushrooms are considered "cleansing," and all except oyster and maitake contain ergothioneine, an amino acid that can help reduce inflammation. They also contain germanium, which improves cellular oxygenation and enhances immunity.

A PREBIOTOIC Eaten raw, mushrooms contain higher levels of prebiotic oligosaccharides, such as chitin and beta-glucan, which feed friendly bacteria in the gut.

A GOOD SOURCE OF VITAMIN D Common white mushrooms are one of the few non-animal sources of vitamin D—essential to bone health, hormone balance, immune defense, and as a cancer preventive.

ANTICANCER PROPERTIES Shiitake contains lentinan, which has anticancer, antiviral, and antibacterial properties. It also boosts the immune system by stimulating the production of white blood cells.

HOW DO I GET THE BEST FROM IT?

CLEANING MUSHROOMS Most store-bought mushrooms have been cleaned, while foraged mushrooms benefit from a brief wash or brush. Their nutrient quality is not affected.

HOW TO COOK IT Cooking mushrooms increases their starch, fiber, and fat content, and frees more antioxidants, including carotenoids and ferulic acid, but does destroy some of their vitamin C content.

HOW DO I USE IT?

DRIED EXOTICS Dried mushrooms have an intense flavor. To reconstitute, soak in boiling water. Reserve the water, which will have leeched some nutrients out of the fungi, to use as a broth or as a stock for soups and stews.

AS A MEAT SUBSTITUTE Mushrooms take on a meaty texture when cooked that can help make a meal more satisfying.

SHIITAKE
Contains lentinan, a substance that has anticancer properties and also keeps the blood from getting "sticky."

REI-SHI
A good general tonic with antiallergic and antiviral properties.

WOOD (JELLY) EAR
Helps control blood sugar levels and has anticancer, anticoagulant, and cholesterol-fighting properties.

WHITE
Even the most unassuming mushrooms have been shown to support immune function.

NUTS

 FIGHTS INFLAMMATORY DISEASES   **HELPS LOWER CHOLESTEROL**   **HELPS KEEP JOINTS SUPPLE**

Some of the highest **antioxidant** levels of all plant foods are found in nuts. Antioxidants are vital for helping to **fight inflammation** and **cell and tissue damage** caused by free radicals (toxic byproducts of metabolism). Nuts are also **rich in fiber**, healthy fats, **vitamins**, and minerals, and research shows they help to **lower cholesterol**, **improve blood vessel function**, and **benefit muscles and joints**, too.

Almonds

ALMONDS

WHAT IS IT GOOD FOR?

LOWERS CHOLESTEROL Almonds are a good source of the minerals zinc, magnesium, and potassium, and are very rich in antioxidant vitamin E, which supports the brain, the cardiovascular and respiratory systems, and helps keep skin healthy. They are especially rich in cholesterol-lowering monounsaturated fatty acids, such as oleic and palmitoleic acids. Their high fiber content also helps regulate blood sugar levels.

HOW DO I USE IT?

A VERSATILE INGREDIENT Eat with their skins on, as the flavonoids in the skins work synergistically with the vitamin E to more than double their antioxidant power. Use ground almonds as a low-starch, gluten-free flour in baking or to make almond milk, a useful alternative to dairy.

Cashews

CASHEWS

WHAT IS IT GOOD FOR?

GOOD FOR BONES A good source of monounsaturated oleic acid and omega-3 alpha linolenic acid (ALA), which are both healthy fats that help protect against heart disease and cancer. Cashews also contain calcium, magnesium, iron, zinc, and folate, making them an excellent source of minerals that contribute to bone health. These nutrients also help with the formation of collagen, which is essential for supporting healthy skin and body tissues.

HOW DO I USE IT?

SWEET AND SAVORY Cashews contain starch so are useful for thickening water-based dishes, such as soups, meat stews, and some Indian milk-based desserts. Cashew cream made from blended soaked cashews can be used as a healthy alternative to dairy cream.

Chestnuts

CHESTNUTS

WHAT IS IT GOOD FOR?

PROTECTS THE HEART Chestnuts can be classed as the only really low-fat nut, because they contain a fraction of the calories of other types of nuts. However, they are high in fiber, beta-carotene, and folate, and are also the only nuts that contain a significant amount of antioxidant vitamin C. In addition, they contain high levels of palmitic acid and oleic acid, the heart-healthy fatty acids found in olive oil.

HOW DO I USE IT?

AN ALTERNATIVE TO WHEAT Eat boiled, puréed, or roasted and added to pastries, soups, poultry, stuffings, casseroles, and appetizers. Chestnut flour is gluten-free and is used in many Italian dishes, such as polenta, gnocchi, sweet breads, and cookies.

Hazelnuts

What Is It Good For?

RICH IN ANTIOXIDANTS High in monounsaturates, which protect the heart and help lower "unhealthy" (LDL) cholesterol levels in the blood, and vitamins E and K. Also a rich source of folate and the B vitamin biotin, which promotes healthy skin and hair, and copper, which helps build red blood cells, protects cells from free-radical damage, and strengthens connective tissues. Eaten with their skins on, hazelnuts contain 3 times as much antioxidant proanthocyanidin, which helps prevent free radicals from damaging organs and cells, as other nuts.

How Do I Use It?

AS A GARNISH Crush and sprinkle over baked fruit, granola, fruit desserts, and savory dishes.

Hazelnuts

Pine Nuts

What Is It Good For?

A GOOD SOURCE OF PROTEIN Contains more vitamin K, which protects bones and arteries, than other nuts. A good source of magnesium and potassium, which help maintain a steady heartbeat, lower blood pressure, and improve circulation. Although higher in fat than other nuts, they are richer in phytosterols, plant hormones that lower "unhealthy" (LDL) cholesterol levels in the blood, reduce the risk of certain types of cancer, and enhance immune function.

How Do I Use It?

ADD A HANDFUL Pine nuts added to a meal can help to create a feeling of fullness and satisfaction. Toss into hot pasta or pilaf or add to stuffed tomatoes, zucchini, or eggplants.

Pine nuts

Pistachio Nuts

What Is It Good For?

ANTI-INFLAMMATORY Their vibrant color indicates a high antioxidant content. Pistachios are also high in beta-carotene and the compound oleanolic acid, both potent anti-inflammatories, and phytosterols, a type of anti-inflammatory plant hormone associated with improved immune function, lower levels of "unhealthy" (LDL) cholesterol, and a reduced risk of cancer. They contain valuable minerals, such as potassium, calcium, zinc, iron, and magnesium.

How Do I Use It?

KEEP IT COOL Heat can reduce their nutritional value so use as a garnish, sprinkle on probiotic yogurt, or combine with nettles, dandelion leaves, and Parmesan cheese to make a detoxifying springtime pesto sauce.

Pistachio nuts

Walnuts

What Is It Good For?

SUPPORTS A HEALTHY HEART A rich source of alpha-linolenic acid (ALA), an omega-3 fatty acid. ALA helps lower "unhealthy" (LDL) cholesterol levels and keeps arteries healthy. Walnuts also contain the antioxidants ellagic acid and a mix of tocopherols (the vitamin-E complex) including alpha, delta, and gamma tocopherol, which help reduce the risk of cancer and heart disease and maintain skin and tissue health. In addition, they contain serotonin, a brain chemical that can help lift depression.

How Do I Use It?

COOKED OR RAW Use in stuffings, baked goods, as a topping for fruit and yogurt, or in salads.

Walnuts

SEEDS AND SPROUTS

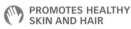 **PROMOTES HEALTHY SKIN AND HAIR**

 HELPS REMOVE TOXINS FROM THE BODY

 SUPPORTS HORMONE BALANCE

 PROTECTS THE HEART AND BLOOD VESSELS

Though tiny, seeds are packed with nutrients such as **protein**, **fiber**, **iron**, **vitamins**, and **omega-3** fatty acids that help promote **healthy skin and hair**, **remove toxins**, **balance hormones**, and support **cardiovascular health**. Sprouting seeds converts their starch to slow-release carbohydrates, releases enzymes that **aid digestion**, and makes their nutrients more **bioavailable** (easily absorbed).

Sesame seeds

SESAME SEEDS

WHAT IS IT GOOD FOR?

HELPS IMPROVE SKIN A good source of vitamin E, which helps improve the condition of the skin as well as strengthen the heart and the nervous system. Also contains the plant hormones sesamin and sesamolin, which have been shown to lower blood pressure and protect the liver from toxic damage. Sesame seeds are very high in calcium, which is necessary for healthy bones and teeth. All varieties—white, brown, and black—are suitable for eating raw or soaking and sprouting.

HOW DO I USE IT?

A VERSATILE SEED Scatter the seeds on steamed vegetables, and add the sprouts to salads, stir-fries, baked goods, sandwiches, and quiches. Ground sesame seeds are the basis of tahini, a sesame paste that can be used in hummus recipes or salad dressings, or simply spread on toast and drizzled with honey or miso.

Sunflower seeds

SUNFLOWER SEEDS

WHAT IS IT GOOD FOR?

MAINTAINS HEALTHY HAIR AND SKIN An excellent source of vitamin E, an antioxidant that helps maintain healthy hair and skin, protects cells from damage, and has anticancer properties. The seeds are an excellent source of B vitamins too, especially folate, which helps support a healthy pregnancy and aids the immune system. They are also rich in protein and heart-healthy fats. Eat raw, or soak and sprout.

HOW DO I USE IT?

AS A SNACK OR IN DISHES Eat a handful as a snack or add to salads, stir-fries, baked goods, and trail mixes. Soaking and sprouting the seeds produce a substantial microgreen (smallest edible plant) that is very nutritious.

Pumpkin seeds

PUMPKIN SEEDS

WHAT IS IT GOOD FOR?

MEN'S HEALTH High in zinc, they are useful for promoting men's fertility and preventing prostate problems.

CARDIOVASCULAR HEALTH A good source of B vitamins, magnesium, iron, and protein. The seeds have high levels of essential fatty acids that help maintain healthy blood vessels and lower "unhealthy" (LDL) cholesterol in the blood. Eat raw or dry-roasted; they are nearly impossible to sprout, but soaking them for 1–2 hours helps release their nutrients.

HOW DO I USE IT?

SOAK THEM Eat the raw, dry-roasted, or soaked seeds on their own as a snack, and use in baking, cooking, as a soup garnish, and with granola.

FLAXSEEDS

WHAT IS IT GOOD FOR?

HEART HEALTH Flaxseeds are a great source of soluble mucilaginous (gumlike) fiber that can lower "unhealthy" (LDL) cholesterol in the blood, balance blood sugar levels, and act as a hunger suppressant. Their high omega-3 fatty acid content can help lower undesirable fats (triglycerides) in the blood, reducing the risk of stroke and heart attack, and is also beneficial to the eyes, joints, and brain health. Flaxseed shells are hard so either grind or sprout the seeds, or buy them ready-cracked, to benefit from their nutrients.

HOW DO I USE IT?

GRIND OR SPROUT If you buy whole flaxseeds, grind as needed and add to yogurt, oatmeal, cereal, smoothies, casseroles, and baked goods. Sprouting flaxseeds releases more of their protein and omega-3 fats.

Flaxseeds

POPPY SEEDS

WHAT IS IT GOOD FOR?

PROTECTS THE HEART The seeds contain both polyunsaturated and monounsaturated fatty acids, which can help protect the heart. They also contain iron, phosphorus, and fiber, as well as an array of B vitamins.

A GENERAL TONIC In traditional Ayurvedic medicine, poppy seeds are considered a general tonic and a remedy for diarrhea. A tea made from the seeds is an age-old remedy for anxiety and nervous tension. Like hemp, most culinary-grade poppy seeds have been sterilized to prevent germination (into the opium poppy), although you cannot get "high" from eating poppy seeds. Because they are too small to chew thoroughly, grind the seeds before use to release their beneficial fats and nutrients, or soak and sprout them.

HOW DO I USE IT?

GRIND OR SPROUT Sprinkle the dried seeds on yogurt and use in savory dishes, such as pasta, fish, and baked goods. If you are able to find unsterilized seeds, soak and sprout them; the sprouts can be eaten raw or incorporated into other foods, such as breads and cakes.

Black poppy seeds

White poppy seeds

HEMP SEEDS

WHAT IS IT GOOD FOR?

BOOSTS HEART HEALTH Contains a perfect balance of omega-3, 6, and 9 fatty acids, which help boost brain and heart health. They are also a source of complete protein and fiber that benefits gastrointestinal and heart health, and a source of phytosterols (plant hormones) that helps lower cholesterol and promote hormonal balance in the body.

ANTI-INFLAMMATORY Hemp seeds also reduce inflammation, and keep skin and joints in good condition. In some countries, selling "live" hemp seed is illegal because the hemp plant is a member of the cannabis family. In these countries, the seeds are sterilized to prevent sprouting. You cannot get "high" from eating hemp seeds or sprouts.

HOW DO I USE IT?

LIVE SEEDS Try scattering hemp seeds on a salad, or use as a topping for yogurt, cereal, or desserts. Where you can buy live seeds, hemp sprouts make a nutritious addition to baked goods and smoothies, as well as to salads and sandwiches.

Hemp seeds

SEEDS AND SPROUTS CONTINUED

Alfalfa seeds

ALFALFA SEEDS

WHAT IS IT GOOD FOR?

DETOXIFIER Rich in nutrients and antioxidants, particularly chlorophyll, which helps remove toxins from the blood. Alfalfa seeds also have a natural diuretic action, which maintains water balance and helps lower blood pressure. In addition, they contain coumarin, a blood thinner that is useful for maintaining good blood circulation and for preventing strokes. They also contain betaine, an enzyme that helps to break down proteins and fats, and so aid good digestion.

WOMEN'S HEALTH Alfalfa seeds are a good source of phytoestrogens and are often used to promote better hormonal balance in women.

HOW DO I USE IT?

HELPS DIGEST PROTEINS Add alfalfa sprouts to any meal to assist digestion. Combine with other diuretic or digestive herbs, such as dandelion, for a synergistic effect.

Chia seeds

CHIA SEEDS

WHAT IS IT GOOD FOR?

HEALTHY HEART High in omega-3 fatty acids, which help lower the undesirable fats (LDL cholesterol and triglycerides) in your blood that can cause heart disease and stroke.

STRONG BONES Chia seeds are high in calcium and magnesium, which promote healthy bones and teeth, and in iron, folate, and soluble fiber.

HEALTHY GUT The mucilaginous (gumlike) fiber in the sprouted seeds promotes bowel regularity and helps stabilize blood sugar levels. Briefly soaking the seeds for 1 hour releases more of their beneficial fiber. Or, leave to soak for longer and sprout the same as you would other seeds.

HOW DO I USE IT?

SOAKED OR SPROUTED Add soaked seeds to yogurt, cereal, and muffin recipes, or scatter on a salad. They are also delicious stirred through warm oatmeal. Chia sprouts can be used the same way as any salad green or sprout. Try adding them to soups or stews as a natural thickening agent. They also add flavor and nutrition to baked goods, such as breads, muffins, and home-made crackers.

Red clover seeds

RED CLOVER SEEDS

WHAT IS IT GOOD FOR?

WOMEN'S HEALTH These seeds are perhaps best known as a source of phytoestrogens (plant hormones) that can help relieve menopausal symptoms, such as hot flashes, water retention, and anxiety. They are also a source of calcium and so can promote strong bones and teeth.

CARDIOVASCULAR HEALTH Contains vitamins C, B-complex, and K, and beta-carotene—all helpful in lowering high blood pressure, improving blood circulation, and reducing the risk of heart disease. Similar in taste to alfalfa seeds, red clover seeds are exclusively for sprouting, not for eating raw.

HOW DO I USE IT?

HEALTHY ADDITION Red clover sprouts add flavor and crunch to food without overloading it with calories. They are best eaten raw, but can be used to add a distinctive flavor to soups and stir-fries.

MEDICINAL HERBS

There are fewer distinctions between culinary and medicinal herbs than we sometimes think; in fact, most medicinal herbs can be incorporated into our daily diet. Their healing benefits are most concentrated as a tincture or tea; they are subtler when used in smaller ratios for cooking. Prolonged exposure to heat is not recommended for any herb, however, so add toward the end of cooking.

Astragalus

ASTRAGALUS

 HELPS BOOST ENERGY LEVELS

WHAT IS IT GOOD FOR?

IMMUNITY ENHANCER A tonic that can help raise your energy levels if you are feeling run down or are recuperating. Astragalus is also useful for enhancing the function and number of white blood cells. It has natural antibiotic properties, so can help increase resistance to viral infections. It is full of antioxidants that protect cells against free-radical damage, and is a natural diuretic.

HOW DO I USE IT?

ADD TO SOUPS AND STOCKS
Astragalus is a healthy ingredient in soups. Try combining ¼–½oz (10–15g) of the herb with shiitake mushrooms, onions, garlic, miso, and carrots, or use as a base for a stock in which to cook rice. To make a tea, steep 2 tsp fresh or 1 tsp dried herb in ¾ cup of boiling water for 5 minutes.

Valerian root

VALERIAN ROOT

 HELPS CALM THE NERVES AND PROMOTE PEACEFUL SLEEP

WHAT IS IT GOOD FOR?

RELIEVES NERVOUS CONDITIONS
Used to treat a variety of conditions including insomnia, anxiety, and nervous restlessness. Sometimes described as "nature's tranquilizer," it has been extensively researched in recent years. Test results suggest it works in a similar way to prescription tranquilizers by increasing gamma aminobutyric acid (GABA)—a substance that has a calming effect on the nervous system—in the brain. Other uses include treating digestive problems, nausea, liver problems, and urinary tract disorders.

HOW DO I USE IT?

TAKE AS A TEA Considered to be inedible raw, valerian root is best taken as a soothing hot tea; combine in equal parts with fresh ginger as a good circulation booster too.

Chamomile

CHAMOMILE

 HAS NATURAL SEDATIVE PROPERTIES

WHAT IS IT GOOD FOR?

RESTORES CALM A classic remedy for anxiety and sleep disturbances. It is excellent for children, for easing colic, teething, restlessness, and hyperactivity. Soothes gastrointestinal cramps, and also inflammation in mucous membranes and the skin. Its antibacterial action helps fight infection, while its sedating qualities benefit the immune system by helping to lower levels of immune-compromising stress hormones.

HOW DO I USE IT?

IN COOKING Its sweet, apple scent makes it a pleasant garnish for salads, rice, or fish dishes. Chop and add to butter or sour cream to top baked potatoes. For bread and cakes, replace the water with a chamomile infusion and add 3 tbsp each of dried chamomile and lavender flowers.

Schisandra

 HELPS BOOST PHYSICAL AND MENTAL ENERGY

What Is It Good For?

RESPONDS TO THE BODY'S NEEDS An adaptogen, it stimulates or calms the body according to its needs. It can help improve physical, mental, or spiritual energy and is a renowned aphrodisiac for men and women.

It supports kidney and lung function and helps improve circulation, which in turn provides benefits for the heart and skin, and may help revive a poor memory and build stamina.

How Do I Use It?

SAVORY AND SWEET A common ingredient in traditional Chinese and Korean cuisines. Add the berries to rice dishes, soups, vegetable patties, jelly, preserves, and even drinks.

Schisandra

Marshmallow Root

 HELPS HEAL STOMACH ULCERS

What Is It Good For?

SOOTHES IRRITATION Rich in mucilaginous (gumlike) fiber, it acts to soothe irritation and inflammation of the mucous membranes, stomach, and intestines. It may be particularly useful for gastric ulcers and irritable bowel syndrome. It can also help heal respiratory and urinary disorders. Its mild laxative effect makes it useful for treating occasional constipation.

How Do I Use It?

DRINK IT Make into a medicinal drink: soak ½ cup of root in 2 cups cold water overnight and strain. The liquid will be very viscous and may need further dilution. Drink small servings throughout the day.

Marshmallow root

Milk Thistle

 SUPPORTS HEALTHY LIVER FUNCTION

What Is It Good For?

SUPPORTS THE LIVER A powerful antioxidant that helps heal the liver and support its ability to break down and metabolize fats and proteins. It is considered a good treatment for gallbladder inflammation, and any premenstrual and menopausal symptoms that are related to liver function. It can also help increase breast milk production.

How Do I Use It?

A SOOTHING BREW Grind 1 tsp of seeds in a coffee grinder and steep in ¾ cup boiling water for 5–10 minutes. Or peel fresh stalks, soak overnight to remove bitterness, boil until just tender, and add butter.

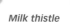
Milk thistle

St. John's Wort

 HELPS LIFT DEPRESSION

What Is It Good For?

FIGHTS DEPRESSION It can help treat mild-to-moderate, but not severe, depression. In many studies it has been shown to work as well as conventional antidepressants. It is also a remedy for seasonal depression, PMS, and depression and anxiety in menopause. Less well known are the herb's antibacterial, anti-inflammatory, and antiviral properties, which make it an effective wound healer when used externally.

How Do I Use It?

USE INSTEAD OF WATER Take as a tea or, like chamomile, substitute water with a strong infusion of the herb in baking or savory broths and stocks.

St. John's wort

CULINARY HERBS

Traditionally, culinary herbs were used not only to add subtle flavor but to preserve and enhance the healthful properties of foods; many have been shown to be concentrated sources of antioxidants and medicinal oils with antibacterial effects. Eaten regularly, herbs can work synergistically with other foods to boost health in many ways, including enhancing digestive health and detoxification.

Basil

BASIL

 AIDS HEALTHY/OPTIMAL DIGESTION

WHAT IS IT GOOD FOR?

EASES DIGESTION Basil fortifies the digestive and nervous systems, and can be a good remedy for headaches and insomnia. Eugenol, a constituent of the oil in the basil leaf, has an anti-inflammatory effect on joints and the digestive tract. It is also a mild diuretic. In addition, it contains a range of natural antioxidants, which can help protect body tissues against free-radical damage.

HOW DO I USE IT?

EAT FRESH Use fresh basil and wait until the last moment to add the leaves to a dish. Scatter onto tomato salads, soups, and egg, rice, and mushroom dishes. Make a pesto sauce or put some fresh leaves into olive oil for a pungent salad dressing (don't worry if they turn black).

Cilantro

CILANTRO

 HELPS REMOVE TOXINS FROM THE BODY

WHAT IS IT GOOD FOR?

DETOXIFYING Contains detoxifying, antibacterial, and immune-enhancing essential oils, and can help remove heavy metals from the body. Cilantro also aids digestion, fights nausea and stomach cramps, balances blood sugar levels, and is mildly laxative.

ANTIOXIDANT The plant's green tops contain a higher concentration of antioxidants, such as quercetin, kaempferol, and apigenin, than the seeds. These substances are known to have cancer-fighting properties.

HOW DO I USE IT?

DON'T COOK IT Cooking destroys cilantro's flavor and essential oils. Use instead as a garnish on rice dishes, salsas, and stir-fries, or juice with celery, cucumber, and carrot in a juicer for a quick detox drink.

Parsley

PARSLEY

SUPPORTS HEALTHY KIDNEYS AND BLADDER

WHAT IS IT GOOD FOR?

DIURETIC AID Parsley has a diuretic action and is rich in antioxidants that can help relieve congestion and inflammation in the kidneys and bladder. It is also an effective treatment for constipation. It has numerous other medicinal uses, including as a general tonic for the body and as a digestive aid. It is also rich in vitamin K, which helps support healthy bones.

HOW DO I USE IT?

A VERSATILE ADDITION Stir into omelets and vegetable and rice dishes, or mix with butter, spread on crusty bread, and broil briefly for a quick snack. Add to mashed potatoes, fish cakes, or meat patties. Chew at the end of a meal to aid digestion and sweeten the breath.

ROSEMARY

 HELPS FIGHT INFLAMMATION

WHAT IS IT GOOD FOR?

A NATURAL ANTISEPTIC Contains caffeic and rosmarinic acids, both potent antioxidant and anti-inflammatory agents that also have strong antiseptic properties. Its antioxidant action can help reduce inflammation, thereby helping to lower the risk of asthma, liver disease, and heart disease. If used in a tea or gargle, it can help fight gum disease and relieve sore throats. It also contains a number of volatile oils, which have a sedative effect that help calm the nerves and ease stomach upsets.

HOW DO I USE IT?

A MEDITERRANEAN STAPLE Use to infuse meats, such as lamb, before or while they cook, add to potatoes before roasting them, to vegetables, such as green beans, peas, and mushrooms, or use to make flavorful salad oils and vinegars. You can even use rosemary to flavor custard. For a medicinal tea, brew 1 tsp dried or 2 tsp fresh rosemary in ¾ cup of boiling water for 5 minutes.

Rosemary

SAGE

 AIDS HORMONAL BALANCE

WHAT IS IT GOOD FOR?

WOMEN'S HEALTH Traditionally used to "normalize" the female reproductive system, sage is useful for helping to treat heavy or irregular periods and relieving menopausal symptoms. Eaten raw, it can also be effective in helping to treat rheumatic conditions, catarrh, excessive sweating, and upset stomachs. In laboratory tests, its antioxidants have shown potential for helping to improve memory and concentration levels in both healthy individuals and those with dementia. It also has a mild diuretic action.

HOW DO I USE IT?

MAKE SAGE HONEY Make a uniquely flavored honey by packing a jar with fresh sage and covering with honey (both are antibacterial). Let it infuse for 2–3 days or longer. Use in herbal teas and sweet dishes for a therapeutic boost. Add the fresh herb to salads, soups, and stuffings for rich meats, such as pork and goose. Make a seasoning by grinding dried sage leaves with coarse sea salt to use on almost any savory dish.

Sage

THYME

 HELPS FIGHT COLDS AND FLU

WHAT IS IT GOOD FOR?

A COLD REMEDY Can help loosen and expel mucus, making it a good choice if you have asthma, bronchitis, a cold, a cough, the flu, or a sinus headache. A general tonic, antioxidant, and aid to digestion, it is also useful for treating colic in babies and excess wind in children and adults. Thymol, a constituent of thyme's essential oil, is an antibacterial that is effective against *Streptococcus mutans*, *E. coli*, *Staphalococcus aureus*, and *Bacillus subtilis*. When made into a tea, thyme can be used to treat sore throats and gum disease.

HOW DO I USE IT?

GREAT WITH MEAT Fresh thyme is best in marinades, sauces, stocks, stuffings, and slow-cooked stews and casseroles. Its high iron content enriches the nutritional value of meat dishes and makes them more digestible. The crushed leaves make excellent herb oils and vinegars. For a medicinal tea, use dried thyme. Brew 1 tsp dried or 2 tsp fresh thyme in ¾ cup boiling water for 5 minutes.

Thyme

CULINARY HERBS CONTINUED

Dill

DILL

HAS A POWERFUL DIURETIC ACTION

WHAT IS IT GOOD FOR?

ANTIBACTERIAL Dill is a natural diuretic and antibacterial that can be effective against cystitis and bladder infections. Its essential oil constituents have a calming, anti-inflammatory effect on the digestive tract, which is why it has long been used as a treatment for stomach upsets and colic. Studies on animals suggest it may also have a useful role to play in helping to regulate blood sugar and cholesterol levels.

HOW DO I USE IT?

SCATTER LIBERALLY Both the seeds and fresh herb have similar benefits. The minty, aniseed flavor of fresh dill goes well with seafood, especially salmon, and makes a pleasant tea, or scatter on salads, new or baked potatoes, and steamed vegetables. Add the seeds to soups or casseroles, or scatter onto vegetables and rice.

Mint

MINT

SOOTHES UPSET STOMACHS

WHAT IS IT GOOD FOR?

RELIEVES INDIGESTION Menthol, the active oil in mint, is responsible for the antiseptic and antibacterial properties that make mint a good choice for relieving indigestion, irritable bowel syndrome, and soothing an upset stomach. Its adaptogenic properties mean it can help balance the body in whatever way is needed, so it can be both invigorating and mildly sedative. It also fortifies the nervous system and helps to relieve headaches.

HOW DO I USE IT?

ALL-ROUNDER Mint sauce is a traditional condiment served with lamb, and helps aid digestion of the meat. Mix into dressings, or chutney or yogurt to serve with spicy foods like curries. Scatter onto new potatoes or peas or, for a tasty salad, mix with cooked bulgur wheat. For tea, steep 1 tsp dried or 2 tsp fresh mint in ¾ cup boiling water for 5 minutes. Drink hot or cold.

Oregano

OREGANO

PROTECTS AGAINST FREE-RADICAL DAMAGE

WHAT IS IT GOOD FOR?

ANTIBACTERIAL Contains the volatile oils thymol and carvacrol, which have an antioxidant effect, helping to protect against the oxidative stress caused by free radicals in the body. These volatile oils have been shown to also inhibit the growth of bacteria, including *Pseudomonas aeruginosa* and *Staphylococcus aureus*, as well as inhibiting the growth of the *Candida albicans* fungus. An analgesic, oregano can ease menstrual cramps and other abdominal pain. It is also a useful diuretic and appetite stimulant and helps clear mucus, so it can be helpful in cases of colds, the flu, headaches, and respiratory illness.

HOW DO I USE IT?

A CLASSIC INGREDIENT Use in pasta sauces and salad dressings, in vegetable, fish, and chicken recipes, or in dishes with eggs and/or cheese. It is a good addition to stews, but add it toward the end of cooking to keep its beneficial oils and resins intact.

Tie a selection of herbs into a bouquet garni to flavor dishes while they cook, and remove the bundle before serving. The classic combination is thyme, parsley, and bay leaf, although you can add other herbs.

Amaranth

 HELPS LOWER CHOLESTEROL

 SUPPORTS CELLULAR METABOLISM

 HELPS PROTECT AGAINST POLLUTION

 HELPS FIGHT INFLAMMATION

Like buckwheat and quinoa, amaranth is actually the seed of a broad-leafed plant rather than a grass. It has been cultivated for 8,000 years, and was a staple of the Aztec diet. Today, both the grain and the leaves, which are high in **antioxidants**, are used in medicinal cooking as a source of **high-quality protein**, **cholesterol-lowering phytosterols**, and **anti-inflammatory phytochemicals**.

Grains
The grains contain phytosterols, plant hormones that help to lower cholesterol

Greens
Nutritionally similar to Swiss chard and spinach, but higher in calcium and 3 times higher in niacin, amaranth greens are worth seeking out in Asian supermarkets

What Is It Good For?

HEART HEALTH Regular consumption of the seeds (or oil) can help reduce blood pressure and "unhealthy" (LDL) cholesterol levels, and improve immunity. Unlike other grains, it is not its fibrous content that protects the heart, but its levels of phytosterols and squalene.

TISSUE GROWTH AND REPAIR A good source of amino acids. In particular, it has good amounts of lysine, an essential amino acid found in limited amounts in other grains and plant sources. Amino acids are the building blocks for proteins in the body. They also aid metabolism and tissue growth and repair.

DETOX Squalene is a strong antioxidant that can help reduce the impact of toxic substances, such as pollution and industrial chemicals, on body systems. It can also improve the symptoms of chronic fatigue.

ANTI-INFLAMMATORY Contains lunasin, an anti-inflammatory substance. In addition to fighting inflammation, lunasin has been shown to halt the growth of cancer cells.

How Do I Get The Best From It?

SPROUT IT The small size of the grains makes them fiddly and difficult to chew thoroughly; whether raw or cooked, a substantial number may pass undigested through the digestive tract with their nutrients unutilized. Instead, sprout them to get all their benefits.

USE THE LEAVES The leaves are a good source of vitamins K and C, iron, calcium, and folate.

How Do I Use It?

ADD TO SALADS Add the sprouted amaranth grains to salads and sandwiches.

FOR BAKING Amaranth flour is gluten-free. On its own it is somewhat bitter, and most recipes recommend that amaranth should comprise no more than 10–15 percent of the total weight of flour in any baked recipe.

QUINOA

 HELPS PREVENT HARDENED ARTERIES

 STRENGTHENS CONNECTIVE TISSUES

 PROTECTS AGAINST FREE-RADICAL DAMAGE

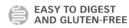 **EASY TO DIGEST AND GLUTEN-FREE**

Easily digestible quinoa (pronounced keen-wah) grains are cooked in the same way as rice, and have a sweet, grassy flavor and texture. Quinoa is a complete **source of protein** and a **good source of anti-inflammatory**, **monounsaturated**, and **omega-3 fatty acids**. A heart-healthy grain, it is known to reduce "unhealthy" (LDL) cholesterol, and contains high levels of **antioxidants**.

WHAT IS IT GOOD FOR?

HEART HEALTH Unlike many other grains, quinoa contains oleic acid, a monounsaturated fatty acid and alpha-linolenic acid (ALA; an omega-3 fatty acid) in useful amounts. This combination can help to reduce "unhealthy" (LDL) cholesterol levels in the blood and fight inflammation that can lead to hardening of the arteries (atherosclerosis).

GOOD SOURCE OF PROTEIN Considered a complete protein because it contains all the essential amino acids; it is particularly high in lysine, important for tissue growth and repair.

ANTIOXIDANTS In addition to a spectrum of E vitamins including alpha-, beta-, gamma-, and delta-tocopherol, quinoa contains two antioxidant flavonoids, quercetin and kaempferol, which fight free radicals and are present in concentrations equal to or higher than high-flavonoid berries, such as cranberries.

DIGESTION Quinoa is easy to digest and doesn't contain gluten, making it suitable for anyone on a gluten-free diet.

HOW DO I GET THE BEST FROM IT?

WHOLE GRAIN The grains cook quickly, usually in 15 minutes, and are ready when translucent and the white germ on each grain has partially separated like a little white tail.

SPROUT IT Sprouting activates the beneficial enzymes in quinoa and boosts its nutrient content. Sprouted quinoa can be used in salads and sandwiches just like alfalfa sprouts.

HOW DO I USE IT?

INSTEAD OF RICE For a nutritious side dish, serve quinoa like rice pilaf, cooked in stock and combined with vegetables. It is also good as a stuffing for squash and bell peppers.

ENRICH YOUR BAKING Add cooked quinoa to muffins, breads, and even pancakes.

WHITE GRAINS
Quinoa grains contain all the essential amino acids (such as lysine), and good quantities of iron, calcium, and phosphorus.

RED GRAINS
The antioxidant pigment betacyanin, which also gives beets their coloring, is responsible for the bright red hue of this variety.

SPELT

 HELPS BALANCE BLOOD SUGAR LEVELS

 HELPS STRENGTHEN THE IMMUNE SYSTEM

 EASY TO DIGEST

An ancient variety of wheat with a subtle sweet, nutty flavor, spelt has a tough outer husk that makes it difficult to process. However, this protective husk helps the grain maintain its nutrient value. It is **high in fiber**, **B vitamins**, and **minerals**, such as copper, iron, zinc, magnesium, and phosphorus. It also contains more **protein** than conventional wheat, and is highly **water-soluble** and **easier to digest**.

GRAINS
Spelt is a good source of B vitamins and certain minerals, and is higher in protein than conventional wheat.

SPROUTED SPELT
Sprouting breaks down indigestible starches into more easily digested sugars.

FLOUR
Though the reasons are not fully understood, some people sensitive to conventional wheat find they can tolerate spelt.

WHAT IS IT GOOD FOR?

METABOLIC SYNDROME Spelt and whole spelt flour offer more soluble fiber than both standard and durum wheat flours. Soluble fiber is particularly beneficial for lowering "unhealthy" (LDL) cholesterol and regulating blood sugar levels.

IMMUNITY It is higher in niacin (B$_3$) than conventional wheat. Like other B vitamins, niacin aids in energy metabolism. It has additional functions, including antibacterial properties that help strengthen the body against disease. It also supports the adrenal glands and helps improve circulation.

DIGESTION Spelt is easily soluble in water and contains less gluten than conventional wheat, making it easier to digest. However, as spelt contains gluten, it is not suitable for celiacs.

HOW DO I GET THE BEST FROM IT?

WHOLE GRAIN Add the whole grain to soups and stews in the same way you would barley, or cook it on its own as an alternative to rice.

FLOUR Spelt flour can be used wherever wheat flour is indicated, though its high water-solubility means you may need to use less liquid than with conventional flours. You can also buy sprouted spelt flour.

SPROUT IT Spelt sprouts are high in vitamins E, C, and B, phosphorus, magnesium, iron, calcium, amino acids, and protein. Select hulled spelt for sprouting.

HOW DO I USE IT?

SPELT RISOTTO Whole grains can be cooked on their own and used as a side dish or combined with vegetables, fresh herbs, and Parmesan cheese to make a risotto.

SPELT PASTA Pasta made from spelt is a delicious alternative to durum wheat pasta, and because of its easy digestibility it may leave you feeling less bloated.

RICE

 HELPS LOWER CHOLESTEROL

 PROTECTS AGAINST COLON CANCER

 HELPS RELEASE CELLULAR ENERGY

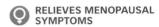 **RELIEVES MENOPAUSAL SYMPTOMS**

Rice is a near-perfect food, and the predominant staple food for around half the world's population. This **cholesterol-lowering** food is available in many varieties and colors and is a good source of thiamine, riboflavin, niacin, and **dietary fiber**. Certain rice varieties help to maintain stable **blood sugar levels**. Rice bran may also help lower the risk of **bowel cancer**.

WHAT IS IT GOOD FOR?

LOWERS CHOLESTEROL The fatty acid content in whole brown rice has cholesterol-lowering properties. It is also rich in magnesium, which has been shown to lower the risk of diabetes.

HEALTHY GUT Brown rice contains fiber and selenium, which help protect the gut. Fiber helps remove waste products efficiently from the body, while the trace mineral selenium has been shown to substantially reduce the risk of colon cancer.

ENERGY RELEASE Rich in manganese, a trace mineral that helps produce energy from protein and carbohydrates. It is also involved in the synthesis of fatty acids, which are important for a healthy nervous system.

HORMONE BALANCE The phytosterols in rice bran oil have been shown to help relieve menopausal symptoms, such as hot flashes.

HOW DO I GET THE BEST FROM IT?

CHOOSE BY COLOR White rice is nutrient-poor, but brown rice is an all-round healthy choice. Its minimal processing preserves the grain's nutritional value and healthy oils, much of which concentrates in the bran. Deeply colored red or black rice has been proven to actively reduce the progress of atherosclerosis (hardening of the arteries).

RICE BRAN OIL This versatile oil is high in monounsaturates and contains the antioxidant y-oryzanol, as well as a range of tocopherols (the vitamin E family) and phytosterols (plant hormones). Heating does not appear to destroy its constituents. Use rice bran oil for cooking, marinades, and dressings.

HOW DO I USE IT?

EXOTIC COCONUT RICE Boil brown rice and grated fresh ginger in unsweetened coconut milk and water. Serve garnished with finely chopped fresh cilantro.

BROWN RICE
This minimally processed rice is one of the most nutritionally dense varieties.

WHITE RICE
Milled or polished white rice has had its hull and bran removed. It is a good source of protein, but most of its other nutrients are removed with the hull.

WILD RICE
Although not a true rice, wild rice is eaten just like one. It contains twice the amount of zinc and 8 times the amount of vitamin E as brown rice.

RED RICE
This variety has the highest iron and zinc content of all commercially available rice. Red rice contains a variety of anthocyanins that give its bran a red or deep purple color.

BULGUR WHEAT

 HELPS FIGHT INFLAMMATION

 PROMOTES BOWEL REGULARITY

 HELPS BUILD STRONG BONES

 HELPS BALANCE BLOOD SUGAR LEVELS

Bulgur wheat is a low-fat whole grain **rich in dietary fiber**. It aids digestion, acts as an **anti-inflammatory**, and **protects against cholesterol** and **gallstones**. It has a characteristic crumbly texture, produced by precooking, drying, and crushing whole grains, often from several varieties of wheat. This process prevents bulgur wheat, one of the world's earliest processed grains, from spoiling.

Wheat berries
In a process discovered 4,000 years ago, wheat berries are parboiled, dried, and ground to produce bulgur wheat grains

Grains
Bulgur wheat is rich in manganese and magnesium, which help keep inflammation at bay and maintain metabolic balance. The grain is a healthy "fast food" that can be prepared in just 20 minutes

WHAT IS IT GOOD FOR?

ANTI-INFLAMMATORY The antioxidant betaine in bulgur wheat is a potent anti-inflammatory. Regular consumption of betaine-rich foods can help prevent the inflammation of joints and arteries by as much as 20 percent.

DIGESTION AND CONSTIPATION High in insoluble fiber, which promotes bowel regularity, and aids the production of butyric acid, which fuels cells that maintain a healthy colon. The carbohydrates in bulgur wheat are absorbed slowly, helping to maintain steady blood sugar levels.

STRONG BONES Around half of all dietary magnesium is required for building healthy bones. As a result, this mineral needs to be constantly replaced and bulgur wheat is a good natural source. Magnesium also relaxes nerves and muscles and maintains the cardiovascular system.

METABOLIC BALANCE High in manganese, a trace mineral with an anti-inflammatory, antioxidant effect essential for most body systems. It supports healthy bones, maintains normal blood sugar levels, helps the body form tissue, and balances sex hormones.

HOW DO I GET THE BEST FROM IT?

A BETTER FAST FOOD Unlike many types of grain, bulgur wheat is quick to prepare. It is a fantastic alternative to rice and potatoes and can be a better choice than a sandwich to maintain energy throughout the day.

HOW DO I USE IT?

BOOST YOUR BREAD Enrich a bread recipe by substituting ⅓ cup of flour with the same amount of reconstituted bulgur wheat.

IN A SALAD Combine cooked bulgur wheat, puy lentils, sliced scallions, radishes, and tomatoes with cumin, and mint and cilantro leaves. Toss in an olive oil and lime dressing.

OATS

 HAS NATURAL SEDATIVE PROPERTIES

 EASY TO DIGEST

 HELPS CONTROL INSULIN SECRETION

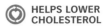 **HELPS LOWER CHOLESTEROL**

Long before we relied on a bowl of sugary instant cereal, breakfast often meant porridge cooked with oats; they can also be used in healthy cereals, snacks, cookies, and breads. Oats contain **multiple nutrients** and a gummy, **water-soluble fiber**, beta-glucan, which helps **reduce "unhealthy" (LDL) cholesterol**. They are also known to be a **natural sedative**, and excellent for **easing indigestion**.

WHAT IS IT GOOD FOR?

SOOTHES NERVES Oats contain the alkaloid gramine, a natural sedative, which can treat depression, anxiety, and insomnia without side effects. Tea made from oat straw is a traditional remedy for anxiety and insomnia.

DIGESTION Oats are easy to digest and useful in diets for recovering patients and for easing upset stomachs. The fact that oats contain more soluble fiber than any other grain also means that they are digested more slowly, creating an extended sensation of fullness.

DIABETES As well helping to prevent big spikes in blood sugar levels, the beta-glucan fiber has beneficial effects for diabetics. Useful amounts of magnesium in the grain also help regulate insulin secretion.

REDUCES CHOLESTEROL Oats, oat bran, and oatmeal contain a specific type of fiber known as beta-glucan, which can quickly help lower "unhealthy" (LDL) cholesterol levels. Studies show that including just ½–¾ cup of oats a day in a low-fat diet can reduce LDL cholesterol by 8–23 percent. In addition, avenanthramides, antioxidant compounds unique to oats, help prevent free radicals from damaging LDL cholesterol, thus reducing the risk of cardiovascular disease.

HOW DO I GET THE BEST FROM IT?

RAW AND COOKED Oats deliver benefits whether eaten raw or cooked.

OAT MILK Made from soaked oat groats, this is a nutritious alternative to dairy milk.

HOW DO I USE IT?

BREW A TEA You can buy oat straw to make a soothing tea for adults and children.

SPROUTED OAT PORRIDGE Use sprouted oats and combine with chopped walnuts, dried fruit, such as raisins or dates, a little cinnamon, and a drizzle of maple syrup.

OAT STRAW
The immature tops of the oat plant can be dried to make a soothing tea that calms the nerves.

WHOLE OATS (ROLLED)
Oats contain more soluble fiber than any other grain.

OAT GROATS
Oat groats are the hulled grains of oats.

OAT MILK
Oat milk naturally contains more calcium than cow's milk.

RYE

 REGULATES APPETITE AND BLOOD SUGAR

 PROMOTES A HEALTHY DIGESTIVE TRACT

 HELPS KEEP BLOOD VESSELS SUPPLE

A hardy, cold-climate grain, rye berries (also known as rye seeds) are a rich and versatile **source of dietary fiber**, especially arabinoxylan, which helps to **balance blood sugar levels** and **lower "unhealthy" (LDL) cholesterol**. They are also **nutrient-dense**, supplying high levels of iron, calcium, potassium, zinc, vitamin E, a variety of B vitamins, and an array of **antioxidant compounds**.

BERRIES
Rye has fewer calories and is higher in soluble fiber than wheat. The whole grains are rich in manganese.

SPROUTED RYE
This form of rye is rich in carbohydrates needed for quick energy and vitality.

FLOUR
Rye flour, which contains gluten, produces a dense, dark, richly flavored bread.

WHAT IS IT GOOD FOR?

BLOOD SUGAR REGULATION A type of fiber in rye, arabinoxylan helps balance blood sugar levels, reducing the risk of type-2 diabetes and heart disease. Whole grain rye bread is the best way of providing this fiber. It also regulates the appetite more effectively than wheat bread, and reduces the signs of inflammation more effectively than potato or wheat bread in people with metabolic syndrome (which can lead to diabetes and heart disease).

DIGESTION Contains mucilaginous (gumlike) fiber, which helps to lubricate the digestive tract and ease gastritis and stomach pain. Its lubricating action is also good for maintaining healthy skin and mucous membranes.

HEART HEALTH Its soluble fiber helps to maintain the elasticity of blood vessels, so lessening the risk of atherosclerosis (hardening of the arteries) and hypertension.

METABOLIC SIGNALING Studies show that rye can actually switch off certain genes involved in metabolic syndrome, including those that regulate insulin, stress response, and overactive immune response.

HOW DO I GET THE BEST FROM IT?

SWITCH TO RYE BREAD Rye bread is a superb dietary aid, helping you feel fuller for longer and ensuring a steady supply of energy.

DRINK IT To make a mildly laxative and energizing drink, boil 2 tbsp of rye berries in 3½ cups of water for 10 minutes. Allow to cool, then strain and add honey and lemon juice to taste.

HOW DO I USE IT?

RYE FLOUR Rye flour can be used for pancakes, muffins, and scones. Use it just as you would use wheat flour, or mix it 50:50 with wheat flour for a lighter result.

MILLET

 HELPS PROMOTE PEACEFUL SLEEP　　 **PROTECTS AGAINST METABOLIC SYNDROME**　　 **HELPS PREVENT GALLSTONES**

Once a staple grain of Africa and India, today millet ranks as the sixth most important grain in the world and sustains around one-third of the global population. It is a **nutritious**, **nonacid-forming** grain considered to be one of the **least allergenic** and **most digestible** grains available. It is **high in protein**, fiber, B-complex vitamins, iron, magnesium, phosphorus, and potassium.

WHAT IS IT GOOD FOR?

PEACEFUL SLEEP Contains substantial amounts of tryptophan, an amino acid that can help induce a good night's sleep.

CONTROLLING METABOLIC SYNDROME The B vitamins in millet, especially niacin (B_3), can help lower "unhealthy" (LDL) cholesterol, while magnesium helps lower blood pressure and reduces the risk of heart attack, especially in people with atherosclerosis (hardening of the arteries) or diabetes. It also helps reduce the severity of asthma and the frequency of migraines. Its high fiber content helps increase insulin sensitivity and reduce levels of blood fats (lipids).

HELPS PREVENT GALLSTONES Evidence shows that eating foods (such as millet) high in insoluble fiber can help prevent gallstones. Insoluble fiber helps to reduce the secretion of bile acids, excessive amounts of which contribute to the formation of gallstones.

HOW DO I GET THE BEST FROM IT?

HULLED MILLET Usually sold with the largely indigestible hull removed. Hulled millet can be used like any other grain.

A LITTLE PREPARATION Presoaking millet shortens its cooking time. Its flavor can be enhanced by lightly roasting the grains in a dry pan before cooking; stir for 3 minutes or until you detect a mild, nutty aroma.

SPROUT IT Millet can also be sprouted to use in salads and sandwiches. Soak the raw, untoasted grains for about 30 minutes, drain, and keep moist until they begin to sprout.

HOW DO I USE IT?

A BETTER BREAKFAST Millet can form the basis of a nutritional porridge. Serve with dried fruit and sliced almonds.

IN A SALAD Use cooked millet instead of rice or pasta in salads to add flavor and nutrition.

FLOUR
This unusual flour can be added to breads to reduce their gluten content

WHOLE GRAINS
Millet seeds are antioxidant-rich and especially high in magnesium, necessary for maintaining healthy nerve and muscle function.

BARLEY

 FEEDS HEALTHY GUT BACTERIA

 HELPS LOWER CHOLESTEROL

 HELPS BALANCE BLOOD SUGAR LEVELS

Barley is a grain with a number of fantastic medicinal properties. Thanks to its **high fiber content**, it is great for **improving digestion** and **lowering cholesterol**, while its low glycemic index is one of a number of its properties that helps to **improve blood sugar levels** and **reduce the risk of diabetes**. It is also versatile, and can be served instead of rice, added to casseroles, or used in baking.

GRAINS
Studies show that whole grain barley can help maintain steady blood sugar levels for up to 10 hours after consumption—much longer than whole grain wheat.

GRASS
Barley grass is an easily digested green food sprouted from barley seeds.

WHAT IS IT GOOD FOR?

DIGESTION AND CONSTIPATION Barley grain has a very high fiber content. One portion provides nearly half the daily recommended amount. Barley fiber feeds good bacteria in the gut, which in turn produce butyric acid, the primary fuel for intestinal cells necessary for maintaining a healthy colon. In addition, barley grass juice has been shown to improve the symptoms of ulcerative colitis.

HEART HEALTH The high levels of soluble fiber in barley help to remove excess fat and cholesterols from the bloodstream, lowering the risk of hypertension and atherosclerosis (hardening of the arteries).

MANAGING BLOOD SUGAR Barley is a slow-release carbohydrate that helps maintain steady blood sugar levels. In addition, barley is abundant in magnesium and manganese, both of which are necessary for carbohydrate metabolism.

HOW DO I GET THE BEST FROM IT?

WHOLE BARLEY When selecting barley, choose whole barley, or pot barley, rather than pearl barley. The husk, which contains much of the grain's nutrients, remains intact in whole barley.

BARLEY GRASS To get the best from the antioxidants in barley grass, juice the young shoots when they are 3–7 days old.

HOW DO I USE IT?

BARLEY RISOTTO Don't simply add barley to casseroles. Whole barley grains make an excellent risotto; the sweet taste of the grain works especially well with mushrooms.

ENRICH YOUR BAKING Barley is low in gluten so use it in baking. Substitute up to half the quantity of regular wheat flour for barley flour. As well as reducing the gluten content, it adds extra flavor and texture.

BUCKWHEAT

 PROTECTS THE HEART AND BLOOD VESSELS

 EASY TO DIGEST

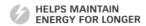 **HELPS MAINTAIN ENERGY FOR LONGER**

Buckwheat is not a true cereal, but is instead related to rhubarb, sorrel, and dock. The grain contains both insoluble and soluble fiber, which help to **lower "unhealthy" (LDL) cholesterol**, **balance blood sugar levels**, and keep the **gut healthy**. Buckwheat is also rich in **antioxidant** flavonoids that help **protect the heart**, and, because it doesn't contain gluten, is ideal for **gluten-free** diets.

WHAT IS IT GOOD FOR?

CIRCULATORY SYSTEM Contains important antioxidant flavonoids: quercetin, thought to have anti-inflammatory and antiallergic properties; and rutin, which strengthens the capillaries and improves circulation, and can help protect against painful varicose veins.

DIGESTION AND CONSTIPATION Its gumlike mucilaginous fiber is lubricating and soothing to the digestive tract. Buckwheat also contains a type of indigestible fiber that acts like a prebiotic, feeding helpful bacteria in the gut.

ENERGY BALANCE The grain contains slow-release carbohydrates that help maintain steady blood sugar levels. It is abundant in magnesium and manganese, both of which are necessary for carbohydrate metabolism.

ANTICANCER Like most whole grains, it contains plant hormones called lignans, which can promote hormone balance in both men and women. One lignan, enterolactone, has been shown to protect against breast and other hormone-dependent cancers.

HOW DO I GET THE BEST FROM IT?

BUCKWHEAT SPROUTS Soak raw, untoasted seeds for 30 minutes, drain, and keep moist until they begin to sprout. (Toasted buckwheat has a golden brown color, whereas raw buckwheat is white or light green.)

BUCKWHEAT FLOUR The flour is gluten-free and can be used in baking. Dark-colored buckwheat flour contains the husk and a greater proportion of protein than the light flour, while sprouted buckwheat flour is even more nutrient-rich.

HOW DO I USE IT?

MAKE A PORRIDGE Soak and sprout the seeds to release their mucilaginous fiber and use to make "porridge" by combining with yogurt or nut milk and fruit.

GRAIN
Buckwheat contains 8 essential amino acids required by the body, as well as high proportions of manganese, magnesium, and fiber.

SPROUTS
Sprouting the grain makes its nutrients more available to the body and activates enzymes, which lower blood pressure.

DRIED BEANS

 PROMOTES BOWEL REGULARITY

 PROTECTS THE HEART AND BLOOD VESSELS

 HELPS BUILD STRONG BONES

Including more dried beans in your diet is a terrific way to **maintain digestive health**, **lower cholesterol levels**, and **regulate blood sugar levels** because they contain **protein** and **fiber**. Most are good sources of **iron**, an integral component of red blood cells, which transport oxygen from the lungs to every cell in the body. Beans are also an excellent choice if you want to cut back your meat intake.

Adzuki beans

ADZUKI BEANS

WHAT IS IT GOOD FOR?

HEART HEALTH Rich in soluble fiber, which is absorbed during digestion and helps maintain "healthy" (HDL) cholesterol levels in the blood. The beans contain potassium and magnesium, which are good for regulating blood pressure and improving blood flow, and essential B vitamins including B_6, B_2, B_1, B_3, and folate—all necessary for the cellular energy production that fuels metabolism. Also a good source of the trace element molybdenum, which aids liver detoxification.

HOW DO I USE IT?

ADZUKI BEAN PATTIES Combine cooked adzuki beans with rice, egg, garlic, onion, and fresh herbs; form into patties and shallow-fry. Or add the beans to casseroles or soups for extra fiber, protein, and flavor, or sprout them and add to salads.

Black beans

BLACK BEANS

WHAT IS IT GOOD FOR?

BLOOD HEALTH Black beans are abundant in both iron and the trace element molybdenum. Iron is essential for carrying oxygen to our red blood cells, and for the production of hemoglobin, a primary component of red blood cells. Molybdenum is essential for healthy liver function and is a key component in chemical reactions that release iron in the body. In addition, the beans are a good source of fiber to help cleanse and protect the colon.

HOW DO I USE IT?

BLACK BEAN SALAD Mix cooked black beans, orange segments, sliced red onion, and cumin seeds with an oil and vinegar dressing. Eating legumes with vitamin-C-rich foods increases iron absorption, as the type of iron (non-heme) in plants is harder to absorb than iron in meat (heme).

Butter beans

BUTTER BEANS

WHAT IS IT GOOD FOR?

BLOOD AND TISSUE HEALTH A milder, creamier relative of the fava bean, butter beans are a good source of potassium, iron, copper, manganese, and soluble fiber—all essential for a healthy cardiovascular system and digestive tract. They also contain molybdenum, which promotes liver health, and are high in tryptophan, an amino acid, and protein, which is necessary for building and repairing tissue and muscle in the body.

HOW DO I USE IT?

BUTTER BEAN HUMMUS Purée cooked butter beans with sautéed onion and garlic, and lemon juice in a food processor or blender. Gradually add enough extra virgin olive oil until the mix reaches a thick but smooth consistency. Season to taste and serve.

CHICKPEAS

WHAT IS IT GOOD FOR?

BONE HEALTH Beyond their fiber content, chickpeas may also be good for bone health. They are rich in manganese, which helps build bones and is necessary for healthy bone structure, and calcium, phosphorus, and magnesium, which are also vital bone-healthy minerals. The fiber in chickpeas has been shown to help reduce levels of "unhealthy" (LDL) cholesterol and help regulate appetite and reduce food cravings.

HOW DO I USE IT?

CHICKPEA GAZPACHO Add chickpeas to gazpacho for a more satisfying dish. The antioxidant lycopene, found in abundance in tomatoes, also works synergistically with chickpeas to reduce oxidative stress (caused by free radicals in the body) on bones.

Chickpeas

KIDNEY BEANS

WHAT IS IT GOOD FOR?

DIGESTION AND BOWEL REGULARITY Kidney beans contain both soluble and insoluble fiber. Soluble fiber can help lower "unhealthy" (LDL) cholesterol; insoluble fiber helps to promote good digestive health and bowel regularity. Also high in blood-building iron, phosphorus—a cofactor in maintaining healthy bones and teeth—and vitamin K, which helps protect the nervous system from free-radical damage and may even have an anticancer effect.

HOW DO I USE IT?

RICE AND BEANS Cooked rice and kidney beans make a complete protein meal. Add sautéed chopped onion, garlic, bell peppers, and tomatoes and season with chili powder, fresh cilantro, thyme, salt, and black pepper to taste.

Kidney beans

LENTILS

WHAT IS IT GOOD FOR?

CARDIOVASCULAR HEALTH Lentils of all types are extremely high in molybdenum and iron, making them an excellent food for helping to oxygenate the blood and aid the release of cellular energy. The insoluble fiber they contain also helps to keep cholesterol at healthy levels. Lentils are also rich in vitamin B$_1$ (thiamine), which helps to regulate the nervous system and maintain a steady heartbeat.

HOW DO I USE IT?

SPROUT IT Dried lentils are deficient in 2 essential amino acids, cysteine and methionine. However, sprouting them increases their levels of all amino acids, including these 2, and produces a food that is a complete protein in its own right.

Red lentils

MUNG BEANS

WHAT IS IT GOOD FOR?

DETOXIFICATION Green mung beans have long been used in traditional Chinese and Indian medicine to keep the body running smoothly due to their detoxifying properties and anti-inflammatory benefits. Mung beans are also rich in fiber and isoflavones and phytosterols (plant hormones) that can help lower cholesterol. In addition, they contain a useful amount of potassium, which can help lower blood pressure.

HOW DO I USE IT?

AS BEAN SPROUTS The beans can be added to stews, but they are usually eaten as bean sprouts. A staple of Chinese cooking, they can be added to any stir-fry, salad, or sandwich.

Mung beans

SPICES

Made from the bark, root, bud, or berry of a plant, spices are generally used **dried** rather than fresh, which means their **essential oil** content is highly concentrated and they have a more **pungent** taste. Research into many common spices has found that they possess **powerful antioxidant** and **antibiotic** qualities, and benefit **digestive health**.

Cardamom

CARDAMOM

 HELPS CLEAR UP CONGESTION

WHAT IS IT GOOD FOR?

METABOLIC BOOSTER A volatile oil constituent called cineol in cardamom can help break up chest congestion, making the spice a good choice for treating bronchitis, laryngitis, and colds. An effective digestive stimulant and diuretic, cardamom boosts the metabolism and helps the body burn fat more efficiently. It is also effective against *H. pylori*, the bacterium that causes ulcers. Studies also show it can help maintain healthy circulation and prevent the free-radical damage that can lead to stroke and atherosclerosis.

HOW DO I USE IT?

USE WHOLE SEEDS Buy the pods or whole green or bleached white seeds to use, lightly crushed, in rice dishes, curries, and meat stews. Freshly ground cardamom can give a surprisingly tangy lift to an everyday fruit salad. It can also be infused in milk to settle the stomach or to make a spicy custard or rice pudding.

Cinnamon

CINNAMON

 HELPS BALANCE BLOOD SUGAR LEVELS

WHAT IS IT GOOD FOR?

ANTISEPTIC Cinnamon is a digestive aid that helps normalize levels of both glucose and triglycerides (a type of fat) in the blood, reducing the risk of diabetes and heart disease. It is also a first-class antiseptic that can help fight bacteria, viruses, and fungal infections. It is rich in antioxidants, which give it a mild analgesic and anti-inflammatory effect, and perhaps this is why it was traditionally used to aid recovery from colds and flu, sore throats, fevers, and headaches. Just smelling cinnamon is said to boost cognitive function and memory.

HOW DO I USE IT?

A VERSATILE FLAVOR For a quick pick-me-up, use a cinnamon stick to stir tea, hot chocolate, or milky coffee. It is equally nice grated or crumbled into savory dishes, such as stews, stuffings, casseroles, pickles, and relishes as it is added to sweet dishes, such as stewed fruits, pies, and rice or milk puddings.

Aromatherapy in your kitchen

Like all plant products, spices contain a wealth of vitamins, minerals, and trace elements. Unlike fresh herbs, spices are generally used in their dried form, and because we use dried spices in such minute amounts in cooking, we benefit less from these nutrients than we do their powerful essential oils, which are highly concentrated. If stored properly—in airtight containers away from light—spices can keep their beneficial properties for a very long time. Wherever possible, buy spices whole and grind or crush them as needed. Their aroma will be stronger and their active ingredients more potent.

CORIANDER

 STIMULATES APPETITE AND AIDS DIGESTION

WHAT IS IT GOOD FOR?

LOWERS CHOLESTEROL Valued in traditional Ayurvedic medicine for its anti-inflammatory properties, modern research shows that coriander has cholesterol-lowering effects. It can stimulate appetite, help increase the secretion of gastric juices, and aid digestion. It is also a diuretic and an antibacterial shown to be effective against salmonella, *E. coli*, and MRSA. Recent studies suggest that the antioxidants in coriander may also have a role to play in protecting the nervous system from free-radical damage. This can help to lower the risk of neurodegenerative illnesses, such as Alzheimer's and Parkinson's diseases.

HOW DO I USE IT?

AN EVERYDAY SPICE The seeds can be used in curries, chutneys, stews, soups, rubs, and marinades. They blend well with smoked meats, game, and even fish. Ground coriander seeds also add an extra dimension to breads, desserts, and sweet pastries.

Coriander

CUMIN

 RICH IN ANTI-INFLAMMATORY ANTIOXIDANTS

WHAT IS IT GOOD FOR?

A POWERFUL ANTIOXIDANT A good general tonic, cumin is also antiseptic and antibacterial, and can help to improve blood circulation. It helps fortify the digestive tract, relieving nausea, bloating, and constipation. Laboratory tests suggest its antioxidant oil content can inhibit the growth of cancer cells. Ordinary cumin seeds are brown in color and contain many beneficial properties. However, black cumin seeds, known as "black seed," have a much higher concentration of these medicinal oils.

HOW DO I USE IT?

USE THE WHOLE SEED Buy the whole seeds and use in pickles or preserves. Add the ground seeds to rubs or marinades, or make a spicy Eastern-style salad with tomatoes, green bell peppers, zucchini, and/or eggplant and then sprinkle a little ground cumin on top.

Cumin

FENUGREEK

 SOOTHES AND PROTECTS THE GUT

WHAT IS IT GOOD FOR?

A METABOLIC BOOST The seeds are a good source of mucilaginous (gumlike) fiber that soothes and protects the digestive tract from free-radical damage. A tonic and antioxidant, fenugreek can also help boost the metabolism, and it is also a traditional remedy for stimulating the production of breast milk. The seeds are rich in diosgenin, a plant estrogen that may boost women's vitality during menopause by easing symptoms including hot flashes, anxiety, and insomnia. In laboratory tests, diosgenin has also demonstrated anticancer effects.

HOW DO I USE IT?

ADD SOME SPICE The seeds have a strong aroma that lifts pickles, dahls, curries, and vegetable and rice dishes. They can be sprouted like bean sprouts and used as a vegetable. A tea made from the seeds mixed with honey and lemon can help soothe flulike symptoms.

Fenugreek

SPICES CONTINUED

Juniper

Licorice

Nutmeg

JUNIPER

 HELPS STIMULATE INSULIN SECRETION

WHAT IS IT GOOD FOR?

A DIABETIC AID Stimulates insulin release, making it a useful aid if you are diabetic. It can also support and, where there has been no permanent damage, help to heal the pancreas. Traditionally, it has been used as a digestive aid, and an antiseptic for treating urinary infections and water retention. Chewing the berries is a traditional remedy for inflamed and infected gums. Essential oils in the berries contain active compounds that help to clear uric acid from the body, making it useful for rheumatic conditions, such as gout.

HOW DO I USE IT?

USE THE FRESH BERRIES Crush the berries lightly and add to meat and game recipes. Combined with garlic and sea salt, they add a wonderful flavor to cabbage and other green vegetables. The fresh berries can also be used in stuffings, sauces, marinades, and pâtés.

LICORICE

 HELPS FIGHT BACTERIAL AND VIRAL INFECTIONS

WHAT IS IT GOOD FOR?

METABOLIC STIMULANT Its antidiabetic and antioxidant properties aid the treatment of metabolic syndrome (a group of risk factors that can lead to diabetes and heart disease). It can help support liver health, and is an antiseptic that helps to calm the stomach. It is also an expectorant and decongestant that can help fight respiratory infections. There is some evidence that licorice in small amounts can be used to decrease sugar cravings. In addition, it can be used as a treatment for low blood pressure.

HOW DO I USE IT?

MAKE A TEA Boil the root to make a tea if you are feeling nauseous or are coming down with a cold. Licorice tea is also good for maintaining dental health; try gargling with the cooled tea. Licorice and soy sauce, which marry well together, help counter the effects of stress, and give a deep, delicious flavor to Asian dishes.

NUTMEG

 FIGHTS THE EFFECTS OF STRESS

WHAT IS IT GOOD FOR?

HELPS YOU ADAPT As an adaptogen, it can be both a stimulant and a sedative, according to the body's needs. In times of stress, it can help lower blood pressure. Conversely, it can lift your mood and acts as a tonic and stimulant, making it beneficial if you are recovering from an illness or overtired. It is also a digestive that can soothe stomachaches, ease wind, and help stop diarrhea. Its volatile oils have anti-inflammatory properties that make it useful for treating joint and muscle pain. In traditional Indian medicine, it is used to calm respiratory problems, such as asthma.

HOW DO I USE IT?

THE ORIGINAL COMFORT FOOD A great addition to cooking when you feel stressed. Use in milk and rice puddings and in white or cheese sauces. It can also transform mashed potatoes and other vegetable dishes. Sprinkle or grate onto hot chocolate or warm milk for a quick pick-me-up.

PEPPERCORNS

 STIMULATES APPETITE AND AIDS DIGESTION

WHAT IS IT GOOD FOR?

DIGESTIVE AID Pepper aids digestion and stimulates the appetite. It has antioxidant and anti-inflammatory properties and is traditionally used to aid detoxification, ease lung and bronchial infections, and relieve shock and stress. In laboratory tests, piperine, a compound found in peppercorns, halted the growth of breast cancer cells. True peppers are green, black or white; pink "peppercorns" are actually from an unrelated species and do not have the same health benefits.

HOW DO I USE IT?

USE THE WHOLE SPICE Always buy whole peppercorns and grind as required; if preground, they quickly lose their active properties. Use in stocks and marinades and grind liberally onto hot vegetable dishes and salads. Crush the peppercorns roughly and use to completely coat meat before grilling, or add to oil and vinegar for a spicy dressing.

Pepper

SAFFRON

 FIGHTS AGE-RELATED VISION LOSS

WHAT IS IT GOOD FOR?

A POTENT ANTIOXIDANT Saffron is actually the dried stigmas of the saffron crocus. It contains the potent antioxidants crocin, safranal, and picrocrocin, which can help delay age-related macular degeneration (loss of vision), help prevent hardening of the arteries (atherosclerosis), and inhibit the growth of cancer cells. Added to tea or milk, it can help treat insomnia and may help lift depression. Its anti-inflammatory properties may be helpful in treating asthma and allergies, and as a stimulant it can help improve the circulation.

HOW DO I USE IT?

USE SPARINGLY Saffron is expensive, but a little goes a long way. Use it to flavor and color dishes, such as paella, risotto, bouillabaisse, spicy lamb, chicken dishes, and even sweet desserts. Mixed with garlic, thyme, and oil it makes an excellent marinade for fish. Saffron can also be used in bread and cake baking.

Saffron

STAR ANISE

 PROTECTS AGAINST COLDS AND FLU

WHAT IS IT GOOD FOR?

ANTIVIRAL Although traditionally used to ease wind, hiccups, and water retention, star anise excels in helping speed recovery from viral infections. Its potent antiviral properties are effective against both the herpes virus and the flu virus—so much so that its constituents have been harnessed by pharmaceutical companies to produce flu medicines, such as Tamiflu. Star anise also contains plant estrogens that can stimulate breast milk supply and help increase vitality in women.

HOW DO I USE IT?

ADD SPICE TO DESSERTS Star anise has a spicy taste that is similar to licorice, and adds an edge to sweet dishes. The seeds go particularly well with figs. Try adding a little ground star anise to ground coffee before brewing, or to some vanilla-flavored yogurt. Add the whole spice or the seeds to fish and vegetable dishes.

Star anise

FATS AND OILS

 ANTI-INFLAMMATORY PROPERTIES

 A READY SOURCE OF ENERGY

 HELPS LOWER CHOLESTEROL

A mixture of different oils and fats in small amounts is crucial for optimal health, **energy**, and **metabolism**. They also help us absorb fat-soluble vitamins D, E, and K, and the carotenoids that we need to make vitamin A. A good balance of polyunsaturates, monounsaturates, and saturated fats (needed for the synthesis of vitamin D) has an **anti-inflammatory** effect and promotes **heart health**.

Butter

Ghee

BUTTER

WHAT IS IT GOOD FOR?

MAINTAINS ENERGY Butter and ghee, a form of clarified butter, have similar properties and are a source of energy. Both contain medium- and short-chain fatty acids, of which one, lauric acid, is a potent antimicrobial and antifungal substance. These fats are not associated with heart disease in the way that long-chain fatty acids (present in some vegetable oils) are, because they are used directly as energy by the body and not stored as fat. Butter supplies saturated fat, but it contains other fats, such as monounsaturates, that help us absorb fat-soluble nutrients. Organic butter has higher levels of these healthy fats.

HOW DO I USE IT?

VERSATILE INGREDIENT Use in moderation as a spread, in baking, and in sauces. Ghee is used in much the same way as butter in cooking.

Olive oil

OLIVE OIL

WHAT IS IT GOOD FOR?

LOWERS CHOLESTEROL Protects against heart disease by raising levels of "healthy" (HDL) cholesterol while keeping levels of "unhealthy" (LDL) cholesterol in check. Contains more monounsaturated fatty acids than any other natural oil. These fatty acids help normalize blood clotting and control blood sugar levels, making olive oil a good choice for helping prevent metabolic syndrome. The oil is easy to digest, which gives it a healing effect on stomach ulcers.

HOW DO I USE IT?

A GOOD ALL-ROUNDER Regular filtered olive oil is better for cooking because it has a higher "smoke point," but it has fewer nutritional benefits. Save cold-pressed extra virgin oil for uncooked dishes and dressings. Store away from heat and light.

Sunflower oil

SUNFLOWER OIL

WHAT IS IT GOOD FOR?

LOWERS BLOOD PRESSURE Sunflower oil is low in saturated fats and high in vitamins E and D and beta-carotene. The best sunflower oils are pressed from plants that have been naturally bred to provide more monounsaturated fat and omega-9 fatty acids, which can help reduce blood pressure, preserve memory, and help prevent cancer. Look for high-oleic content sunflower oil and avoid regular sunflower oil—it is low in monounsaturates and high in omega-6 fatty acids, making it pro-inflammatory.

HOW DO I USE IT?

ALTERNATIVE TO ANIMAL FATS Good for both sweet and savory recipes. Use the nutrient-rich unrefined oil for cold dishes; the refined oil has a higher smoke point that is better for cooking.

FLAXSEED OIL

WHAT IS IT GOOD FOR?

HEART HEALTH Flaxseed oil, which is extracted from flaxseeds, contains the essential fatty acid alpha-linolenic acid (ALA), which can help prevent heart attacks and stroke. Studies suggest ALA may reduce heart disease risk in a variety of ways, including reducing inflammation and excessive blood clotting, promoting blood vessel health, and reducing the risk of arrhythmia (an irregular heartbeat). The oil also contains polyunsaturated omega-3 and omega-6 fatty acids. Consumed daily, it can help improve the dry eyes associated with Sjogren's syndrome.

HOW DO I USE IT?

KEEP IT COOL Flaxseed oil doesn't keep well. Buy in a dark container and store away from light and heat. It's not heat stable, so use it cold. Drizzle on cottage cheese, or scoop out the flesh of a baked potato, mix with quark cheese and flaxseed oil, and replace in the potato skin. Add to juices and smoothies or use to enrich condiments such as ketchup, mayonnaise, and salad dressings.

Flaxseed oil

HEMPSEED OIL

WHAT IS IT GOOD FOR?

ANTI-INFLAMMATORY Hempseed oil contains the highest percentage of essential fatty acids in any oil and contains the perfect ratio of omega-3, -6, and -9 fatty acids, which are crucial for healthy circulation, cell growth, and the immune system. Its high omega-3 content makes it a good vegetarian alternative to fish oil, and means it is both anti-inflammatory and an antioxidant. Including it in your diet will benefit your heart and nervous system as well as improving your skin and helping to maintain healthy joints. A good brain food, hempseed oil can support memory and cognitive function and may help prevent dementia.

HOW DO I USE IT?

KEEP IT SIMPLE Store in a dark container away from heat and light. Look for oils that have not been bleached or deodorized. The oil is not suitable for frying or cooking at high temperatures and should be used cold to enjoy its benefits. Add to juices, smoothies, yogurts, cottage cheese, salad dressings, and steamed vegetables, or use a little on bread instead of butter.

Hempseed oil

BLACK SEED OIL

WHAT IS IT GOOD FOR?

ANTI-INFLAMMATORY Studies show its anti-inflammatory and detoxifying effects can help treat arthritis and rheumatic conditions, and can relieve symptoms in cases of allergic rhinitis (hay fever), eczema, and asthma. It also contains a component called gamma linolenic acid (GLA), which has been shown to reduce the pain associated with diabetic neuropathy (damage to the nerves due to high blood pressure from diabetes). In addition, black seed oil can help raise levels of "healthy" (HDL) cholesterol in the bloodstream.

HOW DO I USE IT?

A HEALTHY ADDITIVE Makes a pungent addition to salad dressings and stir-fries. Mix with honey and garlic to treat allergies and coughs and ward off colds and flu. To treat diarrhea, mix 1 tsp black seed oil with 1 cup of plain probiotic yogurt and eat as needed. Mix 1 tsp of the oil with a glass of orange juice as an energy boost to start the day.

Black seed oil

FERMENTED FOODS

 HELPS STRENGTHEN THE IMMUNE SYSTEM   **FEEDS GOOD BACTERIA IN THE GUT**   **CONTAINS ANTICANCER SUBSTANCES**

The biochemical process of fermentation in foods encourages the growth of friendly bacteria that help maintain a **healthy gut**. It is not an overstatement to say that a healthy gut—one that digests food and nutrients efficiently—is the basis of good health. Healthy and balanced intestinal flora is also a way of **preventing intestinal disorders**, from **irritable bowel syndrome** to **cancer**.

Sauerkraut

SAUERKRAUT

WHAT IS IT GOOD FOR?

INHIBITS CANCER CELLS Laboratory studies show that isothiocyanates, the antioxidant chemicals in fermented cabbage, or sauerkraut, can inhibit the growth of cancer cells

SUPPORTS HEALTHY GUT FLORA Cabbage naturally contains the friendly bacterium *Lactobacilli plantarum*. Fermenting promotes the growth of this organism, which can help balance intestinal flora and inhibit the growth of *E. coli*, salmonella, and candida. It can also help improve the general health of the digestive tract.

HOW DO I USE IT?

A BETTER CONDIMENT Use uncooked as a condiment. Add sauerkraut to a sandwich or bagel instead of lettuce, or serve to accompany rich meats and sausages. Mix 1–2 tbsp into stir-fried brown rice, scrambled eggs, shiitake mushrooms, carrots, or onions, and drizzle with a little soy sauce and sesame oil. Avoid pasteurized brands of sauerkraut because these have fewer nutrients.

Kimchi

KIMCHI

WHAT IS IT GOOD FOR?

ANTICANCER BENEFITS A Korean version of sauerkraut, kimchi is a pungent blend of fermented cabbage, radish, red chiles, garlic, and salt, and is the national dish of Korea. The anticancer and heart-healthy benefits in kimchi derive from the many nutrients in the cruciferous cabbage. The mixture of spices and beneficial bacteria in kimchi is also powerfully antimicrobial against harmful bacteria, such as *Helicobacter pylori*, *Shigella sonnei*, and *Listeria monocytogenes*.

HOW DO I USE IT?

A SPICY SIDE DISH Kimchi can be served not only as a side dish with steamed rice, but also with tempeh, noodles, fish, meat, and vegetables. Use as you would a relish on burgers, roasted meat, and baked potatoes.

The benefits of brine

Vegetables can be preserved in brine using a natural process known as lacto-fermentation. The brine solution allows beneficial bacteria and enzymes to flourish while retarding the growth of harmful organisms. The result is a food with multiple health-giving properties for the digestive tract. However, unlike homemade pickled vegetables, most commercially available kinds are produced using a strong mixture of processed salt and industrial-strength vinegar. This added salt eliminates any health benefits, while the pasteurization (heating) process destroys precious enzymes.

Soy Sauce

What Is It Good For?

SUPPORTS A HEALTHY GUT
Fermenting soybeans to make soy sauce creates unique carbohydrates, called oligosaccharides, which are probiotics that feed friendly bacteria in the gut. Although high in sodium, which could contribute to raised blood pressure in some individuals, recent research suggests that the peptides in soy sauce, created by the fermentation process, help to keep blood pressure low. Soy sauce is rich in antioxidants, which can help protect blood vessels and lower cholesterol. It also contains niacin (B_3) and manganese, which help support an efficient metabolism.

How Do I Use It?

BUY THE BEST QUALITY Look for properly fermented products. If you have a wheat sensitivity, try tamari soy sauce. Use to season sautéed vegetables or combine with garlic and fresh ginger as a marinade for tempeh, fish, or chicken. Use instead of table salt to season foods. Avoid soy sauces containing MSG (monosodium glutamate, a synthetic flavor enhancer), which can cause headaches and rashes.

Soy sauce

Miso

What Is It Good For?

ANTICANCER PROPERTIES Rich in cancer-protective isoflavones, which protect the heart and aid hormone balance in both men and women. Evidence suggests that women who consume 3 or more bowls of miso soup daily have a significantly lower risk of breast cancer.

AIDS DIGESTION Miso is a high-antioxidant fermented food that feeds friendly bacteria in the gut, helping to enhance immunity and aid digestion. It is made from grains, such as barley and rice, or soybeans, and contains all the essential amino acids required by the body, which makes it a complete protein.

How Do I Use It?

AS A VERSATILE PROTEIN Look for organic, naturally aged, nonpasteurized miso, which is sold as a thick paste. The longer it is aged, the darker its color. Use dark miso in a vegetable-bean casserole to supply plenty of high-quality protein, or mix with water to make an energizing, alkalizing broth. Use a light-colored miso as a substitute for milk, butter, and salt in creamed soups, or as a marinade to tenderize meat.

Miso

Tempeh

What Is It Good For?

PHYTOESTROGEN-RICH High in phytoestrogens, tempeh helps protect against heart disease and cancer, regulates immune function, and may help relieve menopausal symptoms. Not to be confused with tofu (which is not fermented), tempeh is made from fermented, lightly cooked soybeans. Fermentation increases its antimicrobial benefits, providing protection against gastrointestinal upsets. Tempeh is rich in dietary fiber, which helps maintain a healthy digestive tract. This fiber also helps remove fats from the blood. It has also been shown to help lower levels of "unhealthy" (LDL) cholesterol while raising levels of "healthy" (HDL) cholesterol.

How Do I Use It?

MEAT SUBSTITUTE Tempeh has a hearty, nutty flavor that makes it a popular meat substitute. It can be baked, sautéed, steamed, or marinated, and used in sandwiches, curries, and salads. Its relatively neutral taste means it absorbs whatever flavors it is cooked in.

Tempeh

MEATS

 PROMOTES TISSUE GROWTH AND REPAIR

 HELPS RELEASE CELLULAR ENERGY

 PROMOTES HEALTHY SKIN AND HAIR

Meat is an important source of nutrients and **bioavailable** (easily absorbed) protein that helps the body repair and **build tissue**, **generate energy**, and maintain **healthy skin and hair**. However, eating too much highly processed, intensively reared meat contributes to health problems, such as heart disease and cancer. Organic meat has a much healthier nutrient profile, particularly in terms of fats.

. Breast meat

. Dark meat

Chicken

CHICKEN

WHAT IS IT GOOD FOR?

IMMUNITY-ENHANCING Chicken contains all the B vitamins, which help the body produce energy and form red blood cells, and also help strengthen the nervous system. Chicken meat is particularly high in the heart-healthy vitamin B_3 (niacin): the dark meat contains double the amount of zinc and iron of the light meat, giving it immune-boosting properties; while the white meat is higher in potassium and phosphorus, helping to build strong bones, teeth, and tissues.

HOW DO I USE IT?

CHICKEN SOUP Laboratory studies suggest that the synergistic action of nutrients in chicken may help halt the spread of infection and fight inflammation. If you have a cold or the flu, a bowl of chicken soup may be your best medicine.

Beef Rolled Rump

BEEF

WHAT IS IT GOOD FOR?

METABOLIC BALANCE A source of high-quality protein, beef also contains B vitamins, which fuel cellular energy production. The iron in beef helps produce more red blood cells that carry oxygen around the body. Beef also contains zinc, which aids cell division and helps in the formation of protein.

CHOLESTEROL HEALTH Stearic acid, a saturated fatty acid that accounts for 50 percent of beef fat, is converted by the body to monounsaturated oleic acid, the main fat in heart-healthy olive oil.

HOW DO I USE IT?

ADD GREEN VEGETABLES Beef can be harder to digest than white meat. Marinating or rubbing raw beef with spices such as rosemary, mustard, black pepper, garlic, onions, or horseradish can aid digestion and prevent the formation of carcinogenic heterocyclic amines—substances that form when red meat is cooked at a high temperature.

Healthy animals produce healthy meat

Outdoor-bred, pasture-fed, organic animals produce meat with lower total fat and higher levels of healthy fats, such as omega-3 fatty acids; they are also less prone to contamination with *E. coli* and other bacteria. Meat does contain cholesterol, but this fat is also an essential nutrient that helps the body synthesize steroid hormones, including those that regulate blood sugar, blood pressure, and sex hormone balance. Eating meat with antioxidant-rich green vegetables, as opposed to starchy ones, can help prevent the free-radical damage to cholesterol that is associated with heart disease.

LAMB

WHAT IS IT GOOD FOR?

HEALTHY NERVOUS SYSTEM Lamb contains good amounts of B vitamins and is particularly rich in B_{12} and folate. These nutrients are necessary for a healthy central nervous system and aid the prevention of heart disease, mood disorders, and dementia, including Alzheimer's disease and vascular dementia in older people. Lamb is one of the few commercial meats that is still mostly pasture fed, which means it is naturally lower in cholesterol than some other meats and contains omega-3 and omega-6 fatty acids and conjugated linolenic acid (CLA).

HOW DO I USE IT?

NONSTARCHY VEGETABLES Animal protein meats, such as lamb, are healthiest and easiest to digest when eaten with nonstarchy vegetables (rather than rice and potatoes). Choose vegetables such as green beans, broccoli, kale, collards, and spinach to serve with lamb.

Leg of lamb

PORK

WHAT IS IT GOOD FOR?

A SOURCE OF GOOD FATS Pork is unique in that it contains more monounsaturated and polyunsaturated fats than saturated fat. This means that, as part of a healthy diet, it has a role to play in lowering cholesterol levels and reducing the risk of stroke and hypertension. Unlike beef and lamb, it is not a source of vitamin A, but it does contain useful amounts of the minerals zinc and iron, which help regulate energy release. It also contains B vitamins, specifically B_1, B_2, and B_3 (thiamine, riboflavin, and niacin), which are also necessary for energy regulation as well as muscle growth and repair.

HOW DO I USE IT?

FRESH CUTS We consume a lot of pork in the form of preserved meat. The link between these processed meats and bowel cancer is now well established, so opt for fresh cuts you can cook yourself. Try eating pork with fermented vegetables, such as sauerkraut, to aid digestion, and feed good bacteria in the gut.

Rolled pork leg joint

TURKEY

WHAT IS IT GOOD FOR?

CONTROLS INSULIN SECRETION Turkey belongs to a small group of high-protein animal foods (which also include tuna and egg whites) that can help keep post-meal insulin levels balanced for longer. The combination of B vitamins and tryptophan amino acid in turkey has a balancing effect on blood sugar levels, helps keep the nerves calm, avoids hypoglycemia and low moods, and has an immune-enhancing effect. It also contains selenium, necessary for the efficient function of the immune system and thyroid. Selenium is an antioxidant that helps combat the oxidative stress caused by free radicals in the body.

HOW DO I USE IT?

EAT THE DARK MEAT As with chicken, there are benefits in choosing the darker meat of the leg and thigh because it contains more metabolism-boosting iron, zinc, and B vitamins than the white meat. Use the dark meat as a filling for a sandwich or wrap with mango chutney and watercress.

Breast meat

Dark meat

Turkey

MEATS CONTINUED

Venison

Quail

Squab

VENISON

WHAT IS IT GOOD FOR?

METABOLIC BOOST Venison is deer meat that is very low in fat. Like other red meats, it is high in protein and iron, which is necessary for efficient metabolism, but is low in saturated fats. It is also rich in potassium, phosphorus, and zinc. Venison contains useful amounts of vitamins B_1 and B_3, which help keep the metabolism in good shape and aid the growth, repair, and detoxification of tissues and bones. It is also a good source of the heart-protective vitamins B_6 and B_{12}, which can help keep arteries healthy.

HOW DO I USE IT?

ANTIOXIDANT-RICH MEAL Many recipes recommend long, slow cooking, although venison is probably best served medium-rare. For an antioxidant-rich meal, cover the raw meat with a dry rub of pepper, paprika, garlic, onion, thyme, and crushed juniper berries, and serve with roasted beets, sweet potatoes, and apple sauce.

QUAIL

WHAT IS IT GOOD FOR?

LOW-FAT ENERGY BOOSTER Quail is lower in fat and higher in protein than chicken. The meat of this small bird has a sweet, delicate taste and is a great source of copper and iron, which are important nutrients for helping to generate energy. Quail also contains vitamin B-complex and vitamins C, E, and K, which help to strengthen the immune system. It is also a great source of iron, which helps transport oxygen throughout the body, and copper which, along with iron, helps prevent anemia and is necessary for healthy joints, skin, hair and connective tissue.

HOW DO I USE IT?

KEEP IT SIMPLE Choose quail that hasn't been intensively farmed. A single quail provides around 3–5oz (85–140g) of meat—essentially a single serving; cook quickly in a moderate oven 350°F (180°C) for 10 minutes only to preserve its moisture and nutrients. Quail quickly absorbs the flavor from marinades, so don't let any strong mixtures overpower its delicate flavor.

SQUAB

WHAT IS IT GOOD FOR?

IMMUNE-BOOSTING A wild bird with a distinctly gamey flavor, squab is high in key immunity-boosting trace elements, such as iron, zinc, and selenium; zinc is particularly important for male prostate health. Squab also contains the highest levels of phosphorous, necessary for healthy bones, tissue repair, and hormone production, of all commonly consumed game. It is low in fat—containing less fat than lamb or duck—and is a better source of blood-building iron than beef.

HOW DO I USE IT?

COOK QUICKLY Squab has a deep crimson color and great depth of flavor. It tastes wonderful in pies or on its own in a red wine sauce. As with quail, it benefits from quick cooking. Try serving hot on a bed of leafy greens or lentils, or in a salad with blackberry vinegar.

WATERFOWL

WHAT IS IT GOOD FOR?

GOOD FATS Duck and goose, known collectively as waterfowl, are particularly good for fueling the metabolic processes. Both are rich in iron and B vitamins, and duck, in particular, can contain up to 3 times more iron than chicken. Although waterfowl is perceived as a fatty meat, both duck and goose have a fat profile that is similar to chicken, meaning that both are high in heart-healthy monounsaturated and polyunsaturated fats. Both meats are also a good source of selenium, an antioxidant mineral that supports a healthy immune system.

HOW DO I USE IT?

NUTRITIOUS VARIETY Try cooking duck breasts instead of chicken breasts to provide variety and extra nutrition, or cook a goose as an alternative to seasonal roasted turkey. Duck and goose fat are very heat-stable alternatives to using olive oil or lard in cooking.

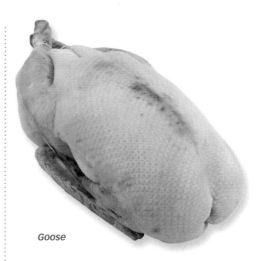

Goose

LIVER

WHAT IS IT GOOD FOR?

BLOOD BUILDER The liver is a storehouse of valuable nutrients for the body. All types of liver provide essential iron and B_{12} to support healthy blood. Whether from mammals or birds (or even fish), liver is also a tremendous source of protein and vitamin A, which is necessary for proper immune function as well as healthy skin, eyes, and mucous membranes. Lamb and calf liver are the richest sources of vitamin A, while chicken livers are a rich source of folate. As long as the animal it comes from was healthy and organic, all types of liver provide a major boost for the immune system, skin, eyes, and lungs.

HOW DO I USE IT?

A CLASSIC DISH Only eat organic liver, and enjoy it in patés or as a main meal. Marinating liver in lemon juice for 1–2 hours to draw out any impurities will give it a better texture. Lightly frying liver so it is still slightly pink in the middle, and serving on a bed of sautéed onions, is a classic way to enjoy this meat.

Pork liver

KIDNEYS

WHAT IS IT GOOD FOR?

ANTIOXIDANT-RICH Kidneys, most often from beef or lamb, are a good source of the antioxidant mineral selenium, which has a role to play in protecting against heart disease and cancer. They also contain moderate amounts of vitamin A, which promotes healthy skin, and large amounts of B vitamins, iron, and zinc. Men benefit from the zinc and selenium in kidneys, both of which help maintain fertility and a healthy prostate, while women of childbearing age will benefit from the iron, which can help replace what is lost during menstruation.

HOW DO I USE IT?

ADD TO CASSEROLES Kidneys add richness to beef and lamb dishes. Before cooking, marinate in lemon juice or brine for 1–2 hours to remove any trace of ammonia and improve their texture. Or cook simply with mushrooms and serve on toast.

Kidneys

OILY FISH

 PROTECTS THE HEART AND BLOOD VESSELS

 SUPPORTS A HEALTHY NERVOUS SYSTEM

HELPS LUBRICATES JOINTS

 SUPPORTS EFFICIENT METABOLISM

This group of fish are unique because their **heart-healthy** fats are distributed through their flesh rather than concentrated in their liver, as with white fish. They are particularly high in certain **omega-3 fatty acids**, which protect the **cardiovascular** and **nervous systems**. The fat-soluble vitamins A, D, E, and K are also abundant, benefitting bone, joint, muscle, skin, and eye health, and metabolic balance.

Salmon

SALMON

WHAT IS IT GOOD FOR?

SUPPORTS HEALTHY AGING Uniquely rich in the omega-3 fatty acids eicosapentaenoic acid (EPA) and decosahexaenoic acid (DHA). In combination with its abundant supply of selenium, these omega-3 fatty acids help lower blood pressure, "unhealthy" (LDL) cholesterol levels in the blood, and inflammation, reducing the risk of heart disease, stroke, and cancer. They also protect the eyes and joints and feed the brain, helping to prevent dementia and loss of mental functions. Salmon is also relatively low in the pro-inflammatory omega-6 fatty acids (already overabundant in the modern diet).

HOW DO I USE IT?

GO WILD Choose wild or organic as farmed salmon can contain residues of veterinary medicines. Grill on a high heat to seal in its nutrient.

Herring

HERRING

WHAT IS IT GOOD FOR?

HEART HEALTH A good source of eicosapentaenoic acid (EPA) and decosahexaenoic acid (DHA), fatty acids that lower hypertension, triglycerides (fatty deposits) in the blood, and inflammation, helping to reduce the risk of heart disease and stroke. It also contains vitamin D, calcium, and phosphorus, which are all important for bone health, and also vitamin B_{12}, which aids the production of cellular energy.

HOW DO I USE IT?

A LIGHT BITE Smoked herring is known as kippers, a delicacy that can be eaten at any meal. Rollmops are pickled herrings. Make your own with subtly flavored vinegar and serve with fresh bread, or cut into chunks and add to potato salad.

Mackerel

MACKEREL

WHAT IS IT GOOD FOR?

HEALTHY AGING Contains an abundance of nutrients, including vitamins A, B-complex, C, D, E, and K, calcium, potassium, selenium, and magnesium, which help regulate the metabolism, including blood sugar and cholesterol levels, and support healthy heart, bones, teeth, nerves, and muscles. It is rich in anti-inflammatory omega-3 fatty acids that keep blood vessels elastic and reduce swollen joints, pain, and stiffness associated with arthritis.

HOW DO I USE IT?

A HEALTHY MEAL Serve warm with asparagus on a bed of noodles and a miso and ginger dressing, or serve cold on a bed of sprouted lentils or other sprouted seeds, walnuts, and chives. To make fish cakes, blend with scallions, lima beans, mustard, parsley, and a little egg.

SARDINES

WHAT IS IT GOOD FOR?

LOWERS CHOLESTEROL Sardines are one of the most concentrated sources of the omega-3 fatty acids EPA and DHA, which have been found to lower triglycerides (fatty deposits) and "unhealthy" (LDL) cholesterol levels in the blood. They are an excellent source of vitamin B_{12} and a great source of vitamin D, which plays an essential role in bone health since it helps to increase the body's absorption of calcium.

HOW DO I USE IT?

QUICK AND CONVENIENT Canned sardines make a convenient and nutritious quick meal served on toast or pasta. Fresh sardines are delicious broiled or grilled. Cooking them quickly in this way keeps their essential nutrients intact.

Sardines

TROUT

WHAT IS IT GOOD FOR?

A GOOD SOURCE OF PROTEIN Lower in fat than some other fish, but still contains good amounts of omega-3 fatty acids. Also a good source of protein, potassium, phosphorus, vitamin B_{12}, and iron, which protect the heart and build healthy bones. Like most oily fish, semi-oily trout contains cholesterol, which is necessary for the synthesis of vitamin D and the production of vital hormones in the body, including the different sex hormones testosterone, progesterone, and estrogen.

HOW DO I USE IT?

MIX WITH FRESH FLAVORS When served with dried beans, oily fish, like trout, help increase the absorption of iron from the beans. Or cook with a lemon and almond crust or a rub of ground dried herbs and garlic mixed in a little olive oil. Grill on high heat.

Trout

SEA BASS

WHAT IS IT GOOD FOR?

IMMUNE ENHANCING An excellent source of high-quality protein and very rich in vitamins A, D, and E, which, with its omega-3 oils, are anti-inflammatory, immune-enhancing, and may help protect against degenerative diseases and cancer. It is also high in phosphorus, potassium, calcium, magnesium, zinc, and selenium. A semi-oily fish, it contains a good balance of fats but in lower quantities than oily fish, so it's a good choice if you want to limit your consumption of total fats.

HOW DO I USE IT?

A LOW-FAT CHOICE Grill simply with lemon and garlic, or spice it up with ginger, chile, and scallions.

Sea bass

TUNA

WHAT IS IT GOOD FOR?

HEART HEALTH Like trout and sea bass, tuna is a semi-oily fish. It is an excellent source of protein, as well as selenium, magnesium, potassium, and omega-3 essential fatty acids. Tuna also contains the B vitamins niacin, B_1, and B_6, and folate; B vitamins help lower levels of homocysteine, which can cause atherosclerosis (hardening of the arteries due to the buildup of plaque).

HOW DO I USE IT?

THINK SMALL Tuna concentrates toxins like mercury. Smaller species like skipjack are safest to eat, but limit consuming any type to once a week. Soy sauce and wasabi makes a good marinade for fresh grilled tuna.

Tuna

ALGAE

 HELPS FIGHT INFECTION　　 **FEEDS GOOD BACTERIA IN THE GUT**　　 **SUPPORTS AND PROTECTS THE LIVER**

This group of aquatic plants is prized by Asian cultures as a delicacy and a rich **source of nutrients** and **antioxidants**, such as beta-carotene and zeaxanthin, **selenium**, zinc, and **vitamins C, E, and B-complex**. It is also rich in **protein** and **amino acids** that help the body to **fight infection,** and a beneficial type of **fiber** that encourages the growth of **good bacteria** in the gut and aids **detox**.

CHLORELLA
Chlorella is a green algae and is one of the richest sources of the detoxifying plant pigment chlorophyll.

SPIRULINA
The most commonly used type of blue-green algae, spirulina is a rich source of beta-carotene and amino acids.

AFA (APHANIZOMENON FLOS-AQUAE)
A unique blue-green algae found in Upper Klamath Lake in Oregon. AFA contains phenylethylamine (PEA), which may help balance mood and improve mental clarity.

WHAT IS IT GOOD FOR?

BOOSTS IMMUNITY Chlorella contains "Chlorella Growth Factor" (CGF), which can enhance immune function and stimulate tissue repair. Laboratory studies suggest that blue-green algae can fight the viruses that cause herpes, HIV, and influenza, though evidence in human beings is still lacking.

PROBIOTIC Helps to promote the growth of friendly bacteria in the gut. It is a good choice after a course of antibiotics, which can kill both good and bad gut flora in the intestines.

DETOX Helps support and protect the liver, and has a laxative effect. Blue-green algae may protect the liver from toxic damage. Chlorella has been shown to help remove heavy metals (such as cadmium and mercury), pesticides, and industrial pollutants from the body.

ANTIOXIDANTS Green and blue-green algae can help fight inflammation and damage to tissues and organs caused by free radicals.

HOW DO I GET THE BEST FROM IT?

DRIED CONCENTRATE Fresh algae doesn't keep well so it is often sold as supplements in a dried, powdered form. Many algae are now farmed rather than wild-gathered; this is not a bad thing, because they can easily become contaminated with waterborne pollutants.

USE IN SMALL QUANTITIES The drying process concentrates the nutrients so a little goes a long way. Mega-dosing with algae can produce uncomfortable stomach cramps.

HOW DO I USE IT?

SALAD DRESSING To give your salad a boost, try mixing 1–2 tsp algae powder into an oil and vinegar salad dressing.

A HEALTHY ADDITIVE Dried algae are versatile and generally have a mild taste ideal for mixing into soups, stir-fries, salsas, guacamoles, smoothies, and vegetable juices.

SEAWEEDS

 ASSISTS WEIGHT MANAGEMENT

 HELPS REMOVE TOXINS FROM THE BODY

 LOWERS RISK OF HEART DISEASE AND STROKE

 FIGHTS THE EFFECTS OF STRESS

Every type of seaweed has a unique taste and texture, but all possess broadly the same nutritional benefits. They are, for instance, **protein-rich** and a source of **iodine**, necessary for **metabolism**. They are also a good source of **fiber** and **chlorophyll**, which help **remove toxins** from the body, and **heart-healthy** magnesium and potassium, which **protect blood vessels** and fight the effects of **stress**.

WHAT IS IT GOOD FOR?

METABOLISM Its high iodine content helps support healthy thyroid function, which in turn helps regulate the metabolism of cells and assists weight management. Brown seaweeds, such as kelp and wakame, contain the antioxidant carotenoid fucoxanthin, which improves insulin resistance and helps metabolize fat more efficiently.

DETOX A source of detoxifying chlorophyll and mucilaginous (gumlike) fiber that helps maintain bowel regularity and binds to and removes toxins and fats from the body.

HEART HEALTH Contains high amounts of magnesium, which lowers blood pressure, and folate, which breaks down homocysteine, a risk factor for heart disease and stroke.

STRESS Magnesium, pantothenic acid, and riboflavin support the health of the adrenal glands, which play a critical role in our response to stress. Without this nutritional support, constant stress can exhaust the adrenal glands, resulting in chronic fatigue, lowered immunity, and mood changes.

HOW DO I GET THE BEST FROM IT?

FRESH OR DRIED Drying does not damage its nutritional content. If you can forage fresh seaweed, make sure you rinse it well.

VEGETABLE PROTEIN If you don't eat meat or want to cut back on animal protein, seaweed provides high-quality vegetable protein.

HOW DO I USE IT?

FLAVOR ENHANCER Use ground seaweed as a flavor enhancer instead of salt, to flavor and thicken stocks, or add to soups, broths, or miso for extra protein and vitamins.

ADD TO BREAD To balance blood sugar levels and add protein, replace half the flour with ground seaweed. Use water, not milk, omit the salt, and add 1 extra tbsp oil or butter.

DULSE
High in protein, dulse contains all the essential trace minerals as well as the antioxidant beta-carotene and vitamins C, E, and B-complex.

KELP
A rich source of iodine and other important trace minerals.

NORI
Particularly high in protein, which makes up 50 percent of its dry weight, and contains a comparable amount of fiber to spinach.

WAKAME
Contains a high amount of magnesium, which improves heart function and acts as a diuretic.

ALOE VERA

 CONTAINS POTENT ANTIVIRAL SUBSTANCES

 HELPS EASE BRONCHIAL COMPLAINTS

 HELPS BALANCE INTESTINAL FLORA

The swordlike leaves of aloe vera contain a clear mucilaginous gel with **detoxifying**, **antiseptic**, and **anti-inflammatory** properties that is used internally and externally to **treat respiratory complaints and aid digestion**. In some Asian countries, the whole leaf, which contains **immunity-boosting** and **antioxidant** beta-carotene and vitamins C, E, many B vitamins, and minerals, is cooked and eaten.

Leaves
The antiviral potential of aloe gel in the leaves has been shown to boost the effectiveness of HIV treatments

ALOE PLANT
Of the 200-plus species of aloe plants, only 2—Aloe Barbadensis Miller and Aloe Arborescens—are grown commercially, with Aloe Barbadensis Miller being the most widely used.

PURE ALOE GEL
Unprocessed aloe gel contains aloin, a powerful laxative. Processed aloe vera juices contain much less of this substance.

WHAT IS IT GOOD FOR?

IMMUNITY STIMULANT Contains a substance called acemannan, an immune stimulant and an antiviral. It is effective against the herpes virus, and in HIV patients it may work synergistically with conventional medicines.

RESPIRATORY EASE Can help soothe coughs and bronchial asthma. Its antiseptic properties can help to heal colds and sore throats.

DIGESTION Helps balance intestinal flora. Can be useful in cases of irritable bowel syndrome, and is a laxative that is reputed to help expel parasites from the digestive tract.

ANTI-INFLAMMATORY Blocks the formation of histamine, which makes it a useful remedy for allergic conditions. Also contains natural salicylic acid, the base material for aspirin, so it is useful for general aches and pains and also conditions such as arthritis. As a gargle, it is also a beneficial treatment for gingivitis, an inflammatory condition of the gums.

HOW DO I GET THE BEST FROM IT?

GROW YOUR OWN Aloe plants are relatively easy to grow, but they don't like cold weather. Plant in pots and bring indoors in winter.

PURE GEL Aloe is most effective if minimally processed. If you can't get fresh aloe, look for 100 percent aloe juice products and pure gels, not extracts from the macerated leaves.

HOW DO I USE IT?

MAKE A FRESH JUICE Cut 1 aloe leaf (10–12in/25–30cm long) into manageable sections, peel like an avocado or mango, and scoop out the clear gel "fillet." Blend in a food processor or blender with 1 cup apple juice and drink while very fresh.

MIX INTO HEALTHY JUICES Aloe juice can be bitter so mix with apple and cucumber juice or fresh pineapple juice and coconut water.

WHEATGRASS

 HELPS REMOVE TOXINS FROM THE BODY

 HELPS BUILD RED BLOOD CELLS

 HEALS AND STRENGTHENS THE GUT

Before they form seed heads, young wheat shoots, called wheatgrass, consist of 70 percent **chlorophyll**. Wheatgrass supports the **immune system**, removes **toxins** from the blood and body tissues, improves **digestion**, is **gluten-free**, unlike other forms of wheat, and is high in vitamins C, E, and B-complex, **beta-carotene**, calcium, magnesium, potassium, iron, natural enzymes, and amino acids.

WHAT IS IT GOOD FOR?

DETOXIFIER Chlorophyll aids detoxification and, along with other plant-based nutrients, is a natural chelator (a substance that helps to draw heavy metals out of the body). In women with breast cancer, wheatgrass juice has been shown to remove the toxic byproducts of chemotherapy from their blood. There is also evidence that chlorophyll helps to protect the liver from toxins.

BLOOD BUILDER Its vitamin C and folate may help treat anemia resulting from deficiencies in these nutrients. Its high chlorophyll content assists in the formation of healthy red blood cells; studies show it reduces the transfusion requirements of people with thalassemia—a genetic disorder in which the body makes an abnormal form of hemoglobin.

DIGESTION Because it contains nutrients but little fiber, wheatgrass juice is a good way to supply nutrition to people with ulcerative colitis. There is also some evidence that daily ingestion of wheatgrass juice can help heal some of the symptoms of ulcerative colitis.

HEART HEALTH Animal studies have shown the juice can help lower total cholesterol and other blood fats, such as triglycerides (a type of fat in the blood), and which can specifically lower "unhealthy" (LDL) cholesterol levels.

HOW DO I GET THE BEST FROM IT?

RINSE WELL It is grown in moist conditions so is prone to mold; wash well before juicing.

ON ITS OWN It doesn't mix with food so take on an empty stomach 1 hour before eating.

HOW DO I USE IT?

AS A SHOT Serve in a shot glass with a slice of orange to help absorb its mineral content.

RECONSTITUTE IT The convenience and consistency of reconstituted dried powders can be a better option than fresh wheatgrass.

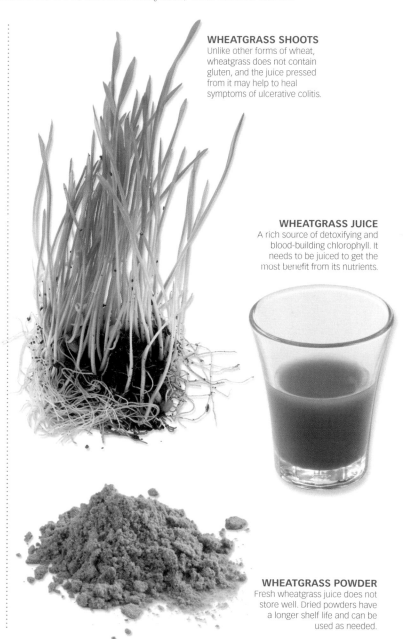

WHEATGRASS SHOOTS
Unlike other forms of wheat, wheatgrass does not contain gluten, and the juice pressed from it may help to heal symptoms of ulcerative colitis.

WHEATGRASS JUICE
A rich source of detoxifying and blood-building chlorophyll. It needs to be juiced to get the most benefit from its nutrients.

WHEATGRASS POWDER
Fresh wheatgrass juice does not store well. Dried powders have a longer shelf life and can be used as needed.

HONEY

 HELPS HEAL ULCERS

 FIGHTS RESPIRATORY INFECTIONS

 HELPS SPEED WOUND HEALING

 PROVIDES SEASONAL ALLERGY RELIEF

Even though honey is made up of mostly simple sugars and water, it has many medicinal properties, including its ability to help **heal skin wounds** and **ulcers**. Its effectiveness lies in its levels of **vitamins C, D, E, K, and B-complex**, and **beta-carotene**, minerals, enzymes, and essential oils. It's also a **natural antibiotic** and rich in **antioxidants**, making it effective at **fighting respiratory infections**.

HONEYCOMB
Raw honey extracted from the honeycomb is not sterilized or pasteurized, leaving its vitamins and enzymes intact and undamaged.

MANUKA HONEY
The antimicrobial properties of this honey (manuka is a wild shrub native to New Zealand) are well known and defined by the Unique Manuka Factor (UMF). A UMF of 10 and above is considered very beneficial.

HONEY
Studies show that honey can be as effective for treating coughs and sore throats as conventional cough syrups.

WHAT IS IT GOOD FOR?

HEALS ULCERS Its antioxidants may help to heal the colon in cases of ulcerative colitis. Manuka honey contains, in addition to hydrogen peroxide, unique antibacterial substances that are useful against *Helicobacter pylori* bacteria, which causes stomach ulcers.

RESPIRATORY INFECTIONS Can be as effective as the cough suppressant diphenhydramine, and may help children sleep better. Types of honey shown to work well for coughs include buckwheat, eucalyptus, citrus, or labiatae (mint family) varieties. The antimicrobial properties of manuka honey make it a good choice if you or your child has a cold.

ANTISEPTIC Contains hydrogen peroxide, one reason why it may be effective at inhibiting bacterial growth in laboratory studies. Used topically, it can help speed wound healing.

ALLERGIES Unfiltered honey, rich in pollen, can relieve the symptoms of seasonal allergies.

HOW DO I GET THE BEST FROM IT?

COLOR COUNTS Choose the darkest honey you can find, because it has more nutrients. Buckwheat, avocado, sagebrush, and tupelo honeys are particularly good choices.

BEWARE OF FAKE HONEY Unpasteurized and unfiltered honey is the most nutritious. Avoid ultrapurified honey, which has had all traces of pollen removed, and cheap fake honeys (often pale in color and sold in squeeze bottles). These have no medicinal benefit.

STORE CAREFULLY Store away from light at room temperature to preserve its properties.

HOW DO I USE IT?

SIMPLE COUGH SYRUP Take 1 tbsp of honey or combine with a little lemon juice and/or grated fresh ginger for a warming cough syrup that will boost your vitamin C intake.

Honey is a powerhouse of healing nutrients and enzymes and is one of the world's oldest natural remedies. The darker the color of the honey, the more concentrated these substances will be.

STEVIA

 HELPS BALANCE BLOOD SUGAR LEVELS

 HELPS FIGHT BACTERIA AND VIRUSES

 PROTECTS HEART AND BLOOD VESSELS

 AIDS HEALTHY DIGESTION

Native to South America, stevia is prized for its naturally sweet taste and medicinal properties. Its leaves contain 2 "glycoside" molecules, stevioside and rebaudioside, which are 300 times sweeter than refined sugar, but contain **no calories** and **do not raise blood sugar levels or cause dental cavities**. These glycosides are also now available as a processed powder or concentrated liquid.

Leaves
Stevia leaves, which have a sweet taste reminiscent of aniseed, can be ground and used in cooking or added whole to teas

Granules
Because it does not contain sugar, stevia is a good alternative sweetener for diabetics

WHAT IS IT GOOD FOR?

ANTIDIABETIC There is evidence to suggest that, for some people, it can improve insulin sensitivity and prevent a postprandial spike in blood sugar levels in type-2 diabetics.

IMMUNITY ENHANCER Inhibits the growth and reproduction of bacteria and other infectious organisms; it has been shown to be effective against *Streptococcus mutans*, *Pseudomonas aeruginosa*, and *Proteus vulgaris*. It is also good as an antiseptic mouthwash and gargle, and studies show regular use can help lower the incidence of dental cavities.

HEART HEALTH Helps strengthen the heart and vascular system. Stevioside, a chemical compound in stevia, is believed to be the active ingredient responsible.

BENEFITS DIGESTION Improves digestion and the overall health of the gastrointestinal tract.

HOW DO I GET THE BEST FROM IT?

AVOID ADDITIVES Look for stevia products with a minimum of additives. Many contain the sweetener maltodextrin or the alcohol sugar erythritol, and bulking and anticaking agents. Use for some, but not all, the same purposes as refined sugar (it won't caramelize and can't be used to make meringues).

FRESH LEAVES Add a fresh leaf to a cup of regular or herbal tea for a hint of sweetness.

HOW DO I USE IT?

MAKE AN EXTRACT Add 1 cup warm water to ⅓ cup fresh, finely chopped stevia leaves. Let infuse for 24 hours, strain into a clean jar or bottle, refrigerate, and use to sweeten drinks. Consume within 1 month.

MAKE A GREEN POWDER Crush dried leaves to a powder in a mortar and pestle, coffee grinder, or herb blender. Store in a clean container to use in baking and other recipes that call for green stevia powder.

Maple Syrup

 HELPS PROTECT THE PROSTATE

 HELPS RELEASE CELLULAR ENERGY

 CONTAINS ANTICANCER SUBSTANCES

 HELPS KEEP BLOOD VESSELS SUPPLE

This natural sweetener is gaining ground as an **energy-boosting**, healthy alternative to refined sugar. Recent studies have found it is rich in **phenolic compounds**, which have **anticancer**, **antibacterial**, and **antidiabetic** properties, and manganese and zinc, making it a good choice for **heart health** and **boosting men's fertility**. In addition, it contains 15 times more calcium than honey, and less sodium.

What Is It Good For?

MEN'S HEALTH Zinc helps support men's reproductive health and protects against prostate enlargement. Its abundant manganese levels also help in the production of sex hormones in both men and women.

SUSTAINED ENERGY Manganese is essential for cellular energy production and the synthesis of fatty acids and cholesterol. Zinc aids cellular metabolism and protein synthesis.

ANTICANCER EFFECTS Laboratory studies show that its antioxidant polyphenols are better than broccoli, blueberries, carrots, and tomatoes at slowing the growth of prostate and lung cancer cells.

HEART The zinc in maple syrup is a useful antioxidant that protects artery walls from free-radical damage and helps prevent hardening of the arteries (atherosclerosis).

BETTER BLOOD SUGAR CONTROL Its antioxidant polyphenols, combined with its plant hormone, abscisic acid, have been shown to improve the body's sensitivity to the blood-sugar-regulating hormone insulin.

How Do I Get The Best From It?

REAL AND ORGANIC Look for 100 percent organic maple syrup; cheap products are simply corn syrup with maple flavoring.

CHOOSE YOUR COLOR Lighter syrups have a mild flavor that suits cereals and coffee. Use dark syrup in baking, marinades, and sauces.

How Do I Use It?

POUR IT ON Add to oatmeal or marinades—it goes well with ginger and soy sauce. Drizzle over broccoli or mix into sweet potato mash.

TO DETOX For a cleansing 1-day fast, mix ¾ cup maple syrup, the juice of 3 small lemons, 2 tsp cayenne pepper, and 7 cups purified water. Drink through the day.

MAPLE SYRUP
Four tablespoons of maple syrup has the same antioxidant capacity as a serving of broccoli or a banana.

MAPLE SUGAR
To make maple sugar, the sap is boiled for longer than it is boiled for making the syrup. It's about twice as sweet as refined sugar and retains most of the minerals of the syrup.

BLACKSTRAP MOLASSES

 **HELPS RELEASE
CELLULAR ENERGY**

 **HELPS STRENGTHEN
BONES AND TEETH**

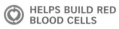 **HELPS BUILD RED
BLOOD CELLS**

 **HELPS EASE
MENSTRUAL CRAMPS**

Unlike refined sugar, corn syrup, and artificial sweeteners, which contain no nutrients and are linked to a variety of health problems, this viscous black-gold residue (produced when sugar cane is turned into refined sugar) is rich in **bone-building** calcium, iron to **enrich the blood**, potassium to **ease muscle cramps**, and B vitamins to fuel efficient **metabolism** and help strengthen the **nervous system**.

BLACKSTRAP MOLASSES
One tablespoon of it contains almost 26 percent of your daily requirement of iron, 20 percent of calcium, and 61 percent of magnesium.

SUGAR CANE
Blackstrap molasses is obtained during the third and final refinement process of boiling sugar syrup derived from sugar cane.

WHAT IS IT GOOD FOR?

ENERGY RELEASE Provides the same quick energy boost as refined sugar. Unlike sugar, it is a source of important nutrients including selenium, manganese, and the B vitamins pyridoxine (B_6) and choline.

STRONG BONES A great source of calcium, which helps build and maintain strong bones and teeth. Calcium also promotes a healthy gut, helps maintain a steady heartbeat, and enhances the function of the nervous system.

HEART HEALTH Choline supports healthy nerve function, strengthens cell membranes, and prevents the buildup of homocysteine, a substance linked to heart disease and osteoporosis. Iron helps build the red blood cells that transport oxygen to all parts of the body, and is necessary for cellular energy production and metabolism.

WOMEN'S HEALTH It is a useful remedy during menstruation. Taking 2–3 tsp daily can help balance any iron lost.

HOW DO I GET THE BEST FROM IT?

IRON TONIC A useful iron supplement for those who cannot tolerate the constipation associated with iron tonics and supplements.

A MORNING ENERGIZER A natural laxative as well as an energy-booster, molasses is best taken first thing in the morning before food.

LOOK FOR UNSULFURED MOLASSES True blackstrap molasses does not need added sulfur as a preservative. If it contains sulfur, it is an inferior product without the nutrients.

HOW DO I USE IT?

GREAT FOR COOKING It gives baked goods, like gingerbread, a distinctive flavor. It is also used in barbecue sauces and baked beans.

MAKE A TEA Add 1 tsp to ginger tea as a remedy for menstrual or abdominal cramps.

CHOCOLATE

 LOWERS RISK OF HEART DISEASE AND STROKE

 PROTECTS AGAINST FREE-RADICAL DAMAGE

 AN EFFECTIVE COUGH SUPPRESSANT

 SOOTHES UPSET STOMACHS

Scientific research into chocolate is turning up some intriguing possibilities about its healthful nutrients, including improved **immunity**, greater **longevity**, and **quicker recovery** from intense exercise. Dark chocolate without unhealthy additives and sugar has been shown to lower the risk of **cancer** and **stroke**, and lowers **blood pressure** as effectively as antioxidant-rich fruit and vegetables.

WHAT IS IT GOOD FOR?

HEART HEALTH Moderate consumption protects the heart by thinning the blood in much the same way as low-dose aspirin, while its beneficial flavanols protect artery walls and lower blood pressure and cholesterol.

IMMUNE SUPPORT Weight for weight it has the same amount of antioxidants as red wine. These support overall immunity and intestinal immunity by boosting the response of antibodies and T-helper cells (a type of blood cell that helps kickstart the immune response), and strengthening the intestinal lining against invading microorganisms.

EASES COUGHS One of the stimulants in cocoa, theobromine, has been shown to be more effective than codeine (a traditional cough suppressant) for soothing a sore throat.

DIGESTION Studies show substances in dark chocolate help ease gastrointestinal upsets.

HOW DO I GET THE BEST FROM IT?

CHOOSE ORGANIC At least 30 pesticides are used in conventional cocoa so opt for organic.

GO DARK For the most antioxidants, choose semisweet or unsweetened chocolate with at least 70 percent cocoa solids and less sugar. Milk chocolate contains fewer antioxidants.

A LITTLE OF THE BEST Eating a little high-quality chocolate will be far more satisfying than a highly processed bar. Avoid bars with hydrogenated or partially hydrogenated oils.

HOW DO I USE IT?

RAW CACAO NIBS The minimally processed nibs contain all the cocoa bean's nutrients. Eat as they are or add to fruit salads or baking.

HOT COCOA Milk inhibits the absorption of cocoa polyphenols, so mix 2 tbsp high-quality cocoa powder with hot water and drink in a demitasse cup as you would an espresso.

COCOA POWDER
Unsweetened cocoa powder has twice the level of antioxidant polyphenols as processed dark chocolate, and 4 times that of milk chocolate (white chocolate contains no antioxidants).

COCOA BEANS
Catechin and epicatechin, the antioxidants found in cocoa beans and cocoa products, are the same as those that give green tea its anticancer properties.

CACAO NIBS
These are dried, roasted, and crushed cacao, or cocoa, beans, which are used to make chocolate. Like cocoa powder, they are high in antioxidants.

DARK CHOCOLATE
Studies show that people who eat dark chocolate regularly have a lower risk of heart disease and stroke.

MILK

 HELPS KEEP BLOOD VESSELS SUPPLE

 HELPS REGULATE SLEEP CYCLES

 HELPS PREVENT METABOLIC SYNDROME

Evidence shows that milk has a place as a healthy food, despite being defamed by food faddists. Its **calcium** and **vitamin D** content helps the body **burn calories** more efficiently and maintain a **steady weight**, while its healthy fats help **lower blood pressure**. Organic and raw milks are higher in these **healthy fats** and **essential cofactors** than cheap milk and so are much better for you.

GOAT MILK
Nutritionally comparable to the milk of a cow, goat milk is higher in B vitamins than either cow or sheep milk. If you are allergic to cow milk, you may be able to tolerate goat or sheep milk.

SHEEP MILK
Milk from sheep is higher in fat than cow and goat milk, but has 40 percent more protein than both. It is also marginally higher in phosphorus, magnesium, zinc, and iron, and is a comparable source of calcium.

COW MILK
A good source of protein and calcium, and is high in phosphorus and vitamin B_{12}.

WHAT IS IT GOOD FOR?

HEART HEALTH Calcium may help reduce the risk of hypertension by keeping blood vessels elastic. Goat and sheep milks contain capric acid, a healthy fat that can help raise levels of "healthy" (HDL) cholesterol. Palmitoleic acid, another healthy fat, protects against insulin resistance and diabetes.

HEALTHY MIND A good source of B vitamins, especially B_{12}, for the healthy functioning of the brain and nervous system, cell metabolism, and for helping to regulate sleep/wake cycles.

METABOLIC BALANCE Can significantly reduce your risk of metabolic syndrome (a group of factors that can lead to diabetes and heart disease) and even some cancers.

WEIGHT CONTROL Contains a novel form of vitamin B_3 (niacin), which may help maintain a steady weight and improve energy expenditure. The calcium in dairy foods also increases the metabolism of fat.

HOW DO I GET THE BEST FROM IT?

HEALTHY FATS Half the fat in milk is saturated fat, but the other half has healthy fat, such as oleic acid (found in olive oil), palmitoleic acid, and conjugated linoleic acid (CLA). Sheep and cow milks are rich sources of CLA.

ORGANIC IS A MUST Milk from grass-fed cows contains CLA. Test-tube studies indicate that CLA helps to kill skin, colorectal, and breast cancer cells. It may also help to lower "unhealthy" (LDL) cholesterol and prevent atherosclerosis (hardening of the arteries).

HOW DO I USE IT?

USE FULL FAT Full-fat milk contains only 4 percent fat; take out the fat, and its fat-soluble vitamins A, D, E, and K are also reduced.

TRY RAW MILK Many nutritionists believe that pasteurizing milk impairs its nutritional value so try unpasteurized, or raw, milk in your diet.

YOGURT

 HELPS STRENGTHEN THE IMMUNE SYSTEM

 ASSISTS WEIGHT MANAGEMENT

 HELPS LOWER BLOOD PRESSURE

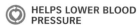 **SOOTHES STOMACH AND BOWEL UPSETS**

The human intestines contain around 400 different species of bacteria, good and bad. Live yogurt, which is colonized by or cultured with certain types of "good" bacteria, can help keep things in balance; good bacteria help to turn organic acids into glucose, **lower cholesterol**, help **metabolize nutrients**, break down the enzymes, proteins, and fibers in food, and help kickstart the **immune system**.

WHAT IS IT GOOD FOR?

IMMUNITY Probiotics in yogurt have a general immunity-boosting effect and inhibit a range of pathogenic bacteria and yeasts in the gut. Probiotics also show potential in preventing allergies, such as eczema, particularly in children. In older or immune-compromised people, live yogurt may help increase resistance to bacterial and viral diseases.

WEIGHT MANAGEMENT Regular consumption of calcium-rich foods is linked to lower body weight in children and adults. Yogurt helps reduce fat around the waistline and retain more lean muscle than diets that don't include it.

LOWERS BLOOD PRESSURE Calcium helps keep blood vessels more supple, enabling them to expand slightly when necessary to keep blood pressure low.

DIGESTIVE HEALTH Gut health is inseparable from the health of the rest of the body. Live cultures in yogurt can improve the microflora of the gut, which in turn helps ease symptoms of inflammatory bowel disease and lowers the incidence of ulcers.

HOW DO I GET THE BEST FROM IT?

CHOOSE LIVE Look for products that state specifically that yogurt is "live" or "probiotic."

KEEP IT NATURAL Avoid yogurts with artificial colors, flavors, thickeners, and sweeteners. Buy a good-quality organic, plain, live yogurt and add your own ingredients.

TRY ALTERNATIVES Sheep- and goat-milk yogurts may be easier for some to digest than cow-milk yogurts. Sheep milk is richer in fat and is a particularly creamy alternative.

HOW DO I USE IT?

AN OMEGA-3 BOOST Stir 1 tbsp ground flaxseed into organic plain yogurt to add both fiber and healthy omega-3 fatty acids.

PLAIN YOGURT
Yogurt is made by culturing milk with a starter culture of friendly bacteria such as *Lactobacillus delbrueckii* subsp. *bulgaricus* and *Streptococcus salivarius* subsp. *thermophilus*. Other beneficial bacteria may be added during the culturing process.

YOGURT DRINK
Flavored yogurt drinks have become a popular way to get concentrated daily "shots" of probiotic cultures, though beware of additives, such as sugar, in the drinks.

GREEK-STYLE YOGURT
This yogurt is strained to remove some of the watery whey. This results in a thicker, creamier yogurt.

KEFIR

 HELPS STRENGTHEN THE IMMUNE SYSTEM
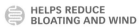 **HELPS REDUCE BLOATING AND WIND**
 CONTAINS ANTICANCER SUBSTANCES
 HELPS LOWER CHOLESTEROL

This probiotic and fermented food is made by culturing fresh milk with kefir "grains"—live colonies of bacteria and yeasts. Kefir is a good source of **calcium**, **protein**, and **potassium**, may have **anticancer** benefits, helps maintain the heath of the **digestive tract,** and **boosts immunity**. Kefir grains, which contain many more live bacteria than yogurt, remain alive indefinitely and can be used repeatedly.

KEFIR GRAINS
These small gelatinous nodules contain colonies of more than 30 bacteria and yeasts that are bound together in a stable, symbiotic relationship. After the grains have fermented milk, they can be filtered out and added to a new batch of milk.

KEFIR CHEESE
Cheese made from kefir contains all the beneficial probiotic microorganisms that kefir is famous for.

KEFIR MILK
Probiotics in kefir can control the growth of harmful bacteria and aid digestion, and some even manufacture vitamins in the gut.

WHAT IS IT GOOD FOR?

IMMUNE SUPPORT Kefiran, an indigestible fiber unique to kefir, has anti-inflammatory and immunity-supporting properties. Regular consumption may increase the activity of the body's natural killer cells and T-helper cells (a type of blood cell that helps kickstart the immune response). Kefir helps maintain the balance of healthy bacteria in the gut necessary to fight harmful fungi, viruses, and bacteria.

DIGESTION By breaking down lactose in milk, kefir may significantly reduce symptoms of lactose intolerance, including bloating and stomach pain, as well as speeding recovery from diarrhea in infants. It may help with other food allergies too, such as those to eggs.

ANTICANCER POTENTIAL Its probiotic properties can have anticancer effects. Laboratory and animal studies have found that kefir can slow breast cancer cell growth.

HEART Various studies have shown that kefir may help lower "unhealthy" (LDL) cholesterol and blood pressure, though results are mixed.

HOW DO I GET THE BEST FROM IT?

MAKE YOUR OWN Many kefir products are mixed with sugars and other additives and don't have the same medicinal benefits. Where possible, make your own kefir (p332).

HOW DO I USE IT?

FOR VEGETARIANS Use kefir grains to ferment nondairy milks, such as almond, soy, coconut, or oat milk.

A VERSATILE INGREDIENT Kefir can be made into a huge variety of products including cheese, spreads, and yogurt. It can also be used in baked goods, and is especially good as a sourdough starter.

TENDERIZES MEATS Kefir's mildly acidic nature can help tenderize meat. Added to sauces, it acts as a thickener.

EGGS

 HELPS PROTECT EYE HEALTH

 HELPS BUILD STRONG BONES AND TEETH

 BOOSTS MENTAL PERFORMANCE

 HELPS PREVENT METABOLIC SYNDROME

Eggs are an excellent source of high-quality **protein**. They contain **vitamin D**, necessary for healthy bones and teeth, and nutrients that help **balance blood sugar levels**, protect against **heart disease**, and support the healthy function of **nerves** and the **brain**. Egg yolks contain cholesterol, but studies show "unhealthy" (LDL) blood cholesterol is raised more by excess saturated fats than it is by eggs.

WHAT IS IT GOOD FOR?

AN ANTIOXIDANT BOOST Egg yolks contain the antioxidants lutein and zeaxanthine, which help protect eyes from age-related macular degeneration (loss of vision), and tryptophan and tyrosine, antioxidant amino acids that help prevent cancer and heart disease.

BONES One of the few food sources of vitamin D, and rich in phosphorus. This combination helps provide the body with the necessary building blocks for healthy bones and teeth.

BRAIN FOOD An excellent source of choline, other B-vitamins, and the mono- and polyunsaturated fats necessary to support a healthy nervous system and brain. Choline helps improve memory, and evidence shows a protein-rich breakfast, such as eggs, improves mental performance throughout the day.

METABOLIC BALANCE Evidence suggests that during digestion, egg proteins are converted into peptides that help lower blood pressure in the same way as conventional drugs, such as ACE inhibitors. In addition, most of the fat in eggs is mono- and polyunsaturated, and other fatty acids called phospholipids help reduce the absorption of cholesterol.

HOW DO I GET THE BEST FROM IT?

FREERANGE AND ORGANIC Organic freerange eggs contain more vitamin A, omega-3 fats, and vitamin E than intensively formed eggs, and less saturated fat.

EASY ON THE HEAT Eggs lose nutritional value when cooked, so try light methods of cooking, such as poaching or soft boiling.

HOW DO I USE IT?

A SIMPLE PROTEIN MEAL Add poached or soft-boiled eggs to salads for a healthy protein-enriched meal.

TRY QUAIL EGGS Substitute 3–4 quail eggs for 1 large chicken egg in salads or on toast.

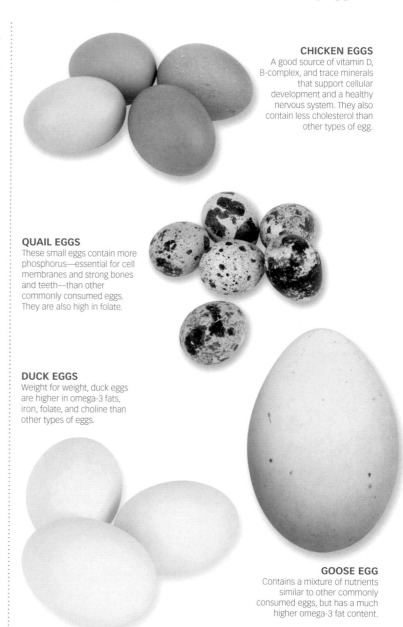

CHICKEN EGGS
A good source of vitamin D, B-complex, and trace minerals that support cellular development and a healthy nervous system. They also contain less cholesterol than other types of egg.

QUAIL EGGS
These small eggs contain more phosphorus—essential for cell membranes and strong bones and teeth—than other commonly consumed eggs. They are also high in folate.

DUCK EGGS
Weight for weight, duck eggs are higher in omega-3 fats, iron, folate, and choline than other types of eggs.

GOOSE EGG
Contains a mixture of nutrients similar to other commonly consumed eggs, but has a much higher omega-3 fat content.

TEA

 ANTIOXIDANT AND ANTIBACTERIAL

 HELPS LOWER CHOLESTEROL

 CONTAINS ANTICANCER SUBSTANCES

 HELPS BUILD STRONG BONES

The average tea leaf contains as much as 30 percent **antioxidant** polyphenols, which help protect against **heart disease** and **cancer** and are **anti-inflammatory,** benefitting joints. Tea also contains **beta-carotene**, vitamins B_2, C, D, and K, and potassium. Even the caffeine in tea, when taken in moderation, has health benefits: it helps **boost metabolism**, **burn fat**, and acts as a **mild diuretic**.

GREEN TEA
This delicate tea is produced by lightly steaming and then drying the freshly cut tea leaves. It is rich in a group of antioxidant polyphenols called catechins.

BLACK TEA
The dominant antioxidant polyphenols in black tea—theaflavins and thearubigins—have been shown to be as beneficial as those in green tea.

OOLONG TEA
Oolong is a semifermented sun-dried black tea rich in the antioxidant polyphenols called theaflavins.

WHITE TEA
Less bitter than green tea, white tea is minimally oxidized but contains similar catechins to green tea.

WHAT IS IT GOOD FOR?

IMMUNE SUPPORT Its powerful antioxidant catechins and theaflavins are antibacterial and antiviral. Studies show they can be effective against the flu virus and common causes of bacterial diarrhea. The catechins in green and oolong teas may also have antiallergy properties, and there is some evidence they can help reduce symptoms of eczema.

HEART Moderate consumption of black and green tea lowers "unhealthy" (LDL) cholesterol, reducing the risk of heart disease and stroke.

ANTICANCER A regular intake of green tea can protect against breast cancer, while tests suggest green and black tea help stop cancer cells from forming and will even kill bone, lung, stomach, and prostate cancer cells. The catechin epigallocatechin-3-gallate (EGCG) in green tea binds to certain carcinogens and helps remove them from the body.

HEALTHY BONES Consumption of green and black tea has been associated with higher bone mineral density in older adults, especially in the lumbar spine region.

ARTHRITIS Green tea polyphenols can prevent the breakdown of collagen and cartilage, so are a useful potential treatment for arthritis.

HOW DO I GET THE BEST FROM IT?

THE PERFECT CUP Use water that has boiled for no more than 10 seconds.

ORGANIC IS BEST Tea is treated with a vast number of pesticides. To avoid a toxic cup of tea, always choose organic.

HOW DO I USE IT?

DECAFFEINATE YOUR OWN TEA Pour boiling water on tea leaves. After 30 seconds discard the liquid to remove roughly 60 percent of the caffeine. Pour on more water and drink. (Waiting longer than 30 seconds destroys many vitamins and polyphenols, and much flavor.)

ROSE

 PROTECTS AGAINST BACTERIAL INFECTION

 HELPS EASE MENSTRUAL CRAMPS

 HAS NATURAL SEDATIVE PROPERTIES

 HELPS EASE JOINT PAIN

A member of the same family as plums, cherries, apricots, and almonds, rose has many of the same benefits. The petals contain volatile oils that help **calm nervous tension** and are **antibacterial**—useful for treating **urinary tract infections** and **digestive upsets**. They are also rich in vitamins C, D, E, and B$_3$, **beta-carotene**, and **antioxidants**, such as lycopene, lutein, and **anti-inflammatory** quercetin.

WHAT IS IT GOOD FOR?

ANTIBACTERIAL Its essential oils have proven antimicrobial properties.

WOMEN'S HEALTH The dried leaves and hips can be used to make an iron-rich tangy tea to make up for lost iron and as a tonic to soothe stomach cramps during menstruation.

STRESS Its scent has been proven to calm breathing and lower blood pressure, while its essential oils have a calming effect on frayed nerves and can lower feelings of anxiety.

ARTHRITIS Rosehips contain flavonoids, such as anthocyanins and quercetin, which have antioxidant properties. With their high vitamin C content, the hips can help decrease inflammation in arthritis and joint pain.

HEART Oil pressed from rosehip seeds is high in vitamin C and linoleic (omega-6) fatty acid and linolenic (omega-3) fatty acids. Eating hips from the *Rosa canina* (dog rose) for just 6 weeks helps reduce both blood pressure and "unhealthy" (LDL) cholesterol in the blood.

HOW DO I GET THE BEST FROM IT?

ORGANIC AND NATURAL Look for organic or wild-crafted sources to avoid a variety of toxic pesticides and fungicides. Choose 100-percent natural rosewater, steam-distilled from rose petals and preservative-free.

ROSEHIP OIL Heart-healthy rosehip oil can be consumed, but it is too delicate to heat. It should make up no more than 20 percent of the total oil content of a salad dressing.

HOW DO I USE IT?

MAKE A TEA For a calming, anti-inflammatory tea, steep rosehips and hibiscus flowers in equal amounts in boiling water for 5 minutes.

ROSEHIPS Can be eaten raw, though some may find the taste too tart so add to jams, jellies, syrups, fruit crisps, and pies.

ROSEHIPS
These fruits are full of vitamin C, and their seeds yield a healthy oil that can help treat inflammation.

DAMASCENA ROSE
The oil from this rose is traditionally used to calm and uplift the mind. It is anti-inflammatory, cooling, and soothing.

ROSEWATER
An extraction of the essential oils found in rose petals, rosewater retains the astringent, toning, soothing, and antiseptic properties of the whole plant.

DRIED ROSES
Rose tea is a traditional remedy for menstrual complaints.

Recipes That Heal

MANY FOODS WORK SYNERGISTICALLY TO BOOST **HEALTH** AND **VITALITY**. DISCOVER THE RIGHT COMBINATIONS WITH THESE **UNIQUE** RECIPES BASED ON THE PRINCIPLES OF TRADITIONAL **HEALING**. IF YOU ARE KEEN TO IMPROVE SPECIFIC HEALTH AREAS, TAKE **INSPIRATION** FROM THE SPECIALLY DESIGNED **A DAY OF...** EATING PLANS.

A Day Of... Heart Health

Many studies have shown that eating a healthy diet and increasing the amount of exercise you get can radically improve your heart health. These cholesterol-lowering recipes are packed with foods to improve your circulation and lower your blood pressure.

Cholesterol-busting Breakfast

Start your day with a steaming bowl of oatmeal, which is full of heart-healthy folate and potassium. This fiber-rich superfood can help lower levels of "unhealthy" (LDL) cholesterol and keep arteries clear. For the tastiest oatmeal, soak the oats in water first, and stir in some freshly grated apple while you cook the oats.

APPLE
Lowers "unhealthy" (LDL) cholesterol and is a source of vitamin C and heart-healthy antioxidants

PLAIN YOGURT
Yogurt is a natural source of calcium, and regular consumption can help prevent high blood pressure, and therefore, lower the risk of heart attack and stroke

OATMEAL
Cooking oats breaks down their phytate content, ensuring that you receive all the benefits of their nutrients

Omega-rich Lunch

Oily fish, such as sardines, are one of the most concentrated sources of the omega-3 fatty acids EPA and DHA, which help lower triglycerides and "unhealthy" (LDL) cholesterol levels.

TO PREPARE THE SARDINES

Mix together 1 tablespoon each of cooked and cooled short-grain rice, toasted pine nuts, and currants, a dash of lemon juice, and 1 teaspoon each of chopped parsley, mint, and dill. Divide among 6 whole, cleaned sardines, packing the stuffing inside each fish. Wrap a vine leaf around each fish to hold it together. Brush with olive oil and broil for 4–5 minutes, turning halfway through. Serve with lemon wedges.

SARDINES
Rich in numerous nutrients, including vitamins B_{12} and D, which have been found to support cardiovascular health

VINE LEAVES
A staple of heart-healthy Mediterranean cuisine; rich in vitamins and minerals

PINE NUTS
Contain an abundance of vitamins and minerals that help maintain normal metabolic functions

LEMON JUICE
Particularly high in magnesium, important for a healthy heart. Its pectin content and limonoid compounds also reduce cholesterol

PARSLEY
Particularly high in vitamin K for heart and circulatory health

HEART-PROTECTIVE DINNER

Dried beans are known to lower the risk of heart attack and strokes because
they help lower "unhealthy" (LDL) cholesterol levels in the blood and balance
blood sugar levels. Recent studies have also proven that shiitake mushrooms
can help protect against cardiovascular diseases.

SEE BEANS BAKED IN A PUMPKIN POT RECIPE *p253*

RED AND YELLOW BELL PEPPERS
Contain vitamins C, E,
and K for heart and
circulation health

SHIITAKE MUSHROOMS
Help keep blood vessels clear and
prevent oxidative stress

BUTTER/LIMA BEANS
Very good source of
cholesterol-
lowering fiber

GARLIC
Cardioprotective by
helping repair damage
to blood vessels

OLIVE OIL
Provides healthy
omega-3, -6, and -9
fatty acids

PUMPKIN
The carotenoids it contains
help to protect the
circulatory system

A Day Of... Good Digestion

In most cultures, good digestion is considered fundamental to general health. Try this plan of eating the right foods at the best time, using ingredients that boost digestive health. To encourage efficient absorption and elimination don't rush, and always chew your food thoroughly.

Balancing Breakfast

Breakfast is a good time to eat a balance of foods: fiber to keep your bowels regular; protein to sustain you; and carbohydrates to give you energy for the day ahead. Top this off with some antioxidant-rich fruit.

BERRIES
A delicious way to boost your vitamin and antioxidant intake

TOASTED FLAKES
Whole grain wheat flakes provide B vitamins and fiber for roughage. To make, toast whole grain flakes in an oven at 350°F (180°C) for 20 minutes, turning occasionally.

SUNFLOWER SEEDS
Good source of pantothenic acid, phosphorus, copper, and manganese

PUMPKIN SEEDS
Contain high levels of essential fatty acids and zinc

PLAIN YOGURT
A natural probiotic to keep gut flora healthy

FLAXSEEDS
Gentle bulk laxative that provides omega-3 and omega-6 fatty acids

Sustaining Lunch

Make lunch your main meal. Chicken provides a low-fat source of protein and assists healthy digestion; here it is rubbed with lime juice, grilled until cooked through, and served with a spicy sauce.

TO MAKE THE SAUCE

Sauté, in olive oil, crushed garlic, a thumb of grated fresh ginger, and chopped scallions and sweet potato, and a spice mix (turmeric, cumin, and coriander seeds) for 10 minutes. Cook until the vegetables are tender, then add 1¼ cups of stock and some lime juice. Purée in a blender.

CHICKEN
Rich in many nutrients including selenium and zinc

LIME JUICE
Excellent source of vitamin C, and can help relieve indigestion

SWEET POTATO
Easily digested source of carotenoids

CUMIN
Stimulates digestive enzymes

TURMERIC
Anti-inflammatory that helps prevent wind

EASILY DIGESTED DINNER

Soup can make an ideal light meal to enjoy in the evening. This carrot soup is easily digested, packed with nutrients, and you can make enough to last for a couple of days. In traditional Chinese medicine, cooked carrots are thought to improve digestion because they contain fiber, thus aiding bowel regularity. The fiber also promotes a feeling of fullness, which is good if you are trying to cut down on calories.

SEE CARROT AND COCONUT SOUP RECIPE *p213*

COCONUT
Helps fight off inflammation and unwanted bacteria

ONION
Provides a source of phytonutrients

CARROT
Easily digested source of carotenoids

CILANTRO
Promotes a healthy digestion

LIME
Source of vitamin C and a digestive tonic

A Day Of... Liver Health

The liver needs all the help it can get—it has the job of breaking down and eliminating every dietary and environmental toxin in our bodies. This 1-day plan will give you an idea of which foods can help stimulate the natural detoxifying processes in the liver and encourage regeneration.

Cleansing Breakfast

Grapefruit is an effective liver-cleansing and antioxidant-rich fruit. Combine it with a detoxifying, freshly juiced fruit and vegetable juice for an invigorating start to your day.

APPLE
Triterpenoids in the skin have potent protective activity for liver cells

CARROT
Its carotenoid content helps prevent oxidative damage inside the body

MINT
An herb with tonic and decongestant properties

GRAPEFRUIT
Contains enzymes that help the liver break down toxins more efficiently

LIVER-BOOSTING LUNCH

Cynarin, an active chemical constituent in globe artichokes, helps improve the proper functioning of both the liver and gallbladder—it causes increased bile flow and is an aid to digestion, making artichokes an ideal food to support the health of the liver.

LEMON
The ultimate liver-cleansing fruit, it is high in vitamin C and bioflavonoids

GLOBE ARTICHOKE
Contains bioactive phytonutrients for liver and gut health

OLIVE OIL
Stimulates activity in the liver, gallbladder, and bile duct

GARLIC
Activates liver enzymes that support detoxification

PARSLEY
A gently stimulating herb that encourages the elimination of toxins; also contains vitamins and minerals

TO MAKE THE HERB ARTICHOKES

Cut off each stalk but leave ¾in (2cm) at the top. Peel the remaining stalk, cutting away the tough exterior. Cut off the top of the cone and scoop out the hairy choke. Squeeze lemon juice into the cavity. Mix 2 chopped garlic cloves, 1 tablespoon of finely chopped mint, and a bunch of finely chopped flat-leaf parsley. Stuff the mix into the cavity. Simmer the artichokes in a pan of water on medium heat for 30 minutes, or until tender. Ensure they stay upright in the pan.

REGENERATIVE DINNER

In traditional Chinese medicine, the liver is strengthened by eating sour-flavored foods and cleansed by green leafy foods. This dish is bursting with ingredients that help the body eliminate toxic substances, clear blood vessels, and enhance bowel movement and urine output.

SEE MUNG BEAN AND BROCCOLI RABE RECIPE *p248*

GREEN MANGO
Its sweet-sour flavor increases liver and gallbladder function

MUNG BEAN SPROUTS
Abundant in minerals and fiber, which are essential for detoxing

CARROTS
Contain antioxidants renowned to enliven the liver

LIME
Source of healing vitamin C and liver tonic

BROCCOLI RABE
Contains sulfur compounds that support the liver's ability to detoxify chemicals in the body

BELGIAN ENDIVE
Traditionally used to cool and cleanse the liver

A DAY OF... SKIN HEALTH

Choosing foods that are packed with the vitamins and minerals your skin needs will, over time, actively nourish your skin and dramatically boost its appearance. Start with this day of delicious meals and build from there, selecting skin-friendly foods and turning them into tasty recipes.

COLLAGEN-BOOSTING BREAKFAST

Eggs are powerhouses of nutrients that are beneficial for the skin. They include collagen-building protein, vitamin A, omega fatty acids, and carotenoids to protect against UV aging. Cook scrambled eggs with chopped fresh herbs to add valuable antioxidants.

CHIVES
Contain detoxifying sulfur and anti-inflammatory quercetin

TURMERIC
Excellent antioxidant properties to prevent free-radical damage

EGGS
Choline and lutein help promote skin elasticity and prevent wrinkles

MARJORAM
Popular Mediterranean herb with antiseptic and anti-inflammatory properties

OMEGA-RICH LUNCH

Oil-rich coldwater fish, such as salmon, are a real superfood when it comes to skin health: their anti-inflammatory properties help to improve dry skin and relieve eczema and psoriasis. Serving baked salmon in a salad with a yogurt dressing is a great way of getting many of the nutrients your skin needs.

TO MAKE THE SALAD DRESSING

Mix together the juice of 1 orange and ½ tablespoon each of chopped hazelnuts, sherry vinegar, plain yogurt, and hazelnut oil.

PLAIN YOGURT
Contains protein and zinc for skin health

HAZELNUTS
Good source of vitamins and minerals for healthy hair, skin, and nails

SALMON
Contains omega oils to keep skin elastic and prevent wrinkles

LAMB'S LETTUCE
Its antioxidants prevent free-radical damage

RADIANCE-BOOSTING DINNER

Eating fresh, young green vegetables regularly is a good way to cleanse the body and keep the complexion clear. Include asparagus because it stimulates the digestion by acting as a prebiotic and contains compounds that have an anti-inflammatory effect and help to prevent the signs of aging.

SEE STIR-FRIED SPRING VEGETABLES RECIPE *p259*

OLIVE OIL
High in polyphenols, known to help postpone aging and boost cell repair......

ASPARAGUS
A storehouse of vitamins and minerals that can benefit the skin...

SNOW PEAS
Good source of vitamins ...A and C for skin health

SPINACH...
Rich in iron and antioxidants, which have anti-inflammatory effects

WILD GARLIC...
Contains sulfur compounds to keep skin blemish-free

A Day Of... Healthy Joints

To reduce the inflammation and pain associated with arthritis and joint problems, switch to a diet that contains foods known to reduce inflammation and cleansing foods, which help remove the toxins that aggravate the problem. Sample this 1-day plan to learn which foods to incorporate into your diet.

Easy-mover Breakfast

Fruit is a source of antioxidants that helps rid the body of cell-damaging free radicals and suppresses inflammation (avoid oranges because they may make some arthritis pain worse). Apple (fresh or dried) is particularly good for joint problems, but keep its skin on—this is what contains many of the best nutrients. Serve with buckwheat grains, toasted in a moderate oven until golden, and plain yogurt.

PLAIN YOGURT
Provides calcium for healthy bones and joints

APPLES
Contain inflammation-fighting antioxidants. Use dried apple rings for extra flavor

DRIED CRANBERRIES
Contain vitamin C to help reduce pain and inflammation

BUCKWHEAT
A highly nutritious, gluten-free grain. Contains quercetin, which has anti-inflammatory properties

DRIED APRICOTS
Good source of anthocyanidins

JOINT-HEALTH LUNCH

Coldwater salmon, tuna, herring, mackerel, and halibut contain omega-3 fatty acids, which are potently anti-inflammatory. Bake in the oven until cooked through and serve cold with an apple cider vinegar dressing.

TO MAKE THE DRESSING

A yogurt-based apple cider vinegar dressing is a great accompaniment to baked salmon. Mix together 2 tablespoons each of apple cider vinegar and finely chopped mint, and ¼ cup Greek yogurt. Drizzle over the cold salmon.

LEMON
A source of vitamin C and bioflavonoids, and can help reduce inflammation

DILL
Good source of calcium to help reduce bone loss, and antioxidants

SALMON
High in protein to help build healthy connective tissue, and in anti-inflammatory omega-3 fatty acids

CUCUMBER
May improve inflamed joints because it helps eliminate uric acid and contains vitamin C

APPLE CIDER VINEGAR
Traditionally used to alkalize the body and relieve the pain of arthritis

ANTI-INFLAMMATORY DINNER

This soup is packed with the powerful anti-inflammatory properties of turmeric and so can help relieve swelling and pain including rheumatic and arthritic pain. Use either dried turmeric or fresh turmeric in your recipes.

SEE PUY LENTIL SOUP WITH FRESH TURMERIC RECIPE *p212*

DRINK

Apple cider vinegar mixed with honey is a traditional remedy for arthritis because the overall effect of apple cider vinegar and honey is alkalizing. To make, add 2 teaspoons each of honey and unpasteurized apple cider vinegar to a glassful of lukewarm water. Drink 2 or 3 times a day before meals.

PUY LENTILS
Vegetarian source of collagen-building protein

TURMERIC
Contains curcumin, a potent anti-inflammatory

GINGER
Zingibain suppresses substances that trigger pain and cause tissues to swell

ONIONS
Source of quercetin, which reduces inflammation

CILANTRO
Source of vitamins A, C, and K for healthy bones and joints

A Day Of... Boosted Energy

Great energy comes from a good balance of rest, exercise, and eating foods that are packed with nutrients to strengthen reserves and provide vitality. This 1-day plan provides an introduction to some of the foods that are known to act as a tonic for the body.

Power Breakfast

Quail eggs are renowned in China for invigorating and strengthening the body. They are a rich source of protein, iron, potassium, and B vitamins, and taste delicious scrambled with lightly fried chopped tomatoes.

TOMATOES
A superfood containing antioxidants, such as lycopene and vitamin C

PARSLEY
Contains energy-promoting iron and vitamins A, C, and K

QUAIL EGGS
Packed with 3–4 times the energy-boosting nutrients of the egg of a chicken

BLACK PEPPER
Volatile oils stimulate digestion to promote the absorption of all nutrients from food

RYE BREAD
A rich source of magnesium, promoting enzymes involved in the body's use of glucose and insulin secretion

Vitality Lunch

Asparagus is packed with energy-promoting nutrients. Stir-fry with other vegetables, such as immune-boosting broccoli and carrots, adding the ones that need the most cooking to the wok first. Combine with protein-rich shrimp and cleansing, anti-inflammatory fresh ginger for an easy yet revitalizing feast.

RED BELL PEPPER
A gently stimulating vegetable full of essential nutrients

SHRIMP
A warming, nourishing food high in protein and carotenoids, such as astaxanthin

CHIVES
A simple way to add stimulating qualities to a dish, chives also promote a healthy appetite

ASPARAGUS
A source of the essential energy nutrients potassium and B vitamins

BROCCOLI
Enhances detoxification, which helps enhance energy

CARROTS
Root vegetables help boost reserves of energy and are a source of beta-carotene

ENERGY-SUSTAINING DINNER

To support long-term energy, eat a light cooked meal in the evening. Squab is tasty, tender, and nutritious, and is regarded as an excellent kidney and energy tonic. Goji berries are added to give a metabolic boost.

SEE SQUAB BREASTS WITH GOJI BERRIES RECIPE *p260*

SQUAB
Excellent source of
iron and B vitamins
for energy

CHILE
Stimulating to taste buds
and improves energy levels

ONION
A warming and
nourishing source
of phytonutrients to
boost good health

**SHIITAKE
MUSHROOMS**
Considered a good
general tonic that boosts
various body systems

GOJI BERRIES
A superfood packed
with essential nutrients

CARROTS
Good source of slow-
release energy

A Day Of... Stress Relief

Traditionally, many foods have been known to support the nervous system during times of stress. Today we understand that in fact these foods have an effect on neurotransmitters in the body, such as the hormone serotonin, which is why they generate a "feel-good" factor.

Positive Breakfast

Eating a healthy breakfast can set the scene for a positive attitude through the day and sustained energy levels. This combination of granola, fresh fruits, and honey provides many nutrients to support the sense of well-being.

TO MAKE THE GRANOLA

On an oiled baking sheet, drizzle rolled oats with honey. Toast in the oven at 350°F (180°C) until golden. Remove and let cool. Mix with ingredients, such as pine nuts, pumpkin seeds, dried fruits, corn flakes, and bran flakes, to taste.

ROLLED OATS
A traditional remedy to support a stressed nervous system

BANANA
Contains potassium to regulate nerve function

PUMPKIN SEEDS
Full of stress-busting magnesium, B vitamins, and serotonin

GOLDEN RAISINS
Good source of energy, vitamins, minerals, and antioxidants

HONEY
A sweet source of antioxidants to protect cells from oxidative damage

STRESS-BUSTING LUNCH

Sustain your body and mind with foods packed with the nutrients you need to fight stress, such as this fish soup, full of B vitamins, magnesium, and phytonutrient-rich herbs and spices.

TO MAKE THE SOUP

Fry 1 chopped onion in olive oil over medium heat until soft. Add 1 crushed garlic clove and 1 finely chopped fennel bulb, and cook until the fennel softens. Stir in 1 minced red chile, a splash of white wine, a 14oz can of tomatoes, 3 cups hot fish stock, and a pinch of saffron. Bring to a boil, then reduce to a simmer for 45 minutes. Purée to a smooth soup. Pour into a clean saucepan and add 1¼ cups hot water. Simmer gently. Add 7oz (200g) cubed monkfish and haddock loin and cook over low heat for 6–10 minutes.

MONKFISH
An excellent source of B vitamins, important for alleviating stress

CHILE
A warming, stimulating source of nutrients for optimal health

TOMATOES
Source of carotenoids and potassium, for good nerve health

HADDOCK
Rich in magnesium, the antistress mineral

FENNEL
Strong antioxidant that contains cell-protective components

SAFFRON
Used in herbal medicine for its antidepressant properties

RECOVERY DINNER

Shiitake mushrooms are renowned for being adaptogenic, which means they help the body recover quickly from all kinds of stress. Marinated tofu, which is made from soybeans, is easy to digest.

SEE MARINATED TOFU WITH SHIITAKE AND NOODLES RECIPE *p258*

SESAME SEEDS
Rich in beneficial minerals

SHIITAKE MUSHROOMS
Potent phytonutrients increase resistance to stress and fatigue

SNOW PEAS
Its B vitamins help produce the hormones necessary to fight stress

TOFU
A good source of tryptophan for stress relief and better sleep

MUNG BEAN SPROUTS
Contain B vitamins and magnesium to manage stress symptoms

A Day Of... Men's Health

To enhance men's health, choose foods that improve vitality, support the body's energy levels, and are good for the heart and circulation. Men also benefit from a diet rich in antioxidants, essential fatty acids, strengthening minerals, and protein. Try this menu for a day of health-boosting benefits.

Fuel-up Breakfast

Start the day with a combination of fresh fruit, seeds, and yogurt—good for your vitamin and mineral intake—or try buckwheat pancakes or oatmeal with fresh fruit. Other suitable options for breakfast are eggs or fish.

PUMPKIN SEEDS
An excellent source of zinc—essential for reproductive system and prostate health

BLUEBERRIES
An immune-boosting superfood packed with antioxidants for the prevention of cancer

SUNFLOWER SEEDS
A rich source of omega oils and B vitamins for both heart and brain health

PLAIN YOGURT
Good source of calcium, and enhances gut health

Active-life Lunch

Coldwater oily fish, such as salmon, mackerel, and herring, are rich in omega-3 and other essential fatty acids good for heart and brain health and for keeping joints flexible. Mix cured or pickled herring with cooked root vegetables, such as potato (capable of building reserves of energy) and beets (particularly good for the heart and circulation).

TO MAKE THE DRESSING

Mix ⅔ cup of mayonnaise, 1 tablespoon of creamed horseradish, and 1–2 teaspoons of Dijon mustard with lemon juice.

HERRING
A very good source of protein, vitamin B_{12}, selenium for longevity, and EPA and DHA

BEETS
Highly nutritious source of magnesium, iron, and betaine for cardiovascular health

POTATOES
Good source of fiber, and rich in vitamins C and B_6 and potassium

ONIONS
Phytochemical compounds allium and allyl disulfide have anticancer and blood-sugar-regulating properties, while quercetin helps prevent heart disease

HORSERADISH
Naturally antibiotic and anticatarrhal herb with decongestant properties

PROTEIN-PACKED DINNER

Quinoa provides important protein with essential amino acids and helps build muscle, while tomatoes contain lycopene, which aids healthy circulation. The addition of strength-building walnuts makes this a great meal for active men.

SEE SAVOY CABBAGE PARCELS RECIPE *p265*

CABBAGE
Good source of detoxifying and anticancer compounds

TOMATOES
Great source of lycopene for heart health

QUINOA
One of the best cereal-sources of protein

WALNUTS
Renowned in China for improving men's health and stamina

CRANBERRIES
Contain proanthocyanidins, which help cells resist bacterial infection

A Day Of... Women's Health

It's much easier to cope with the demands of modern life if you eat healthy meals that boost your energy levels and sense of well-being. Here are foods that are particularly suitable for women's health, and known for their anticancer, antistress, nourishing, and balancing benefits.

Balancing Breakfast

Choose a breakfast of ingredients that are full of essential nutrients, such as iron, calcium, and the antioxidant vitamin C. Eating plenty of soluble fiber-rich dried fruits, such as prunes and apricots, will also help balance blood sugar levels and prevent constipation.

PLAIN YOGURT
Contains probiotics for gut health and calcium for bones

ORANGE
Excellent source of vitamin C and bioflavonoids to support the circulation

APRICOTS
Rich in fiber, vitamin A, carotenoids, and iron to to promote better digestion, improve eyesight, and build red blood cells

PRUNES
Source of fiber and antioxidant phytonutrients

Hormone-protective Lunch

Research has confirmed watercress as a true superfood. It contains an abundance of phytonutrients including substances renowned for their anticancer properties, and also iron and vitamin K to help prevent osteoporosis. Try this light yet filling watercress soup.

ONION
Its phytochemical compounds contribute to healthy skin and help prevent infections

WATERCRESS
Contains gluconasturtin with potent cancer-inhibiting properties

PEARS
Low in calories and high in dietary fiber and antioxidants

CRÈME FRAÎCHE
Good source of calcium for bone health

OLIVE OIL
Mediterranean diet staple containing omega-3, -6, and -9 fatty acids

HOW TO MAKE THE SOUP

Fry 1 onion in butter until soft, stirring to prevent burning. Add the stalks of a large bunch of watercress, 3 chopped pears, and 3½ cups vegetable stock and season. Simmer for 15 minutes. Remove from the heat, add the watercress leaves, and purée. Add 1 cup crème fraîche and the juice of ½ lemon. Garnish with Parmesan to serve.

IMMUNITY-ENHANCING DINNER

Chicken is particularly suitable for women in terms of nourishment and rejuvenation because it has immune-boosting properties and high B vitamin levels to help the body produce energy. Eat with stress-reducing potatoes and salad.

SEE GINGER CHICKEN RECIPE *p261*

CHICKEN
Low-fat protein and selenium for metabolic and thyroid health

GARLIC
Contains compounds to protect the heart and prevent infection

LIME
Excellent source of vitamin C

HONEY
This antioxidant-rich elixir protects heart and waistline

GINGER
Improves digestion and protects against aging

POTATOES
Source of vitamins B and C to protect against stress

A DAY OF... HEALTHY PREGNANCY

While you are pregnant, eat foods that are packed with as much nourishment as possible for you and for your growing baby. It is particularly important to concentrate on foods that contain abundant minerals, such as calcium and iron. Consume as few additives as possible, so eat organic if you can.

DIGESTION-FRIENDLY BREAKFAST

Ease yourself into the day with foods that are nourishing and easily digested. This smoothie of fresh fruits, crushed flaxseeds, and orange juice is the perfect choice. Eggs are also a good breakfast option.

APRICOTS
Good source of fiber, iron, and antioxidants

PAPAYA
Contains enzymes that assist the digestive system

ORANGE JUICE
Rich in vitamin C and bioflavonoids to help prevent varicose veins

FLAXSEEDS
Help prevent constipation and a good source of omega-3 fatty acids

OAT CRACKERS
A slow-release carbohydrate to balance blood sugar levels, and easily digested

NUTRITIOUS LUNCH

Lunch is a good time to have a protein-rich meal to benefit you and your baby. Chicken contains B vitamins that help the body cope with stress, release energy, and form DNA. This lunch includes chicken shaken in a spicy toasted coconut mix, stir-fried, and served with a tropical salad.

TO MAKE THE SALAD

Put 2 tablespoons of toasted coconut, 1 teaspoon each of ground ginger and cinnamon, a pinch of ground nutmeg, and zest of ½ lemon in a food bag. Seal and shake to mix. Add 1 chicken breast cut into strips. Season and shake well to coat the chicken. Stir-fry the coated chicken for 3–4 minutes in olive oil. Mix with the salad ingredients and add lemon juice.

GINGER
One of nature's best antinausea remedies, ginger also stimulates digestion

AVOCADO
Rich source of omega fatty acids, vitamin K, and fiber

COCONUT
Contains manganese and healthy essential fatty acids

ARUGULA
Source of folate and antioxidant phytonutrients

CHICKEN
Source of protein and tryptophan to help the body cope with stress

MANGO
Prebiotic qualities, plus fiber, vitamins B$_6$, and C

SUSTAINING DINNER

Sweet potatoes are both nourishing and easy to digest, making them a great food to eat in the evening. They are combined here with eggplant and sweet bell peppers—all good sources of phytonutrients known to be beneficial for the healthy development of new cells.

SEE VEGETABLE MOUSSAKA RECIPE *p278*

EGGPLANT
Anthocyanins in the skin of the eggplant help brain cell development

CHEESE
Good source of calcium to build strong bones and teeth, and for muscle and nerve function

RED BELL PEPPERS
Contains carotenoids for healthy heart and eyes

SWEET POTATO
Contains nutrients that act as antioxidants, and are anti-inflammatory and blood-sugar regulating

ZUCCHINI
Source of B vitamins including folate

RECIPE CHOOSER

◉ HEART AND CIRCULATION

Mushroom Frittata with Cherry Tomatoes and Basil p236

Spicy Raw Vegetable Spaghetti p246

URINARY

RESPIRATORY

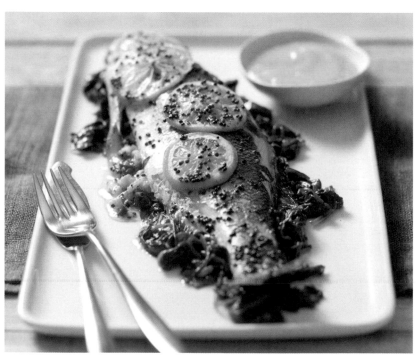

Sea Bass with Spinach and Mango p250

DETOX

Quail Egg and Endive Salad p224

METABOLIC BALANCE

Chanterelles and Chiles with Pasta p267

Cherry Strudel p293

⊜) IMMUNE SUPPORT

⚡ ENERGY BOOST

Butternut Squash Soup p219

MUSCLES AND JOINTS

SNACKS

Butternut Squash and Walnut Bites p200

Mushroom and Chestnut Bites p202

SOUPS

Puy Lentil Soup with Fresh Turmeric p212

Carrot and Coconut Soup p213

Sweet Potato and Celeriac Soup p216

LIGHT MEALS AND SALADS

Mushroom Frittata with Cherry Tomatoes and Basil p236

MAIN MEALS

Savoy Cabbage Parcels p265

Broiled Mackerel with Chard p275

Grilled Sardines with Tomato Salsa p276

Barlotto with Chestnut Purée p281

SWEET TREATS

Nutty Sugar Loaf p289

Cherry Strudel p293

Baked Quince p294

Sesame Heart Cookies p299

DRINKS

Barley Grass and Barley Lemonade p306

Sour Cherry Drink p308

Deep Cleansing Tea p322

OILS, DRESSINGS, AND EXTRAS

Flatbread with Sweet Potato and Coriander p327

Sourdough Rye Bread p328

SKIN AND HAIR

BREAKFASTS

Feta and Oregano Squares p180

Almond Porridge with Apricots p188

SNACKS

Sprouted Medley p204

Tomato Crackers p205

SOUPS

Carrot and Coconut Soup p213

LIGHT MEALS AND SALADS

Spinach and Ricotta Filo Rolls p230

Buckwheat Pancakes with Nettles and Feta Cheese p238

Artichokes in a Sweet Spicy Sauce p239

MAIN MEALS

Spicy Raw Vegetable Spaghetti p246

Chanterelles and Chiles with Pasta p267

SWEET TREATS

Sesame Heart Cookies p299

DRINKS

Five-Flavor Juice p312

Marshmallow and Licorice Tea p320

Deep Cleansing Tea p322

Deep Nurture Tea p322

OILS, DRESSINGS, AND EXTRAS

Sourdough Rye Bread p328

Rose and Fennel Seed Oil p333

Rose and Raspberry Vinegar p334

Blackberry Vinegar p334

MIND AND EMOTIONS

BREAKFASTS

Poached Eggs and Spinach p182

Quail Eggs on Rye Bread p184

Kefir Cheese with Flaxseed and Berries p184

Baked Oatmeal with Goji Berries and Cinnamon p187

Sweet Saffron Rice With Cardamom p191

SNACKS

Butternut Squash and Walnut Bites p200

Mushroom and Chestnut Bites p202

Spicy Crackers p207

SOUPS

Raw Tomato Soup p210

Quail Soup p217

Butternut Squash Soup p219

LIGHT MEALS AND SALADS

Nori Vegetable Roll p234

Fresh Cilantro Leaf Pesto with Pasta p241

Braised Red Chicory and Celery Heart Salad p243

MAIN MEALS

Vegetable Hot Pot p256

Sauerkraut Parcels p264

Savoy Cabbage Parcels p265

Grilled Sardines with Tomato Salsa p276

Fragrant Rice and Millet p283

SWEET TREATS

Fresh Fig Delight with Pear and Red Wine Sauce p285

Almond and Raspberry Cake p286

Nutty Sugar Loaf p289

Warm Fruit Salad in Sweet Wine Sauce p290

Cherry Strudel p293

Rose Petal and White Wine Sorbet p295

Mediterranean Nut Squares in Rose and Cardamom Syrup p298

Almond and Pistachio Macaroons p300

Poppy Seed and Walnut Roulade p302

Dried Fruit and Nut Roll p303

DRINKS

Sour Cherry Drink p308

Alert and Joyful Juice p313

Valentine's Special p315

Rose Syrup p315

A Cup of Happiness p317

Mint and Friends Tea p318

Marshmallow and Licorice Tea p320

Deep Sleep Tea p321

Astragalus and Schisandra Broth p324

Seaweed and Miso Broth p325

Venison Casserole with Cranberries p270

Blackberry Lemonade p306

BREAKFASTS

DON'T SKIMP ON THE MOST **IMPORTANT MEAL** OF THE DAY. FRESH FRUIT, WHOLE GRAINS, AND HIGH-QUALITY PROTEIN SET THE TONE FOR YOUR DAY WITH **BALANCING AND SUSTAINING** MEALS THAT FEED YOUR **BODY AND MIND**.

BUCKWHEAT AND BLACKBERRY CREAM

 PROTECTS THE HEART AND BLOOD VESSELS

 CONTAINS SLOW-RELEASE SUGARS

 HELPS ALLEVIATE HEAVY PERIODS

 EASY TO DIGEST AND GLUTEN-FREE

This is a quick, antioxidant-rich porridge recipe. Both blackberries and roasted buckwheat help strengthen the heart, lower cholesterol, and have hemostatic properties, meaning that they help reduce the flow of blood. This makes it a good choice for women who suffer from heavy bleeding during menstruation. It can also be beneficial for men with prostate discharge.

SERVES 4

½ cup buckwheat grains
3½ cups almond milk
a large pinch of salt
4 tsp vanilla extract
2¾ cups blackberries

1 To toast the buckwheat, preheat the oven to 350°F (180°C). Spread the buckwheat grains thinly over some baking sheets and toast in the oven until they are golden. Shake the baking sheets occasionally to stop the grains from burning. Remove from the oven.

2 Place a handful of roasted buckwheat in a coffee grinder or a powerful food processor or blender, and grind into a fine meal. Repeat with the rest of the roasted buckwheat. Pour the almond milk into a small saucepan and heat it gently over low heat. Spoon in the buckwheat, add the salt and vanilla extract, and whisk thoroughly until the mixture is smooth. Cook for 5 minutes, adding more almond milk, if necessary, until you achieve the consistency you prefer.

3 Meanwhile, place the blackberries in the clean food processor or blender and purée to a smooth sauce.

4 Remove the pan from the heat and pour the buckwheat cream into 4 serving bowls. Pour the blackberry sauce on top and serve.

Blackberries (p30) need to be fresh, because nutrients can deteriorate with age. They contain salicylic acid, which helps protect against heart disease.

BUCKWHEAT PANCAKES WITH FRESH BERRY SAUCE

 HELPS KEEP BLOOD VESSELS SUPPLE

 PROMOTES A HEALTHY DIGESTIVE TRACT

 PROTECTS AGAINST FREE-RADICAL DAMAGE

This antioxidant-rich breakfast dish is heart-healthy and full of beneficial fiber, and contains warming cinnamon, which has antiseptic properties. For the maximum nutrients, why not grind your own flour (see Tip below); use either raw buckwheat or roasted buckwheat grains. Raspberries, cranberries, and blueberries are ideal, either on their own or in combination.

SERVES 4–6

1¼ cups fresh berries, such as raspberries, cranberries, and blueberries

1¾ cups organic buckwheat flour

1 tsp baking powder

¼ tsp rou gui (Chinese cinnamon bark) or ½ tsp ground cinnamon

a pinch of salt

1¼ cups rice milk (or milk if dairy is not an issue)

1 large egg

1–2 tbsp ghee

3 tbsp maple syrup, to serve

1 Place the fresh berries in a food processor or blender, and purée until smooth (avoid puréeing blueberries, if using, because their flavor is lost when blended with other berries). If you want the sauce to be free from seeds, strain it through a fine sieve. Set the sauce aside while you make the pancakes.

2 Mix together the buckwheat flour, baking powder, rou gui or cinnamon, and salt in a mixing bowl. In another bowl, whisk together the rice milk and egg. Gradually pour the egg mixture into the dry ingredients, whisking constantly as you do so, to form a smooth batter.

3 Heat a skillet, brush the base and sides with a knob of ghee, then ladle a little of the pancake mixture into the pan to make a thin pancake. Fry for 2–3 minutes, then toss or turn the pancake and cook it on the other side. Keep the cooked pancakes hot by stacking them on a plate set over a bowl of very hot water while you repeat with the rest of the batter.

4 Stir the blueberries, if using, into the berry sauce. Drizzle the pancakes with maple syrup and serve with the berry sauce.

TIP: Grinding your own flour is always a healthier choice because once the grains are crushed, their nutrients begin to deteriorate quickly. As a result, whole grains have a much longer shelf life than ready-milled flour, which may already be up to 1 year old by the time you buy it. Buckwheat is a soft grain (it has had the hull, or bran, already removed), so it is easy to turn into flour. Simply grind a few handfuls of grain at a time in a coffee grinder (or use a powerful food processor or blender).

Cassia bark or "rou gui" (Cinnamon cassia or Cortex Cinnamoni) is a pungent variety of Chinese cinnamon, with properties similar to culinary cinnamon (Cinnamon zeylanicum).

Feta And Oregano Squares

 INVIGORATES THE BODY   **LUBRICATES THE INTESTINES**   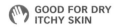 **GOOD FOR DRY ITCHY SKIN**

These individual savory filled breads are a great centerpiece for breakfast or brunch. Salty feta cheese and black sesame seeds supply sustained energy and help lubricate the gut, improving digestion. Sesame seeds are especially beneficial for dry, itchy skin. The addition of a little oregano helps stimulate appetite. They are best served warm.

MAKES 12

¾oz (20g) fresh yeast

1 tbsp sugar

¼ cup olive oil, plus extra for frying

¾ cup plain yogurt

3 cups all-purpose flour, plus extra for dusting

1 tsp salt

oil, for greasing

For the filling

7oz (200g) feta cheese, crumbled

1 large egg, beaten

1 tsp dried oregano

1 tbsp black sesame seeds

1 Dissolve the fresh yeast in ¾ cup of warm water along with the sugar. Once it has dissolved, add the olive oil and yogurt and stir.

2 In a large bowl, sift the flour and salt together and create a well in the center. Add the yeasty liquid slowly, gently stirring it with a wooden spoon as you pour to gradually incorporate the flour.

3 Turn the dough out onto a lightly floured surfaced and knead gently. Place the dough back in the bowl and cover with a clean cloth. Set the bowl aside in a warm place for the dough to rise until it is doubled in size, about 1 hour.

4 To make the filling, put the feta cheese in a bowl. Add the egg, oregano, and black sesame seeds and combine well.

5 Punch the dough down, knead again, and divide into 12 equal pieces. Take a piece of dough and, on a lightly floured surface, roll it out thinly. Spread 1 teaspoonful of the feta cheese filling over it.

6 To fold the flattened dough into a square, pick up the edge nearest to you and fold it over into the center. Then fold the opposite edge into the center to align with the first fold and create a rectangular shape. Fold over the left and right sides in the same way so they meet in the center, then fold the dough in half to make a square. Roll the rolling pin gently over the square parcel to flatten it and encourage the layers of dough to stick together.

7 Repeat with the remaining pieces of dough and using the rest of the filling until you have 12 squares. Put the squares on a greased tray, cover, and set aside for 15–20 minutes in a warm place to let the dough rise again.

8 Heat a little olive oil in a skillet over medium heat and fry each square for 2–3 minutes on each side until golden. Remove from the skillet and place on paper towels to absorb any excess oil. Serve warm.

BLACKCURRANT SMOOTHIE

 AIDS HEALTHY DIGESTION

 HELPS COMBAT FATIGUE

 HELPS STRENGTHEN THE IMMUNE SYSTEM

PROTECTS THE HEART AND BLOOD VESSELS

The high levels of vitamin C and antioxidants in blackcurrants make them a useful food to eat if you have intestinal problems, a buildup of toxins or fats in the blood and liver, or if you feel tired and run down. Flaxseeds, hemp, and chia seeds, which are full of omega-3 fatty acids and soluble fiber, support intestinal health, too, and help address issues related to cardiovascular health.

SERVES 2

1 tbsp flaxseeds
2 cups blackcurrants
2 tbsp hemp seeds
1 tbsp chia seeds
1 tsp clear honey

1 Place the flaxseeds in a blender or food processor and pulse briefly to a coarse powder.

2 Add the fresh blackcurrants, the hemp and chia seeds, and the honey and purée all the ingredients to a smooth paste. Stir in enough water to achieve the consistency you prefer. Pour the smoothie into 2 tall glasses and serve immediately.

Blackcurrants (p31) help to strengthen the immune system because of their vitamin C content.

POACHED EGGS AND SPINACH

 BOOSTS IRON STORES TO COMBAT FATIGUE   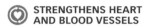 **STRENGTHENS HEART AND BLOOD VESSELS**   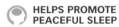 **HELPS PROMOTE PEACEFUL SLEEP**

Organic, freerange eggs are high-quality foods that, when prepared correctly by poaching or soft-boiling, provide complete nutrition. Traditionally, egg yolks are considered nourishing to the liver, heart, and kidneys, and are known to contain antioxidant amino acids that protect against heart disease. They can also help combat anemia, diarrhea or constipation, and even insomnia.

SERVES 4

1 tbsp olive oil

4 shallots, finely chopped

1 chile, seeded and minced

1 tsp ground turmeric

2 garlic cloves, crushed

¼ cup coconut cream

7oz (200g) spinach, chopped

salt and freshly ground black pepper

1 tbsp white wine vinegar

4 chicken or duck eggs

4 slices of whole wheat toast, or some cooked millet, to serve

a bunch of cilantro leaves, finely chopped, to garnish (optional)

1 Heat a tablespoon of water with the olive oil in a small saucepan over low heat. Add the shallots and chile, and cook until the vegetables are soft. Stir in the turmeric, then add the garlic and coconut cream. Cook until the coconut cream is heated through, and then add the spinach. Stir the mixture until the spinach wilts then remove from the heat. Add a pinch of salt and sprinkle with black pepper.

2 Heat a wide, shallow pan filled with water until tiny bubbles appear on the bottom (don't allow the water to boil before adding the eggs). Add the vinegar to the water to help keep the egg protein from disintegrating (the acid in the vinegar acts as a coagulant). Give the water a few swirls with a spoon, which will keep the eggs in the center of the pan. Crack each egg into a small plate or ramekin and slide into the water, just below the surface. The egg will sink to the bottom and rise as it cooks. Poach the eggs for about 3 minutes.

3 Place a piece of whole wheat toast on each plate, or fill a cook's ring with a ¾in (2cm) layer of cooked millet, and spoon some of the spinach on top. Remove the ring, if using. Place a poached egg on top of each stack and scatter with cilantro leaves, if using. Season with a little black pepper and serve immediately.

Duck eggs (p143) are traditionally believed to have a cooling, anti-inflammatory effect on the lungs, which makes them useful for asthma, dry coughs, and sore throat.

Quail Eggs On Rye Bread

 HELPS MAINTAIN ENERGY LEVELS   **PROMOTES A SENSE OF WELL-BEING**

As a hearty breakfast or brunch on cold winter mornings, this recipe is ideal. Quail eggs, which are considered to be an energizing food in traditional Chinese medicine, are combined here with bell peppers, chile, garlic, and chives, which have warming properties. This dish is particularly beneficial if you need to regain your strength after a prolonged illness, surgery, or childbirth.

SERVES 4–6

2 tbsp olive oil

1 small onion, finely chopped

½ red chile, minced

1 large yellow bell pepper, seeded, skinned (optional), and finely chopped

2 large tomatoes, skinned (optional), and finely chopped

1 garlic clove, crushed

salt and freshly ground black pepper

6 slices of rye bread

1 tbsp ghee, or clarified butter

6 quail eggs

1 tbsp chopped chives

1 Heat the olive oil in a medium saucepan over medium heat and sauté the onion and chile for 2–3 minutes, or until the onions soften. Add the yellow pepper and continue stirring for 2–3 minutes, then add the tomatoes, crushed garlic, and 2 tablespoons water. Cook over low heat until the mixture thickens. Remove from the heat and season with salt and black pepper.

2 Meanwhile, toast the rye bread and heat the ghee in a medium skillet. Break the eggs into the pan and fry them, removing them as soon as the whites are cooked and while the egg yolks are still soft.

3 Divide the slices of toast between 4 or 6 hot serving plates. Top each slice of toast with a spoonful of sautéed vegetables and an egg. Garnish with the chopped chives, and serve while hot.

Kefir Cheese With Flaxseed And Berries

 HELPS FIGHT INFLAMMATION   **HELPS IMPROVE CIRCULATION**   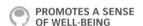 **PROMOTES A SENSE OF WELL-BEING**

This pairing of high-quality dairy produce and anti-inflammatory, omega-3-rich flaxseed oil is a twist on a healing regimen, the Budwig Diet, which helps to counter the effects of modern diets that are high in unhealthy fats. The diet has been used to treat and help prevent heart disease, diabetes, arthritis, and even cancer. The probiotic kefir cheese also helps to boost immunity.

SERVES 2

¼ cup flaxseeds

heaped ⅓ cup organic kefir cheese (p332), or use quark or cottage cheese

⅓ cup flaxseed oil

about 1⅔ cups soft berries

1 Place the flaxseeds in a food processor or blender and pulse briefly to crush them roughly.

2 Add the kefir cheese and flaxseed oil to the food processor and pulse again until combined. Transfer the mixture to 2 serving bowls.

3 Add the berries to the food processor and purée until smooth. Spoon the berry sauce onto the kefir cheese mixture in the bowls, and serve.

MILLET AND QUINOA PORRIDGE WITH PLUM COMPOTE

 PROMOTES BOWEL REGULARITY　　 **PROMOTES METABOLIC BALANCE**　　 **SUPPORTS HEALTHY LIVER FUNCTION**　　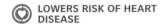 **LOWERS RISK OF HEART DISEASE**

Plums are often used in the treatment of diabetes and liver conditions—and stewed plums also help relieve constipation—while millet and quinoa benefit the metabolic balance. Although millet is one of the most easily digestible grains, sprouting it and the other grains and seeds enhances their digestibility further, and therefore the body's ability to assimilate the nutrients they provide.

SERVES 4

¼ cup quinoa, sprouted
¼ cup millet, sprouted
2 cups organic rice milk
12 purple plums, cut in half with the pit removed
1 small cinnamon stick (optional)

1 Heat the sprouted quinoa and millet with the rice milk in a small saucepan over medium heat. Bring to a boil, reduce the heat, and simmer for 10–12 minutes.

2 Meanwhile, place the plums and cinnamon stick, if using, in a separate pan, add water to cover, and simmer over low heat for 10–12 minutes.

3 Remove the cinnamon stick and discard. Divide the porridge among 4 serving bowls, spoon the plum compôte on top, and serve.

MILLET AND PEARS WITH CARDAMOM

 HELPS BALANCE BODY pH　　 **RELIEVES VOMITING AND DIARRHEA**　　 **SUPPORTS HEALTHY KIDNEY FUNCTION**　　 **HELPS ALLEVIATE MORNING SICKNESS**

The soothing properties of millet, cooling pears, mind-enhancing cardamom seeds, and energy-boosting pistachio nuts are united in this comforting recipe. It's a perfect breakfast if you are suffering from acidosis (excessive acid buildup in the body), but you can enjoy its benefits any time. It is also a useful dish to eat in the days before embarking on a detox regime.

SERVES 4

1lb 2oz (500g) millet
a pinch of salt
3 pears, peeled, cored, and sliced
1 tbsp raisins
¼ tsp cardamom seeds
1 tbsp kudzu (an Asian thickener), or all-purpose flour or cornstarch
1 tsp vanilla extract
2 tbsp maple syrup
1 tbsp chopped pistachio nuts

1 Rinse the millet in cold water and drain thoroughly. Transfer to a skillet and dry-fry over medium heat until it releases a fragrant aroma.

2 Bring 2½ cups water to a boil in a medium saucepan. Add the millet and salt, reduce the heat, and simmer for 10 minutes.

3 Add the pears, raisins, and cardamom seeds to the millet and cook for 15 minutes more over low heat.

4 Dissolve the kudzu in 2 tablespoons water and add to the millet. Stir in the vanilla extract and keep stirring until the mixture thickens. Divide among 4 serving bowls, drizzle with the maple syrup, scatter the pistachio nuts on top, and serve.

BAKED OATMEAL WITH GOJI BERRIES AND CINNAMON

 EASY TO DIGEST   **HELPS MAINTAIN ENERGY LEVELS**   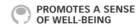 **PROMOTES A SENSE OF WELL-BEING**

Oats and goji berries are full of slow-release energy and fiber, and both contain nutrients to help support a healthy nervous system. They are also considered to be natural sedatives, helping to lift low moods and calm the nerves. The addition of cinnamon and black sesame seeds provides a warming quality that makes this an excellent dish if you are feeling weak or are recuperating.

SERVES 4

butter, for greasing
2½ cups rolled oats (not instant)
2¾ cups rice or cow milk
1 tbsp maple syrup
¼ cup goji berries
1 tsp ground cinnamon
½ cup sunflower seeds
2 tbsp black sesame seeds
a pinch of salt

1 Preheat the oven to 375°F (190°C). Generously grease a glass or ceramic ovenproof dish with the butter. Place all the ingredients in the dish, stir well to combine, and bake in the oven for 30 minutes. After 15 minutes, check the oatmeal and give it a stir, adding some hot water or more milk if it is sticking or becoming too thick and solid.

2 Remove from the oven, divide among 4 serving bowls, and serve with warmed milk.

Almond Porridge With Apricots

 HELPS LOWER CHOLESTEROL

 PROMOTES HEALTHY SKIN AND HAIR

REPLACES IRON LOST IN MENSTRUATION

HELPS BALANCE BLOOD SUGAR LEVELS

This simple breakfast is a good source of iron, which helps build red blood cells so they can carry more oxygen around the body to benefit your heart, skin, hair, and general health. It is also good for replenishing iron lost during menstruation. If you don't want to prepare ahead and soak the almonds overnight first, simply grind the dry raw nuts coarsely and use store-bought almond milk.

SERVES 4

1 cup raw almonds

1 tsp vanilla extract

12 apricots, halved, with pit removed

2 tbsp maple syrup

2 tbsp chia seeds

2 tbsp flaxseeds, crushed in a mortar and pestle

1 Rinse the almonds, add them to a bowl, and pour in twice the amount of water to cover, so the nuts can swell and still remain submerged. Leave to soak overnight.

2 Strain the soaked almonds, rinse, and place in a blender or food processor. Add 2 cups water and the vanilla extract, and purée until the ingredients turn into a milky liquid.

3 Strain the liquid through a sieve, reserving the almond milk and leaving the almond meal in the sieve to drip-dry.

4 Pour enough water into a medium saucepan to cover the bottom of the pan. Add the apricots and cook over medium-high heat for 15–20 minutes, or until they soften, adding a little more water if necessary. When the apricots are soft, but not mushy, add the maple syrup, stir to combine, and remove the pan from the heat.

5 To serve, put 2 tablespoons of almond meal into each serving bowl and sprinkle each portion with ½ tablespoon each of chia seeds and crushed flaxseeds. Put some of the apricots and maple syrup on top and pour in a little of the reserved almond milk to serve.

Flaxseeds (p95) are a great source of soluble fiber that help balance blood sugar levels and suppress hunger.

PRESOAKED BARLEY BREAKFAST

 HELPS MAINTAIN ENERGY LEVELS

 HELPS EASE CONSTIPATION

 RELIEVES FLUID RETENTION

 LOWERS RISK OF HEART DISEASE

Make this "instant" energizing breakfast cereal of toasted barley before you go to bed at night and it will be ready when you get up in the morning. It is a great way to set you up for an active day. Barley is often used as a traditional remedy for nonspecific inflammatory conditions of the urinary system and, together with prunes, helps maintain bowel regularity and blood pressure.

SERVES 4

¾ cup toasted barley

2 tsp vanilla extract

¼ cup soft prunes, chopped

¼ cup maple syrup

¼ cup toasted pumpkin seeds

1 Place the toasted barley in a large heatproof resealable container (which can hold 2½–3½ cups to accommodate the threefold increase in the volume of barley grains). Add the vanilla extract and pour 1¾ cups boiling water over the barley. Seal the container and leave overnight.

2 In the morning, empty the soaked barley into a mixing bowl, stir in the soft prunes, divide the mixture among 4 serving bowls, drizzle with maple syrup, scatter with toasted pumpkin seeds, and serve.

Prunes (p24) are renowned for promoting bowel regularity, but their high fiber content also helps to balance blood sugar levels.

SWEET SAFFRON RICE WITH CARDAMOM

HELPS IMPROVE CIRCULATION

FIGHTS AGE-RELATED VISION LOSS

ENHANCES MEMORY AND SENSE OF WELL-BEING

This is a version of desi, a sweet rice eaten on the first morning of the new year by Buddhist communities to symbolize their hopes and expectations for a new cycle of life. Supported by cardamom, the yellow pigments in saffron aid memory retention and recall, help slow age-related macular degeneration, improve blood circulation, and impart a sense of well-being.

SERVES 4–6

¾ cup jasmine or basmati rice

a pinch of salt

2in (5cm) piece of cinnamon stick

¼ cup milk

a pinch of saffron strands

2 tbsp butter, melted

1 tbsp brown sugar

½ tsp cardamom pods, crushed

zest of 1 orange

1 tbsp raisins

3 tbsp pistachio nuts, plus a few extra to garnish

2 tbsp almonds

1 Rinse the rice in a sieve under cold running water, then place in a bowl. Pour in enough water to cover, and set aside to soak for 30 minutes.

2 Drain the rice, place it in a medium saucepan, and add 1¼ cups water, the salt, and the cinnamon stick. Bring to a boil, turn the heat down, and simmer for 10–12 minutes.

3 Meanwhile, place the milk and saffron in a separate saucepan and warm gently over low heat. Add the melted butter and sugar and stir until the sugar dissolves. Add the cardamom pods and orange zest and allow all the ingredients to infuse for 2–3 minutes on very low heat.

4 Using a thick-bottomed medium saucepan, toast the raisins over medium heat for 1–2 minutes. Remove from the heat and set aside, then add the nuts, toast until golden, and remove from the heat.

5 When the rice is cooked and the water has been absorbed, add the toasted raisins and nuts and combine well. Pour in the infused milk, stir well, and cook over low heat for 1–2 minutes until the aromas and saffron color have suffused the rice.

6 Transfer to small serving bowls, heaping up the mixture to symbolize prosperity, and serve with few pistachio nuts scattered on top.

Saffron threads (p119) have long been used in traditional medicines for their stimulating and mood-lifting qualities.

WARM CHICKEN CONGEE

 SOOTHES UPSET STOMACHS   **HELPS MAINTAIN ENERGY LEVELS**

Congee is a soothing, nourishing food for anyone recovering from gastric upsets or recuperating from exhaustion and illness. This Chinese dish is traditionally made by gently simmering rice and water on the lowest possible heat for up to 6 hours, stirring regularly to prevent it from sticking. This recipe is an adaptation of the original and cooks in half the time or less.

SERVES 4–6

1 organic free-range chicken, about 3¼lb (1.5kg)

1 cup long grain or basmati brown rice

2in (5cm) piece of fresh ginger, grated

1 tbsp tamari soy sauce

1 tbsp sesame seed oil (toasted sesame seed oil is fine)

sea salt and freshly ground black pepper

2 tbsp finely chopped scallions, to garnish

2 tbsp finely chopped cilantro leaves, to garnish

1 Place the chicken, rice, and ginger in a large, heavy saucepan with a lid. Cover the ingredients with water and bring to a boil. Then reduce the heat to low and gently simmer for 1½–3 hours, or until the chicken meat is falling off the bones and the rice is soft. Add more water if necessary during cooking to prevent the congee from boiling dry. Congee should have a thick souplike consistency.

2 Remove the pan from the heat, transfer the chicken to a plate, and carefully remove the bones and skin. Shred the chicken meat and return it to the pan. Add the tamari soy sauce, sesame oil, and sea salt and black pepper to taste, and stir to combine.

3 Divide the congee among 4 serving bowls, garnish with the scallions and cilantro leaves, and serve.

TIP: Tamari is a type of soy sauce that contains little or no wheat, making it a good, gluten-free choice.

SNACKS

WHY WASTE TIME ON EMPTY CALORIES? THESE **NUTRIENT-DENSE** NIBBLES ARE GREAT ON THEIR OWN OR FOR DAYS WHEN YOU NEED SOMETHING EXTRA TO **SUSTAIN YOU**. YOU COULD ALSO TRY THEM AS DELICIOUS SIDE DISHES.

Ezze

HELPS IMPROVE CIRCULATION **AIDS HEALTHY/OPTIMAL DIGESTION** **HELPS STRENGTHEN THE IMMUNE SYSTEM**

This hot Bhutanese relish brings together the therapeutic properties of chiles, onions, garlic, cilantro, and tomatoes to help stimulate blood circulation and enhance the digestive system. It is also a good food to eat in winter to bolster your immune system. The large chiles used here are not as hot as some smaller varieties, but if you prefer a milder relish, substitute them for bell peppers.

SERVES 4

3 large tomatoes

5 large red chiles, seeded and minced

5 large green chiles, seeded and minced

1 large red onion, finely chopped

3 garlic cloves, crushed

a small bunch of cilantro leaves, chopped

juice of ½ lime

1 tbsp extra virgin olive oil

salt and freshly ground black pepper

1 Cut a cross on the top of each tomato with a sharp knife, then dip the tomatoes in a bowl of boiling water for 20 seconds. Remove with a slotted spoon and, when cool enough to handle, remove the skins and finely chop the flesh. Transfer to a large bowl.

2 Add the chiles, onion, garlic, cilantro leaves, and lime juice to the mixing bowl. Pour in the olive oil, mix well, and season to taste with salt and black pepper. Serve with Cabbage Momos (p235), or with other snacks as a sauce.

Chiles (p56) have antioxidant and anti-inflammatory properties, which means they can help lower cholesterol and balance blood sugar levels.

HUMMUS WITH CORIANDER

 HELPS EASE CONSTIPATION   **HELPS BALANCE BLOOD SUGAR LEVELS**   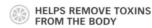 **HELPS REMOVE TOXINS FROM THE BODY**

The high-fiber chickpeas in hummus benefit gut health, while sesame seeds act as a general tonic. For the best flavor and the most antioxidants, choose a dark variety of dried chickpeas and soak and cook them yourself; otherwise canned chickpeas are fine. Store any leftover garlic purée under a layer of olive oil in a tightly sealed jar. Refrigerate and use within 2 weeks.

MAKES 1LB (450G)

14oz (400g) chickpeas, cooked, drained, and rinsed, or 14oz can chickpeas, drained and rinsed

3 tbsp dark tahini paste

juice of ½ lemon

1 tsp coriander seeds, very finely crushed

½ tsp smoked paprika

1 tbsp extra-virgin olive oil

salt and freshly ground black pepper

2 tsp black sesame seeds (or use white sesame seeds instead)

1 tbsp pomegranate seeds, to garnish

a small bunch of cilantro leaves, finely chopped, to garnish (optional)

For the garlic purée

2 heads garlic, cloves separated and peeled

½ cup olive oil

1 tbsp white wine

½ tsp chopped thyme leaves

½ tsp chopped rosemary leaves

1 Preheat the oven to 325°F (170°C). To make the garlic purée, place the garlic cloves in a small baking dish, add the olive oil, wine, thyme, and rosemary, cover the dish with a lid or foil, and bake for 40 minutes, or until the garlic cloves are soft. Pulse the softened mixture briefly in a food processor or blender to make a purée.

2 To make the hummus, put 1 tablespoon of the garlic purée and the rest of the ingredients except the sesame seeds in a food processor or blender, and pulse to a semicoarse paste. Add the sesame seeds, taste the hummus, and add more seasoning and/or lemon juice if needed. If the mixture is quite dry, add a little water to loosen it. If you prefer a very smooth texture, use a hand-held stick blender and add the sesame seeds along with the rest of the ingredients. Serve in a bowl scattered with pomegranate seeds and garnished with cilantro leaves, if using.

AJVAR

 HELPS REMOVE TOXINS FROM THE BLOOD

 HELPS EASE MENSTRUAL CRAMPS

 AIDS HEALTHY DIGESTION

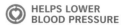 **HELPS LOWER BLOOD PRESSURE**

This traditional relish is popular in southeastern Europe. It contains bell peppers and eggplants, which boost blood circulation and help alleviate period cramps and water retention, together with chile peppers, which aid detoxification, help to lower blood pressure, and protect the heart. The bell peppers and eggplants are traditionally baked in the ashes of a barbecue.

MAKES 1LB 2OZ (500G)

6 large red bell peppers, stems removed

2 large eggplants, stems removed (and cut in half lengthwise if very wide)

½ cup olive oil

1 red chile, seeded and minced

juice of 1 lemon

2–3 garlic cloves, minced

salt and freshly ground black pepper

2 tbsp chopped cilantro leaves, to garnish (optional)

1 Preheat the oven to 450°F (230°C), if not using a barbecue. Place the peppers and eggplants on a baking sheet and bake for 25–30 minutes, or until their skins are blistering and turning black.

2 Remove from the oven, transfer to a ceramic bowl, cover with plastic wrap, and leave to sweat (so the blackened skins can be removed more easily). When cool enough to handle, remove the skins, core, and seed the peppers, and peel the eggplants. Reserve the juices in the ceramic bowl and drain the peeled eggplants in a colander to remove some excess juice, which can be discarded.

3 Transfer the peppers and eggplants to a blender or food processor and pulse to a coarse or smooth texture, depending on your preference.

4 Heat 2–4 tablespoons of the olive oil with some of the reserved juices in a large heavy saucepan over medium heat. Add the chile and then the pepper and eggplant mixture. Simmer over low heat for 30 minutes, or until the juices have thickened. Occasionally add a little more oil (retaining about 1 tablespoon) to stop the mixture from sticking to the bottom of the pan. When the mixture has thickened, add the lemon juice and garlic, let them heat through, season with salt and black pepper, and remove the pan from the heat. If eating immediately, transfer to a serving bowl and garnish with the chopped cilantro leaves. Serve with Rye Sourdough Bread (p328) as a snack or as a part of a mezze.

5 To store the relish instead, transfer to a hot, sterilized glass jar. Pour 1 tablespoon of the olive oil on top to seal the relish, fasten the lid on, label, and set aside to cool. Store in the refrigerator and use within 1 week.

6 LARGE RED BELL PEPPERS

2 LARGE EGGPLANTS

1 RED CHILE

BOOST CIRCULATION

BELL PEPPERS AND EGGPLANT ENCOURAGE BLOOD CIRCULATION— HELPING TO SOOTHE MENSTRUAL CRAMPS AND RELIEVE COLD EXTREMETIES OR PINS AND NEEDLES.

EGGPLANT DIP

 HELPS REMOVE TOXINS FROM THE BLOOD   **HELPS EASE MENSTRUAL CRAMPS**   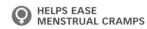 **HAS A DIURETIC ACTION**

The eggplant in this dip is rich in dietary fiber, which can help to remove toxins from the blood. Eggplant is also great for easing premenstrual and menstrual symptoms, and the addition of fatty-acid rich Rose and Fennel Seed Oil (p333) makes this dish a particularly good choice for abdominal cramps and water retention. Serve with Ajvar (opposite) as part of a mezze, if you like.

SERVES 4–6 AS PART OF A MEZZE

3–4 large eggplants (total weight approximately 2¼lb/1kg)

1 medium onion, chopped

4 garlic cloves, crushed

½ tsp chili flakes

1 tbsp olive oil, or Rose and Fennel Seed Oil (p333)

½ cup sour cream

2 tbsp chopped cilantro leaves, to garnish

1 Preheat the oven to 350°F (180°C). Prick the eggplants all over with a fork. Place on a baking sheet and bake for 1 hour or until tender and the skins are blackened. Remove from the oven, transfer to a ceramic bowl, cover with plastic wrap, and leave to sweat (so the blackened skins can be removed more easily). When cool enough to handle, remove the skins and roughly chop the cooked flesh. Place in a colander to drain— there will be a lot of excess juice. Leave to drain while you prepare the other ingredients and when you are ready to use them, press the eggplant pieces down gently to remove the last of the juices (too much liquid will result in a watery dish).

2 Heat 3 tablespoons of water in a skillet, add the onion and garlic, and sauté over medium heat for 3–4 minutes, or until the onion is soft and translucent, adding a dash of water if necessary. Add the chili flakes and olive oil or Rose and Fennel Seed Oil blend, stir well, and transfer the mixture to a mixing bowl or a blender or food processor (you can use a hand-held immersion blender if you have one, to blend the ingredients in the bowl). Add the chopped eggplants and sour cream and mix or purée to a smooth paste.

3 Transfer to a serving bowl, garnish with the chopped cilantro leaves. This dip is good served as part of a mezze, with chunks of French bread and a green salad for lunch, or with melba toast as a starter.

BUTTERNUT SQUASH AND WALNUT BITES

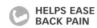 **PROMOTES A SENSE OF WELL-BEING**

 HELPS EASE BACK PAIN

AIDS HEALTHY DIGESTION

HELPS MAINTAIN WATER BALANCE

Astringent walnuts and creamy butternut squash promote a sense of well-being, support bone and muscle health, and benefit the digestive and urinary systems. Tamari sauce—a Japanese dark soy sauce—helps give these bites a complex depth of flavor. You can turn this into a light meal for four people, if you like, by simply tossing the cooked bites in some salad leaves.

SERVES 8–10 (ABOUT 30 BITES)

½ cup walnut halves

1 medium-sized butternut squash, peeled and seeded

2 garlic cloves, minced

2 tbsp olive oil

2 tbsp tamari soy sauce

1 Count how many walnut halves you have, then cut the squash into the same number of small cubes, making sure each cube is just big enough for a walnut half to sit on top of it. Place the cubed squash in a bowl. Add the walnuts, garlic, olive oil, tamari soy sauce, and 1 tablespoon of water, and mix well. Set aside to marinate for 1–2 hours.

2 Preheat the oven to 350°F (180°C). Transfer the marinated squash and walnuts to a baking dish arranging them in a single layer. Cover with foil and bake in the oven for 20–30 minutes.

3 Arrange the squash cubes on a serving dish, decorate each with a walnut half, and serve as a finger food with drinks.

Walnuts (p93) contain beneficial oils that promote healthy skin and hair.

MUSHROOM AND CHESTNUT BITES

 STRENGTHENS KNEES AND LOWER BACK

 PROMOTES A SENSE OF WELL-BEING

PROMOTES A HEALTHY DIGESTIVE TRACT

These bites make great party canapés and are a tasty vegetarian alternative to sausage rolls. Chestnuts and hazelnuts are traditionally considered to be a tonic for the body, including muscles and joints. Shallots, oregano, and parsley bring the added benefit of helping to boost energy levels. Oregano and shallots can aid the body's digestion of the puff pastry in this recipe, too.

MAKES 24

1 tbsp olive oil, plus extra for greasing

5 small shallots, finely chopped

heaped ½ cup hazelnuts, toasted, finely chopped

3½oz (110g) chestnuts, cooked, peeled, and finely chopped

6oz (175g) button mushrooms, chopped

salt and freshly ground black pepper

1 tbsp chopped parsley leaves

½ tsp dried oregano

12oz (350g) store-bought puff pastry

1 large egg, beaten

1 Preheat the oven to 400°F (200°C). Place the olive oil in a medium skillet and heat gently. Add the shallots and cook over medium heat until soft and translucent. Add the hazelnuts, chestnuts, and a dash of water and mix well.

2 In a separate skillet, dry-fry the mushrooms, stirring constantly to prevent them from sticking to the bottom of the pan and burning. This process help to dry them out and concentrates their flavor. When all the mushroom juices have been released and have evaporated, transfer the mushrooms to the shallot and nut mixture, season with salt and black pepper, add the parsley and oregano, and combine all the ingredients.

3 Roll out the puff pastry to 5mm and cut it into 3 long strips, each 3in (7.5cm) wide. Spoon the mixture down the center of each strip. Brush the edges with beaten egg, roll up the pastry strips lengthwise to make long sausage shapes, and seal the edges well. Slash the top of each pastry roll with a sharp knife in criss-cross shapes and cut each roll into 8 pieces. Arrange the bites on an oiled baking sheet and bake in the oven for 10 minutes, or until golden. Serve warm or cold.

Hazelnuts (p93) are a good source of biotin, a B vitamin that supports musculoskeletal health by strengthening connective tissues.

KALE CHIPS

 PROMOTES A HEALTHY DIGESTIVE TRACT   **HELPS LOWER CHOLESTEROL** 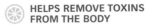 **HELPS REMOVE TOXINS FROM THE BODY**

Kale, which retains its vibrant color when dried (rather than baked), supports the body's detoxification processes and helps to lower levels of "unhealthy" (LDL) cholesterol in the blood. Its high fiber content also improves digestion and benefits intestinal health. Drizzling lemon juice on the leaves and leaving them to stand enhances their concentration of phytonutrients.

MAKES 3½OZ (100G)

1lb 2oz (500g) kale, tough stems removed, and the leaves torn into bite-sized pieces

juice of 1 lemon

1 tbsp extra virgin olive oil

¼ tsp salt

½ tsp garlic powder

1 Place the kale in a large bowl, add the lemon juice, and set aside for 30 minutes. Add the olive oil, salt, and garlic powder and combine well.

2 If you have a dehydrator, set it to 104°F (40°C). Cover the silicone sheets with parchment paper and arrange the leaves on top, ensuring they don't touch. Dehydrate for 6–8 hours, turning them halfway through. When dry, store in an airtight jar and consume within 2 days.

3 Otherwise, preheat the oven to its lowest setting—120°F (50°C) or lower. Arrange the leaves on large rimmed baking sheets, making sure they don't overlap. If they won't all fit, make the chips in batches. Dry in the oven for 1–2 hours or until the leaves are dry and crisp, switching the baking sheets from back to front and top to bottom halfway through, and turning the leaves over if needed.

YELLOW SUMMER SQUASH CHIPS

 HAS A DIURETIC ACTION   **AIDS HEALTHY DIGESTION**   **HELPS PREVENT BLOOD VESSEL DAMAGE**

Yellow squash, like other summer squashes, have cooling, refreshing properties, and are a mild diuretic. Here they are marinated in warming, heart-friendly spices and then dried to make healthy snacks. The trick is to slice them thinly so that they dry out more quickly and turn crisp. Smaller summer squash with mild-tasting yellow skins are best, but any summer squash will work well.

MAKES 1LB (450G)

juice of 3 lemons

3 medium yellow squash, thinly sliced

For the spice powder

1 tsp coriander seeds

1 tsp cumin seeds

¼ tsp ground turmeric powder

¼ tsp chili powder

¼ tsp ground ginger

¼ tsp garlic powder

½ tsp Himalayan pink salt, or sea salt

1 For the spice powder, dry-fry the coriander and cumin seeds over medium heat until their aromas develop. Transfer to a mortar and pestle, grind to a powder, and combine with the spice powders and salt.

2 Pour the lemon juice into a large bowl, add 1½ tsp of the spice powder, and mix to a thin consistency, adding more lemon juice if necessary. Add the squash and combine well. Set aside for 1 hour.

3 Cover silicone sheets or baking sheets with parchment paper and arrange the squash slices on top. If using a dehydrator, set it to 104°F (40°C) and dry the slices for 10–12 hours, turning them halfway through.

4 Otherwise, preheat the oven to its lowest setting—120°F (50°C) or lower—and dry the slices for 1–2 hours or until crisp, turning them halfway through. Store in an airtight jar and consume within 1 week.

SPROUTED MEDLEY

 PROMOTES HEALTHY SKIN
 PROMOTES EFFICIENT METABOLISM
 HELPS MAINTAIN ENERGY LEVELS
 AIDS HEALTHY DIGESTION

This healthy snack is full of enzymes, flavor, and vital nutrients: germinated seeds provide amino acids to support skin and cell regeneration in the body and boost energy levels and digestion. They may also help fight the signs and symptoms of premature aging. For this dish, prepare a little ahead—3 types of sprouts are used and they all take different amounts of time to sprout.

SERVES 6

1 tbsp alfalfa seeds
½ tbsp celery seeds
1 tbsp clover seeds
½ tbsp radish seeds
¼ cup green or Puy lentils
¼ cup mung beans
2 tbsp millet
2 tbsp wheat grain
2 tbsp quinoa
¼ cup sunflower seeds

For the dressing

2 tbsp chopped lemon thyme leaves
3 tbsp toasted sesame oil
2 tbsp orange juice
1 tbsp tamari soy sauce
1 tsp honey

1 When you sprout each type of seed, legume, or grain, put it into a separate 3½–5½-cup wide-mouthed jar and cover with cheesecloth, securing the cloth in place with a rubber band. To drain the water from a jar, pour it out through the cheesecloth cover. Pour fresh tepid water into the jar through the cloth, and drain in the same way.

2 Half-fill the jars of alfalfa, celery, clover, and radish seeds with tepid water and place them away from direct sunlight at room temperature for 5 hours. Drain, rinse, and drain again, then let the seeds stand without water for 8–12 hours. Rinse and drain the seeds twice a day for the next 6 days. On the seventh day, rinse and drain the seeds and leave the jars in broad daylight for 12 hours to increase their chlorophyll content. The sprouted seeds should have expanded to 8 times their original size.

3 Half-fill the jars of lentils and mung beans with tepid water, place the jars away from direct sunlight at room temperature, and let soak overnight. Drain, then rinse and drain twice a day for 3 days. The sprouted legumes will expand to 2–3 times their original size.

4 Half-fill the jars of millet, wheat, and quinoa with tepid water, place the jars away from direct sunlight at room temperature, and let soak overnight. Drain, then rinse and drain twice a day for 2 days, or until they sprout small "tails" no bigger than the grains themselves.

5 Half-fill the jar of sunflower seeds with tepid water, place the jar away from direct sunlight at room temperature, and let soak overnight. Drain, then rinse and drain the seeds twice at 6-hourly intervals. Sunflower seeds have a delicate filmlike skin that detaches from the seed during sprouting. Remove the cheeecloth cover and skim as many of these skins off the surface of the water as you can while you rinse the seeds, because they quickly spoil and can cause the sprouts to rot. Leave to sprout for 18 hours or until the seeds have a ¼–½in (5mm–1cm) long "tail" and a crunchy texture.

6 Mix all the ingredients for the dressing together in a small bowl. Drain the sprouts and serve them as 3 different medleys in separate serving bowls: alfalfa, celery, clover, and radish sprouts in the first; lentil and mung bean sprouts in the second; and sunflower, quinoa, wheat, and millet sprouts in the third. Combine each of these medleys with one-third of the dressing, and invite the guests to graze.

TOMATO CRACKERS

 HELPS KEEP BLOOD VESSELS SUPPLE   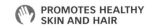 **PROMOTES HEALTHY SKIN AND HAIR**   **AIDS HEALTHY DIGESTION**

These crackers are a great substitute for other savory snacks, and are full of health benefits. Flaxseed and tomatoes help improve blood circulation and maintain the health of blood vessels. They also help nourish the skin, help restore dull, unruly hair, and soften and strengthen dry, brittle nails. Chew the crackers well to benefit from the rich healing oil in the flaxseeds.

MAKES 50

1½ cups whole flaxseeds

1 tsp dried oregano

heaped 1 cup sun-dried tomatoes (not in oil)

⅓ cup cracked flaxseeds

10oz (300g) tomatoes

salt and freshly ground black pepper

1 Take ⅓ cup of the whole flaxseeds, place them in a food processor or blender, add the oregano, grind to a fine consistency, and empty into a bowl. Add the sun-dried tomatoes to the food processor, pulse to fine pieces, and transfer to the bowl. Add the rest of the whole and the cracked flaxseeds to the bowl and mix.

2 Add the fresh tomatoes to the food processor and pulse. Add the puréed tomatoes to the dry ingredients, season with the salt and pepper, and mix everything together well with a wooden spoon.

3 Taste and adjust the seasoning as required, then set the mixture aside for 2–3 hours for the seeds to partly absorb the liquid. When the mixture has thickened and is sufficiently dry yet pliable, divide into 3 equal parts.

4 Spread the cracker mixture thinly (⅛–¼in/2–4mm thick) over 3 silicone sheets or sheets of parchment paper. Score the surface of the cracker mixture into small triangles, squares, or rectangles with a sharp knife to define the shape and size of the crackers.

5 If you have a dehydrator, set it to 113°F (45°C) and dry the crackers for 6–7 hours, turning them halfway through. Otherwise, preheat the oven to its lowest setting—120°F (50°C) or lower. Cover the top of the cracker layer with another sheet of parchment paper and bake for 2 hours. Carefully turn each cracker layer over, remove the parchment paper or silicone sheets, place the cracker sheets directly onto the oven racks, and bake for 1 hour more. Remove from the oven and allow to cool for 6–7 hours, turning the cracker sheets over halfway through so they dry out completely.

6 Once cool, break along the scored lines to make individual crackers. Store in an airtight container and consume within 1–2 weeks.

SPICY CRACKERS

 PROMOTES BOWEL REGULARITY

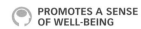 **PROMOTES A SENSE OF WELL-BEING**

Seeds are packed with protein for energy and fiber to boost digestive health. Here flaxseeds, chia seeds, and black and white sesame seeds (ingredients in furikake, a dried Japanese condiment) are enlivened by flavorsome tomatoes, spices, and herbs. Drying or baking the seed mixture on very low heat to make "raw" crackers means the seeds retain more of their beneficial nutrients.

MAKES 50 CRACKERS

1¼ cups whole flaxseeds

⅓ cup cracked flaxseeds

⅓ cup whole chia seeds

2 tablespoons furikake (or black and white sesame seeds)

¼ cup sun-dried tomatoes (not in oil) or tomato paste

salt and freshly ground black pepper

chili flakes, to taste

1 tsp dried Italian seasoning (basil, thyme, and garlic powder), or similar mixed herbs

10oz (300g) tomatoes

1 Mix the seeds and furikake together in a bowl. Pulse the sun-dried tomatoes, if using, to fine pieces in a food processor or blender. Add the tomato pieces or the tomato paste to the seeds and season with salt, black pepper, chili flakes, and the dried mixed herb seasoning. Mix everything thoroughly, taste, and adjust the seasoning if necessary.

2 Place the fresh tomatoes in a food processor or blender and pulse to a fine purée. Gradually mix this fresh tomato purée into the dry seed mixture with a wooden spoon.

3 Divide the cracker mixture into 3 equal batches and spread it thinly (⅛–¼in/2–4mm thick) onto 3 silicone baking mats or sheets of parchment paper. Score the surface of the seed mixture into small triangles, squares, or rectangles to define the shape and size of the crackers.

4 If you have a dehydrator, place the crackers in it and dry at 113°F (45°C) for 6–7 hours, turning them halfway through. If you don't have a dehydrator, preheat the oven to 120°F (50°C). If using parchment paper or silicone baking mats, cover the top of the cracker layer with another sheet of parchment. Place the crackers in their parchment or on the silicone baking mats onto cookie sheets and bake for 2 hours. Remove the cookie sheets from the oven and carefully turn each cracker layer over to dry out the bottom. Remove from the parchment paper or silicone baking mats, place the cracker layers directly on the oven racks, and bake for a further 1 hour. Remove from the oven and allow to cool.

5 Once cool, break along the scored lines to make individual crackers. Store in airtight containers. They will keep for up to 2 weeks.

TIP: Rather than choosing sun-dried tomatoes stored in oil, look for ones that are packaged like dried fruit; they have a drier texture that is excellent for this recipe.

SOUPS

EVEN THE **SIMPLEST** INGREDIENTS CAN BE QUICKLY
TRANSFORMED INTO EASY-TO-DIGEST SOUPS THAT
STIMULATE, **PROTECT**, **DETOX**, AND **STRENGTHEN**.
WARM YOURSELF UP—OR COOL YOURSELF DOWN—
WITH THESE SATISFYING BLENDS.

Mung Bean And Spinach Soup

⊙ **HELPS LOWER BLOOD PRESSURE**   ⊛ **AIDS DETOXIFICATION SYSTEM**   ⊜ **HELPS EASE CONSTIPATION**

If you suffer from high blood pressure, headaches, or constipation, or are in need of a detox, try this soup. Mung beans contain lots of fiber and potassium, both of which help lower blood pressure. They also have detoxifying properties and are anti-inflammatory, as is iron-rich spinach. Plan ahead and soak the beans overnight or sprout them for 3 days before cooking.

SERVES 4

1 cup mung beans

5 small shallots, finely chopped

¾in (2cm) piece fresh ginger, finely chopped

2 garlic cloves, finely chopped

½ tsp turmeric powder

½ tsp crushed coriander seeds

1 tbsp olive oil

3½ cups vegetable stock, or your choice of broth (pp323–325), or water

3 cups baby spinach leaves

juice of 1 small lime

salt and freshly ground black pepper

2 tbsp chopped cilantro leaves, to garnish

1 Soak the beans following package directions or sprout them for 3 days (p204).

2 Pour a thin layer of water into a medium saucepan, set over medium heat, and bring to a simmer. Reduce the heat, add the shallots, ginger, garlic, turmeric powder, and coriander seeds, and cook over low heat, stirring occasionally and adding a little more water if necessary. Meanwhile, drain and rinse the beans.

3 When the shallots have softened, add a dash of water, the olive oil, and the beans to the pan. Pour in the vegetable stock, increase the heat, and bring to a simmer. If you are using sprouted beans, let the soup simmer gently for 20–25 minutes, or until the sprouts are soft. Otherwise, simmer for 30–40 minutes, or until the cooked soaked beans fall apart. Stir in the baby spinach leaves and add the lime juice.

4 Serve the soup as it is, or purée to a smooth consistency using an immersion hand blender or in a food processor or blender. Add salt and black pepper to taste just before serving (adding salt to beans while you cook them makes them harder), then transfer to 4 serving bowls and garnish with the chopped cilantro leaves.

Limes (p40) *contain high levels of vitamin K, which stimulates the liver to support blood coagulation.*

RAW TOMATO SOUP

 HELPS LOWER BLOOD PRESSURE

 TONES AND CLEANSES THE LIVER

 HELPS CLEAR CONGESTION

 HAS AN UPLIFTING EFFECT

Comprising more than 90 percent water and rich in antioxidants, tomatoes cleanse the liver, purify the blood, and are cooling and hydrating. They are useful in treating high blood pressure accompanied by red eyes and headaches. The freshly juiced basil in this recipe enhances digestion, helps clear respiratory congestion and phlegm, and can lift the mood.

SERVES 4

8 large ripe tomatoes
2 stems of basil
8 celery stalks
1 red chile, seeded and minced
2 small garlic cloves, roughly chopped
2 tbsp extra virgin olive oil
salt and freshly ground black pepper

1 Using a sharp knife, cut a light cross through the skin at the top of each tomato, then place the tomatoes in a bowl and cover with hot water. Let the water cool a little, then drain. Peel the skins off the tomatoes, cut into quarters, and remove the seeds. Dice the flesh and place it in a blender or food processor.

2 Remove the basil leaves from their stems and reserve the leaves as a garnish. Juice the basil stems with the celery stalks in a juicer and add the juice to the blender, along with the chile and garlic.

3 Blend the ingredients until smooth. Add the olive oil, season to taste, and blend once more. Pour the soup into 4 serving bowls. Garnish with the basil leaves, tearing them roughly with your fingers if they are large, or leaving them whole if they are small, and serve.

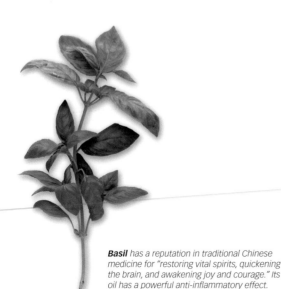

Basil *has a reputation in traditional Chinese medicine for "restoring vital spirits, quickening the brain, and awakening joy and courage." Its oil has a powerful anti-inflammatory effect.*

Puy Lentil Soup With Fresh Turmeric

 HELPS EASE JOINT INFLAMMATION

 HELPS LOWER CHOLESTEROL

HELPS BALANCE BLOOD SUGAR LEVELS

 AIDS HEALTHY DIGESTION

The ingredients in this soup have anti-inflammatory properties, helping to relieve the swelling and pain associated with rheumatic and arthritic pain. Lentils help to lower "unhealthy" (LDL) cholesterol levels and balance blood sugar levels too, and turmeric helps to improve digestion.

SERVES 4

1¼ cups puy lentils

2 tbsp sesame oil

4 banana shallots, finely chopped

salt

1¼in (3cm) piece each fresh ginger and turmeric, peeled and sliced

1 chile, seeded and minced

2 tsp cumin seeds, crushed

½ tsp coriander seeds, crushed

½ tsp ground turmeric

2 garlic cloves, crushed

2½ cups vegetable stock

¼ cup chopped cilantro leaves

1 Although puy lentils can be cooked without soaking, it's worth doing so for at least 2 hours to make them more easily digestible. Rinse thoroughly afterward.

2 Heat the sesame oil with 3 tablespoons of water in a Dutch oven over medium heat. Add the shallots and a pinch of salt and cook until they have softened. Add the fresh ginger and fresh turmeric, followed by the chile, cumin seeds, coriander seeds, ground turmeric, and garlic.

3 Add the lentils and stir until coated. Cook for 1–2 minutes to let them absorb the flavors of the spices and shallots, then pour in the stock and bring to a boil. Reduce the heat and let the lentils simmer for about 20 minutes. Scatter with the chopped cilantro and serve with Flat Bread with Sweet Potato (p327) on the side.

Watercress And Flaxseed Soup

 AIDS HEALTHY DIGESTION

 HELPS CLEAR CONGESTION

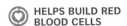 **HELPS BUILD RED BLOOD CELLS**

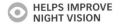 **HELPS IMPROVE NIGHT VISION**

Pungent, bittersweet watercress is an excellent digestive and is most beneficial when eaten raw or in soups. It also helps moisten the respiratory tract, making this warming soup an excellent remedy if you have a sore throat or lung infection. Eaten regularly, this soup can help boost iron levels, improve night vision, support healthy kidney function, and improve skin condition.

SERVES 4

1 leek, finely chopped

2 small zucchini, diced

1 garlic clove

salt and freshly ground black pepper

5½oz (150g) watercress

3 level tbsp flaxseeds and 1 tsp coriander seeds, crushed to a powder in a coffee grinder or blender

2 tbsp extra virgin olive oil

¼ cup Greek-style yogurt (optional)

1 Place the leek and zucchini in a medium saucepan with enough water to cover the bottom of the pan. Sweat for 5–10 minutes over low heat, stirring occasionally, and adding more water if needed to prevent the vegetables from sticking to the bottom of the pan.

2 When the vegetables are tender, add the garlic and salt. Transfer the mixture to a blender or food processor, add 2 cups hot but not boiling water, and purée.

3 Add the watercress, 1 tablespoon of the flaxseed and coriander seed powder, and the extra virgin olive oil, and purée until smooth. Season to taste, then transfer the soup to 4 serving bowls, add a spoonful of yogurt to each, if using, sprinkle with the remaining seed powder, and serve.

CARROT AND COCONUT SOUP

 AIDS HEALTHY DIGESTION

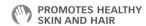 **PROMOTES HEALTHY SKIN AND HAIR**

 HELPS EASE RHEUMATIC PAIN

 HELPS STRENGTHEN THE IMMUNE SYSTEM

With the combined powers of carrot and coconut, this soup enhances the digestive system, soothes inflammation, and protects against premature aging and degenerative diseases. Carrots are also a traditional remedy for conditions such as acne and rheumatism, while coconuts promote a healthy complexion, glossy hair, and support the health of the immune system.

SERVES 4

1 tbsp coconut oil

3 shallots, chopped

½lb (250g) carrots, chopped

2 garlic cloves, crushed

3 cups coconut water

juice and zest of ½ lime

salt and freshly ground black pepper

4 tsp coconut milk

a small handful of cilantro leaves, chopped, to garnish

1 Heat the coconut oil in a saucepan over medium heat, add the shallots, and cook until translucent. Add 3 tablespoons water and the carrots and sweat for 2–3 minutes. Add the garlic and cook for 15 more minutes or until the carrots are soft. Add more water if needed.

2 Pour the contents of the saucepan into a blender or food processor, add 2 cups of the coconut water, and blend. Return the blended soup to the pan and add more coconut water until you achieve a consistency you like. Heat the soup through gently (there is no need to bring it to a boil). Add the lime juice and zest, season with salt and black pepper to taste, and divide among 4 serving bowls. Swirl a teaspoon of coconut milk into each portion and garnish with the chopped cilantro leaves.

BEET SOUP

 HELPS LOWER BLOOD PRESSURE

 PROMOTES A HEALTHY DIGESTIVE TRACT

 BOOSTS IRON STORES TO COMBAT FATIGUE

 HELPS STRENGTHEN THE IMMUNE SYSTEM

Good for balancing blood pressure, this soup also enhances circulation and relieves constipation. Antioxidant-rich beets are traditionally used in many parts of Europe as a nourishing food for patients who are recovering, to help combat fatigue, improve digestion, and support healthy immunity. Lemon thyme is antibacterial and helps to combat lingering infections.

SERVES 4–6

3 tbsp olive oil

1 medium onion, minced

salt and freshly ground black pepper

1 medium leek, cut in short thin strips

3 medium beets, peeled and grated

1 large carrot, grated

2 garlic cloves, crushed

3½ cups hot vegetable stock

2–3 tsp chopped lemon thyme leaves

2 tbsp plain yogurt

1 Heat the olive oil in a large saucepan over medium heat, add the onion along with a pinch of salt, and cook until translucent. Add the leek and let soften, then add the other vegetables and garlic and cook for a further 2–3 minutes.

2 Add the stock and simmer for about 20 minutes, or until the vegetables are soft. Add the thyme 5 minutes before the end of cooking and season to taste. Divide the soup among 4 serving bowls and swirl a little yogurt into each portion just before serving.

WILD GARLIC SOUP

 **HELPS STRENGTHEN
THE IMMUNE SYSTEM**

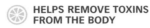 **HELPS REMOVE TOXINS
FROM THE BODY**

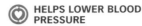 **HELPS LOWER BLOOD
PRESSURE**

Sweet potato, wheatgrass, and wild garlic, all have anti-inflammatory and cleansing properties, so this is the perfect soup if you are feeling the cold or your immune system is sluggish after any winter bugs or illnesses. Wild garlic are only available in spring, so if you want to make this soup at other times of the year, substitute it with a mixture of wild arugula and spinach.

SERVES 4

1 tbsp sunflower or vegetable oil

4 medium shallots, chopped

1 medium sweet potato
(about 14oz/ 400g), peeled and
chopped into small cubes

2½ cups vegetable stock

1 tbsp wheatgrass juice or 1 tsp
wheatgrass powder (optional)

¼ cup crème fraîche or plain yogurt,
to serve (optional)

7oz (200g) wild garlic leaves

salt and freshly ground black pepper

1 Heat the oil in a medium saucepan over low heat, add the shallots and a little water, and allow the shallots to soften. Add the sweet potato and sauté for 5 minutes. Pour in the hot vegetable stock, bring to a boil, and simmer for about 15 minutes, or until the sweet potato softens.

2 Meanwhile, if using the wheatgrass juice or powder, mix it with the crème fraîche or yogurt in a small bowl.

3 Remove the pan from the heat, pour the mixture into a blender or food processor, and purée until smooth. Add the wild garlic and purée again until smooth. Season to taste. Pour the soup into 4 individual serving bowls, swirl a tablespoon of crème fraîche or yogurt into each portion, and serve.

Wild garlic *(p82) is a seasonal leafy
food that is easy to digest and
can be eaten cooked or raw.*

Sweet Potato And Celeriac Soup

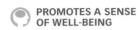 **PROMOTES A SENSE OF WELL-BEING**

 HELPS MAINTAIN ENERGY LEVELS

 HELPS IMPROVE CIRCULATION

 SUPPORTS HEALTHY KIDNEY FUNCTION

Root vegetables and spices are the essential ingredients in this comforting, warming, and healthy soup. These foods increase your energy levels, boost the circulatory system, aid digestion by promoting bowel regularity. They also strengthen the kidneys and enhance urine output. Turmeric also benefits muscles and joints and helps to alleviate any inflammation.

SERVES 6

1 tbsp ghee, or clarified butter

1 onion, finely chopped

1 garlic clove, chopped

1 tsp coriander seeds, crushed

½ tsp turmeric powder or ground turmeric root

½ tsp chili flakes

2 sweet potatoes (9oz/250g total weight), peeled and diced

1 celeriac (14oz/400g total weight), peeled and diced

4 cups vegetable stock

salt and freshly ground black pepper

⅓ cup natural yogurt

2 tbsp pumpkin oil

a small handful of cilantro leaves, chopped

1 Melt the ghee and a little water in a large, heavy saucepan with a lid over medium heat, then add the onion and cook until soft. Add the garlic, coriander seeds, turmeric powder, and chili flakes and stir. Add the sweet potato and celeriac, cover, reduce the heat, and let sweat for 5 minutes, making sure they don't discolor. Add the stock and bring to a boil, then reduce the heat, cover, and simmer over low heat for 30 minutes, or until the vegetables are tender.

2 Remove the pan from the heat, let the soup cool slightly, season with salt and black pepper to taste, and use an electric hand blender to blend to a smooth consistency. Alternatively, purée the soup in several batches in a food processor or blender.

3 Transfer the soup to 6 serving bowls, stir a spoonful of yogurt into each portion, drizzle each with a little pumpkin oil, scatter with cilantro, and serve.

QUAIL SOUP

⚡ **BOOSTS IRON STORES TO COMBAT FATIGUE**   ♥ **HELPS IMPROVE CIRCULATION**   △ **PROMOTES EFFICIENT METABOLISM**   ⊃ **HELPS STRENGTHEN THE IMMUNE SYSTEM**

This cold-weather soup is best eaten at lunchtime; quail meat, shiitake mushrooms, goji berries, and astragalus root are all well known for being traditional tonics that help boost energy levels and improve circulation. They can also support the lungs, spleen, and kidneys, building resistance to infections, lowering the rate of perspiration, and reducing water retention.

SERVES 4–6

2 quails

¼oz (10g) astragalus root, or astragalus root powder

6 shallots, trimmed but with skins on

3 garlic cloves, with skins on

1 large carrot, sliced

10 black peppercorns

½oz (15g) goji berries, washed

7oz (200g) shiitake mushrooms, sliced

a large piece of wakame or nori seaweed, cut into small pieces

1 tbsp barley miso paste

1¾oz (50g) buckwheat noodles, to thicken

a large sprig of flat-leaf parsley, finely chopped

1 Place the quails in a large Dutch oven, add the astragalus root, shallots, garlic, carrot, and peppercorns, cover with water, and bring to a boil. Turn the heat down, half-cover the pot with the lid, and simmer on very low heat for 1½ hours.

2 Remove the pot from the heat, remove the quails, and set aside to cool slightly. Strain the soup through a sieve and reserve the liquid. Discard the astragalus root and carrot slices and reserve the rest of the ingredients in the sieve. Measure the soup and return it to the pot.

3 When the quails are cool enough to handle, carefully remove the meat from the bone, shred it with 2 forks, and return it to the pot. If the birds are from wild stock, look for lead shot and discard any shot you find while you shred the meat. Squeeze the garlic cloves and shallots from their skins directly into the soup.

4 Adjust the quantity of soup by adding more water if needed to make 3½ cups of soup. Bring the soup back to a boil, add the goji berries, and lower the heat to a simmer.

5 Add the shiitake mushrooms, followed by the wakame seaweed and barley miso paste. Let the soup simmer for 10 minutes, then add the buckwheat noodles and let them cook through for 5–7 minutes.

6 Pour into serving bowls, garnish with the parsley, and serve with some rye bread on the side.

QUAIL
copper and iron

SHIITAKE MUSHROOMS
panthothenic acid (vitamin B$_5$)

GOJI BERRIES
pyridoxine (vitamin B$_6$)

INCREASE YOUR ENERGY

THESE THREE FOODS, ARMED WITH THEIR RESPECTIVE NUTRIENTS, HELP BOOST THE METABOLISM'S ABILITY TO GENERATE ENERGY.

BUTTERNUT SQUASH SOUP

AIDS HEALTHY DIGESTION

SUPPORTS HEALTHY LUNG FUNCTION

HELPS STRENGTHEN THE IMMUNE SYSTEM

PROMOTES A SENSE OF WELL-BEING

Squash has fiber, which benefits the stomach and digestive system. It's a good choice if you have allergies or food sensitivities, because it's nonallergenic. Squash is also rich in beta-carotene to strengthen lungs, pancreas, and spleen. Combined with garlic, onions, and spices, this makes an immune-boosting meal. Both lemongrass and coconut milk add a mental and emotional uplift.

SERVES 6

2 tbsp olive oil

3 small onions, finely chopped

2¼lb (1kg) butternut squash, seeded and cut into small chunks

5½ cups vegetable stock

4 kaffir lime leaves

1 stalk lemongrass, bruised

2 garlic cloves

¾ cup coconut milk

zest and juice of 1 lime

salt and freshly ground black pepper

a few sprigs of cilantro leaves, to garnish

1 lime, cut into 6 wedges with a cut across the center of each wedge, to serve

1 Heat the olive oil in a large saucepan, add the onions, and sauté over low heat for 2–3 minutes, or until they are translucent. Add the squash and cook over medium heat, stirring occasionally until the vegetables are softened at the edges. Add the stock, kaffir lime leaves, lemongrass, and garlic. Bring to a boil, then lower the heat. Simmer for 30 minutes or so, or until the squash is cooked through, but still retains some shape.

2 Remove the kaffir lime leaves and lemongrass and discard. Add the coconut milk and bring back to a boil. Remove from the heat, add the lime zest, and season with salt and black pepper to taste. Pour the soup into a food processor or blender, and purée to a smooth consistency. Add some fresh lime juice to taste, pour into bowls, and garnish with the fresh cilantro. Just before serving, fix a lime wedge to the rim of every bowl for each person to add a little extra lime juice, if they like.

TIP: Keep the skin on the butternut squash to take advantage of the extra fiber, especially if it is a young one. Once cooked and blended the texture will become smooth.

Coconut milk (p49) *is rich in antioxidants, such as beta-carotene, and bowel-healthy fiber.*

ADZUKI BEAN SOUP

 HAS A DIURETIC ACTION   **AIDS HEALTHY DIGESTION**   **HELPS MAINTAIN ENERGY LEVELS**

Tangerine peel is thought to aid digestion and so is excellent in combination with adzuki beans, which are also known to benefit digestive health, eliminate toxins, and reduce water retention, particularly in women who are menstruating. They also help sustain energy levels. This is an unblended, chunky soup, so it's up to you how small you want to chop the vegetables.

SERVES 4–6

1 tangerine or orange

4oz (115g) adzuki beans

2 tbsp olive oil

4 shallots, finely chopped

1 medium leek, chopped

2 carrots, finely diced

2 garlic cloves, crushed

2 celery stalks, finely diced

4 medium tomatoes, skinned and finely chopped

1 tsp tomato paste

2½–3 cups chicken or vegetable stock

2 bay leaves

2 zucchini, finely diced

2 tbsp finely chopped parsley

salt and freshly ground black pepper

2 tbsp finely chopped basil leaves, to garnish

1 Using a potato peeler, remove the peel from the tangerine or orange and arrange it on a baking sheet. Leave the sheet in the oven on a low temperature (225°F/110°C) for 1 hour, or until the skin has dried. Grind the peel to a powder in a pestle and mortar, or leave whole and remove at the end of cooking.

2 If you are using dried adzuki beans, soak them following package instructions, then drain, discarding the soaking water. Place the beans in a saucepan, cover with fresh water, bring to a boil, simmer for 15 minutes, and drain. If using canned beans, simply drain and rinse.

3 Meanwhile, heat the olive oil in another large saucepan and sauté the shallots over low heat until they soften. Add the leek, carrots, and garlic, stir, and cook for 2–3 minutes. Add the celery, allow to soften, then add the tomatoes and tomato paste. Cook for 5–10 minutes, or until soft. Add the adzuki beans to the onion and tomato mixture.

4 Pour in the stock, add the bay leaves and dried tangerine peel, and bring to a boil. Reduce the heat immediately and let simmer slowly for 30 minutes, then add the zucchini and parsley. Simmer for a further 10 minutes, then remove the bay leaves and whole peel, if using. Season with salt and black pepper to taste, and serve in bowls garnished with the basil. Serve with rye bread on the side.

Light Meals and Salads

LIGHT DOESN'T HAVE TO MEAN INSUBSTANTIAL. ENJOY A FUSION OF **FRESH** INGREDIENTS, **THERAPEUTIC** HERBS, AND FLAVORFUL SPICES THAT **HEAL** AND SATISFY YOUR NEED FOR **SUSTAINED ENERGY**.

Raw Curly Kale Salad

 HAS ANTICANCER PROPERTIES   **HELPS REMOVE TOXINS FROM THE BODY**   **PROTECTS AGAINST COLDS AND FLU**   **HELPS IMPROVE CIRCULATION**

Kale is rich in antioxidant, anti-inflammatory, and anticancer nutrients. It also contains sulfur, making it an ideal food to help detox the body, and is known to help lower "unhealthy" (LDL) cholesterol levels in the blood. Leaving the dressed leaves to stand for 30 minutes softens them and makes cooking unnecessary, but if they are large and tough, steam them first for just 5 minutes.

SERVES 2

1lb 2oz (500g) kale, stems removed
juice of 1 lemon
2 tsp coriander seeds
¼ small lemon (with peel on)
2 avocados, pits removed, peeled
2 tbsp olive oil
salt and freshly ground black pepper
1 red chile, seeded and minced
4 garlic cloves, minced

1 Place the kale in a large bowl and sprinkle with the lemon juice. Using your hands, toss the leaves to coat them thoroughly in the lemon juice. Set aside for 30 minutes to let the kale soften.

2 Place the coriander seeds and lemon quarter in a blender or food processor and pulse briefly. Add the avocados, olive oil, salt, and black pepper and purée to a paste.

3 Transfer to the large bowl. Add the minced chile and garlic, and stir until well combined and the kale is thoroughly coated. Set aside for 15–30 minutes for the flavors to develop fully and to enhance the availability of the nutrients. Serve.

Avocados (p50) contain healthy monounsaturated fat, which helps in lowering blood pressure and lubricating joints.

QUAIL EGG AND ENDIVE SALAD

 HELPS MAINTAIN ENERGY LEVELS

 TONES AND CLEANSES THE LIVER

 HELPS IMPROVE CIRCULATION

Known in the East as "animal ginseng," quail eggs have a sweet flavor and are very nutritious. They are an excellent energy-giving food, helping to improve the circulatory system, which in turn strengthens muscles and bones. Here the eggs are combined with Belgian endive leaves, which have a slightly bitter taste and act as a gentle stimulant and tonic for the liver.

SERVES 4

12 quail eggs

salt and freshly ground black pepper

5½oz (150g) assorted lettuce leaves

1 medium avocado, peeled and sliced

2 medium heads of Belgian endive, leaves separated

1½ cups cherry tomatoes, halved

a large handful of cilantro leaves, roughly chopped

For the dressing

2oz (60g) feta cheese

¼ cup extra virgin olive oil

1 large garlic clove, crushed

2 tbsp lemon juice

1 tsp green peppercorns in brine, drained, with a little extra brine

2 tbsp roughly chopped parsley leaves

1 To make the dressing, cut the feta cheese into small cubes and place them in a small bowl or screwtop glass jar. Pour over the olive oil, garlic, and lemon juice. Add the green peppercorns together with a little of their brine and the chopped parsley. Stir gently to combine well and leave for 3–4 hours for the flavors to develop.

2 Put the quail eggs in a saucepan, cover with water, add a pinch of salt, and bring to a boil. Cook in the boiling water for 3 minutes, then drain and rinse under cold water to prevent the yolks from discoloring. Remove the eggshells.

3 Arrange the lettuce, avocado slices, endive leaves, and cherry tomatoes on 4 serving plates. Slice the eggs in half and divide them among each portion. Spoon the feta cheese dressing over the salad, garnish with the chopped cilantro leaves, season with salt and black pepper, and serve.

Quail eggs *are high in phosphorus— essential for cell membranes, and strong bones and teeth.*

Adzuki And Mung Bean Salad

 HELPS MAINTAIN WATER BALANCE

 PROTECTS THE HEART AND BLOOD VESSELS

 HELPS REMOVE TOXINS FROM THE BODY

 HELPS CONTROL BODY TEMPERATURE

Both adzuki and mung beans have diuretic properties and can help reduce water retention, particularly in the lower abdomen and legs. In addition, they can benefit the heart and vascular systems, and help the body eliminate toxins. Mung beans are also known to cool the body's internal temperature, so they are a useful food to eat if you are suffering from heatstroke.

SERVES 4

³/₄ cup dried adzuki beans

³/₄ cup dried mung beans

6 garlic cloves with skins on

1 lemon, sliced in half

2 bay leaves

1¹/₃ cups cherry tomatoes, sliced in half

a pinch of salt

For the dressing

2 garlic cloves, peeled

juice of ½ lemon

juice of ½ lime

¹/₃ cup extra virgin olive oil

a handful of basil leaves, coarsely torn into shreds

a handful of flat-leaf parsley leaves, chopped

a handful of mint leaves, chopped

1 Soak the beans following package directions, then drain and rinse in cold water. Transfer to a large saucepan and add the garlic, lemon, and bay leaves. Pour over plenty of water, bring to a boil, and simmer for about 1 hour over low heat until the beans are cooked.

2 Meanwhile, preheat the oven to 350°F (180°C). Arrange the tomato halves on a greased baking sheet, sprinkle with a little salt, and roast in the oven for 15–20 minutes.

3 To make the dressing, pound the garlic with the lemon and lime juices using a mortar and pestle. Slowly add the extra virgin olive oil and herbs until all the ingredients are combined. Keep the dressing ready to pour over the hot beans as soon as they are cooked.

4 Drain the beans and remove the lemon, garlic, and bay leaves. Reserve the garlic cloves, if you like, and squeeze the softened garlic paste into the dressing. Discard the rest of the flavorings. Toss the hot beans in the dressing, add the tomatoes, and set aside until cool to serve as a light summer salad.

SUPPORT YOUR HEART

THE GARLIC CLOVES IN THIS RECIPE PROVIDE A HIGH DOSE OF THE COMPOUND ALLICIN, WHICH CAN HELP LOWER CHOLESTEROL AND PROMOTE HEART HEALTH.

Herring With Cucumber And Seaweed Salad

 HAS A DIURETIC ACTION   **HELPS REMOVE TOXINS FROM THE BODY**   **HELPS IMPROVE CIRCULATION**   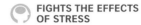 **FIGHTS THE EFFECTS OF STRESS**

This dish offers the health-boosting properties of seaweed and oily fish. Seaweed has a diuretic effect, helping to detoxify the body, and also helps protect blood vessels and fight the effects of stress. The omega-3 fatty acids and vitamin D in herring benefit the heart and blood circulation, too. If you can't find a packaged seaweed mix, try using nori and dulse seaweeds.

SERVES 4

1 package of dried mixed seaweed vegetables (approximately scant 1oz/25g)

½ cup dry white wine

juice of 2 limes

1 tsp coriander seeds, crushed

1 tbsp white wine vinegar

½ tsp salt

2 kaffir lime leaves

4 fresh herring fillets, about 3½oz (100g) each

1 cucumber, thinly sliced

3½oz (100g) red clover sprouts

1 carrot, peeled and julienned

4 lemon wedges, to garnish.

For the dressing

1 tbsp tamari soy sauce

1 tsp honey

2 tsp rice vinegar

2 tbsp finely chopped dill leaves, plus extra to garnish

1 Rinse the seaweed vegetables in a colander under running water, place in a bowl, and cover with tepid water. Set aside to reconstitute for at least 15 minutes or until soft, then drain.

2 Place the white wine, lime juice, coriander seeds, white wine vinegar, salt, kaffir lime leaves, and ½ cup water in a medium saucepan and bring to a slow boil. Turn the heat down low, let the ingredients simmer for 2–3 minutes, then turn the heat down again to its lowest setting, add the herring fillets, and let them poach for 10–12 minutes, or until cooked through. The fish are cooked when their flesh is opaque. If you like, you can reserve the poaching liquid, thicken it with 1 tablespoon of kudzu (a popular Asian thickener) or all-purpose flour or cornstarch, and serve it as a warm sauce to pour over the fish and seaweed and vegetable salad.

3 Meanwhile, combine all the ingredients for the dressing in a small bowl. Place the reconstituted seaweed, cucumber slices, red clover sprouts, and julienned carrot in a large bowl, pour over the dressing, and mix well.

4 Divide the salad among 4 serving plates and place a herring fillet on top of each. Garnish with a little more dill and the lemon wedges.

Swiss Chard And Sweet Potato

 HELPS FIGHT INFLAMMATION　　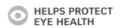 **HELPS MAINTAIN WATER BALANCE**　　 **HELPS PROTECT EYE HEALTH**　　 **AIDS HEALTHY DIGESTION**

Here's a different way of serving leafy, fiber-rich Swiss chard, which is high in vitamin K and antioxidant carotenoids. Its slightly bitter taste fades with cooking, and marries well with the sweet potato in a dish that helps relieve inflammation and dryness in the body, for instance in the mouth, skin, nose, and lungs, supports eye health, and improves digestion. This also makes a great side dish.

SERVES 4

1 tbsp olive oil, plus extra to drizzle

2 shallots, peeled and finely chopped

1 tsp coriander seeds, crushed

1 chile, seeded and finely chopped

2 garlic cloves, minced

2 large sweet potatoes, peeled and cubed

9oz (250g) Swiss chard, stalks removed and finely chopped, and leaves finely sliced

salt and freshly ground black pepper

1 Heat the olive oil with a tablespoon of water over low heat in a medium saucepan with a lid. Add the shallots and coriander seeds and cook, stirring occasionally, until the shallots have softened.

2 Add the chile and garlic, and cook for 1 minute. Add the sweet potato and cook over medium heat for about 5 minutes, adding a dash of water if necessary. Then add the chopped chard stalks, cover with the lid, and cook for 10 minutes.

3 When the sweet potato is almost cooked, add the shredded chard leaves, cover, and let them wilt for about 3 minutes. Season with salt and black pepper, drizzle over a few drops of olive oil, and serve.

Swiss chard *is a good source of phytonutrients that help protect the pancreas and balance blood sugar.*

SPINACH AND RICOTTA FILO ROLLS

 HELPS COMBAT ANEMIA   **AIDS HEALTHY DIGESTION**   **HELPS PROTECT EYE HEALTH**   **HELPS RELIEVE DRYNESS AND ITCHING**

The primary therapeutic benefit of this iron-rich dish is to help build the red blood cells that carry oxygen throughout the body and help improve anemia. It can also assist digestion and help moisten the lungs and colon. Spinach is often recommended in cases of night blindness and hypertension while soft cheese also has a moistening effect on dry, itchy skin.

SERVES 4

1lb 2oz (500g) ricotta cheese

5 large eggs

a pinch of salt

1lb 2oz (500g) young spinach leaves, roughly chopped

½ cup crème fraîche

2 tbsp olive oil

1 package store-bought filo pastry

thick or Greek-style yogurt, to serve

1 Preheat the oven to 400°F (200°C). In a large bowl, mix the ricotta cheese with the eggs and salt. Add the spinach and crème fraîche and mix well.

2 Grease a square baking dish with a little olive oil. Lay a large piece of parchment paper on a flat surface and place a sheet of filo pastry on it with one of the longer edges facing you. Drizzle the pastry with a few drops of olive oil and spread a thin layer of the spinach, egg, and cheese filling over it. Roll up the pastry sheet into a neat roll, pushing it away from you, and using the parchment paper to help you. Transfer the roll to the baking dish, curving the ends up if the dish is smaller than the length of the pastry sheet.

3 Repeat with the rest of the filo pastry sheets and filling. Drizzle a few drops of olive oil over the rolls and bake for 30–40 minutes, or until the rolls are golden on top and the filling is cooked through. Serve with some thick yogurt on the side.

Spinach (p67) is famous for its iron content, which is more easily absorbed by the body when cooked.

TROUT AND LETTUCE WRAPS

 AIDS HEALTHY DIGESTION   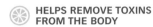 **HELPS REMOVE TOXINS FROM THE BODY**   **HELPS LOWER CHOLESTEROL**

This dish enhances digestion and can aid weight reduction. In addition, cooling lettuce has detoxifying properties and mangoes can help relieve symptoms of motion sickness, while the omega-3 fatty acids in trout bring cardiovascular benefits. Using a bed of fresh rosemary, fennel, or dill leaves on which to broil the trout gives them a fragrant, smoky aroma.

SERVES 4

8 large lettuce leaves, such as romaine, butter, escarole, or iceberg, or use 12 leaves of Little Gem lettuce

2 trout (12oz/350g each), filleted

a bunch of rosemary sprigs

a bunch of fennel or dill fronds

a dash of olive oil

a pinch of salt

2 tbsp pumpkin seeds

For the filling

1 large mango, peeled, seed removed and discarded, flesh cubed

a bunch of cilantro leaves, chopped

3 tbsp scallions, finely chopped

1¾ cups cherry tomatoes, halved

1 small chile, seeded and minced

1 tbsp olive oil

½ tbsp lemon juice

salt and freshly ground black pepper

1 If using large lettuce leaves, remove any thick veins so they can be folded over without breaking.

2 Preheat the broiler to high. Score the trout fillets with several diagonal cuts through the skin along their length to prevent them curling up while being broiled. Line the broiler pan with sprigs of rosemary and large fronds of fennel or dill. Arrange the trout fillets skin-side up on top and drizzle with olive oil rubbing it into the skins. Season the fish with salt and place under the hot broiler. Broil for 4–5 minutes, or until the skin is crisp and the flesh is cooked through and flakes when tested with a fork. Remove the fillets from the broiler and allow to cool.

3 To make the filling, combine the mango cubes, cilantro leaves, scallions, tomatoes, and chile in a bowl. Add the olive oil, lemon juice, and salt and black pepper, mix together gently, and set aside.

4 To toast the pumpkin seeds, heat a small saucepan over medium heat. Add the pumpkin seeds and dry-fry for 2–3 minutes, or until they darken slightly and give off a fragrant aroma. Shake the pan regularly and stir the seeds with a wooden spoon as you heat them. Cut the cooled trout fillets into squares and gently fold them into the filling.

5 To make the wraps, divide the filling between the lettuce leaves, placing a little in the middle of each leaf. Sprinkle some toasted pumpkin seeds on top and fold the edges of each lettuce leaf up and over the filling. Use a toothpick to secure each wrap. If using small leaves, such as Little Gem lettuce, don't wrap the filling but use the leaves like a scoop to enjoy the filling. Arrange the wraps on a plate to serve.

Stuffed Vine Leaves

 AIDS HEALTHY DIGESTION

 HAS A DIURETIC ACTION

Dark green vine leaves contain fiber, vitamins, and minerals, including vitamins C and K, folate, and manganese. These nutrients help reduce water retention and benefit the urinary system, and together with pine nuts, almonds, and mint they also benefit the digestive system. The leaves have a subtle acidic flavor and soft texture similar to spinach once cooked.

SERVES 4

30 vine leaves, or Swiss chard leaves, stalks removed

¾ cup white or brown basmati rice

4 shallots, minced

3 tbsp olive oil

2 tbsp pine nuts, toasted

2 tbsp sliced almonds, toasted

2 tbsp raisins

2 tbsp finely chopped mild mint leaves

1 tsp smoked paprika

salt and freshly ground black pepper

2½ cups vegetable stock or broth

1 tbsp tomato paste

1 tbsp lemon juice

thin lemon wedges, to serve

1 Preheat the oven to 350°F (180°C). Blanch the vine leaves by immersing them in a large saucepan of boiling salted water for 30 seconds, then quickly rinse in cold water to halt the cooking process, drain, and set aside. Cook the rice following package directions.

2 Heat a thin layer of water in a saucepan, add the shallots, and stir for about 5 minutes until they have softened. Stir in the cooked rice, olive oil, pine nuts, sliced almonds, raisins, mint, and smoked paprika, and season with salt and black pepper. Remove from the heat and allow the mixture to cool before handling it.

3 Arrange some of the vine leaves, vein-side up, on a flat surface. Place a small ball of the filling at one end of each leaf, fold 3 sides of the leaf up over the filling, and roll into a cylindrical parcel. Place each parcel, with the loose end of the vine leaf facing down, in an ovenproof dish with a lid. Repeat with the rest of the vine leaves and filling. Arrange the parcels tightly together to stop them from unfolding while cooking.

4 Heat the stock in a small saucepan, add the tomato paste and lemon juice, mix well, bring to a boil, and gently pour the hot stock over the stuffed vine leaves. Cover them with a small ovenproof plate to keep them in place and then cover with the lid. Cook in the oven for 1 hour, or until all the liquid has been soaked up. Transfer the stuffed vine leaves to a serving dish, decorate with lemon wedges, and serve.

Vine leaves are rich in antioxidants and are a traditional remedy for pain and inflammation.

NORI VEGETABLE ROLL

 HAS NATURAL SEDATIVE PROPERTIES   **PROMOTES BOWEL REGULARITY**   **HELPS MAINTAIN ENERGY LEVELS** 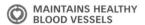 **MAINTAINS HEALTHY BLOOD VESSELS**

Brown rice and red quinoa, which both have a nutty flavor, are known to have a calming effect on the nervous system. The high fiber content of brown rice also benefits digestion. Nori, like quinoa, is high in protein, keeping your energy levels higher for longer. It also helps strengthen blood vessels. This wholesome dish is a practical food to eat on the go or serve as a picnic snack.

SERVES 4–6

¾ cup short grain brown rice

scant 1 cup red quinoa

¼ tsp Himalayan pink salt or other natural salt

1 tbsp rice vinegar

1 tbsp mirin sauce

1–2 tbsp sesame seeds

6–8 sheets of nori, toasted

1–2 tbsp toasted sesame oil

For the dipping sauce

1 tbsp tamari soy sauce

juice of 1 orange

For the filling

1 large avocado, pit removed, peeled, and cut into strips

1 carrot, peeled and julienned

¾in (2cm) fresh ginger, peeled and julienned

1 small chile, seeded and julienned

1 red bell pepper, seeded and julienned

1 celery stalk, julienned

1 small leek, white part only, julienned

1 Place the rice and quinoa in a large saucepan, add 2½ cups water and bring to a boil. Reduce the heat, cover, and simmer for 1 hour, or until the water is absorbed.

2 Remove the pan from the heat and add the Himalayan pink salt, rice vinegar, and mirin sauce. Combine well and set aside to infuse.

3 Meanwhile, toast the sesame seeds by dry-frying them in a saucepan until they turn golden, then set aside to cool. Combine the ingredients for the dipping sauce in a small bowl and set aside.

4 If you don't have a sushi roll mat, use a sheet of parchment paper slightly larger than the nori sheets (which will enable you to store the rolls for a few hours before serving) or you might find it just as easy to roll without either. To assemble a roll, place a sheet of nori, shiny-side down, on a clean, flat surface. Spread a thin layer of rice, about 2in (5cm) thick, on top of the sheet. Scatter with toasted sesame seeds and drizzle over a few drops of toasted sesame oil. Carefully arrange one or two of each of the sliced vegetables at one end of the nori sheet so that they all lie horizontally across the rice. Fold the nori sheet over the vegetables and continue to roll it up. Seal the end of the nori sheet by running a little water along the seam side with your finger. Repeat this process until you have the desired amount of rolls.

5 To serve, dip a serrated knife into water and slice the nori rolls into bite-sized pieces. Stand the rolls upright on a serving plate with the bowl of dipping sauce on the side.

CABBAGE MOMOS

 AIDS HEALTHY DIGESTION

 HELPS STRENGTHEN THE IMMUNE SYSTEM

 SUPPORTS HEALTHY LIVER FUNCTION

These dumplings, known as momos, are traditionally served at Bhutanese social gatherings. They can be filled with either meat or vegetables, but they are always served with a hot chile relish locally known as ezze (p195). Both cabbage and warming chile stimulate the digestion, help strengthen the immune system, combat seasonal infections, and cleanse the liver.

MAKES 24 MOMOS

For the filling

¼ medium cabbage, finely chopped

3 large onions, finely chopped

3 carrots, finely chopped

1 tbsp chopped lovage or celery leaves

1 tbsp chopped parsley or cilantro leaves

olive oil, for frying

¾ cup cream cheese (preferably home-made kefir cheese, p332)

2 garlic cloves, very finely crushed or powdered

1 tbsp soy sauce

¼ tsp salt

For the dough

2¾ cups whole wheat flour

2 large eggs, beaten

2 tsp baking powder

1 tsp salt

1 For the filling, fry the chopped vegetables, lovage or celery, and parsley or cilantro, in a very little olive oil over medium heat in a heated wok for 5–6 minutes. Stir in the cream or kefir cheese, garlic, soy sauce, and salt and set aside.

2 Make the dough for the momos by sifting the flour into a large bowl, adding the beaten eggs, and mixing lightly. Stir in ⅔ cup water and the baking powder and salt. Combine the ingredients well, then transfer the dough to a floured surface. Knead the dough lightly until smooth. Cover with a damp cloth and set aside for 5–10 minutes. This will allow the baking powder time to activate so that the momos swell when steaming.

3 Roll the dough into a large sausage and cut into 24 evenly sized pieces. Roll each piece into a thin circle 4in (9–10cm) wide. Place a tablespoonful of the filling in the center of the dough circle, gather the edges of the circle together, pinch the edges together with your fingers, and twist to seal. Repeat with the rest of the dough circles and filling.

4 Stand the momos in an oiled steaming basket. Place over a large saucepan of simmering water, cover, and steam for 12–14 minutes. If you don't own a steaming basket, place the momos in a heatproof colander or sieve over a saucepan filled with a 2in (5cm) layer of water; the base should not touch the water. Cover with the lid and bring the water to the boil; steam for 12–14 minutes. Serve the momos with Ezze relish (p195).

MUSHROOM FRITTATA WITH CHERRY TOMATOES AND BASIL

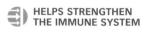 **HELPS STRENGTHEN THE IMMUNE SYSTEM**
 AIDS HEALTHY DIGESTION
 HELPS EASE RHEUMATIC PAIN
 PROTECTS THE HEART AND BLOOD VESSELS

This is an ideal meal if you are recuperating. Like other mushrooms, morels (*Morchella esculenta*) are rich in the essential amino acids the body needs to build protein, while shiitake and crimini mushrooms help improve digestion and have anti-inflammatory properties. Wash the morels thoroughly under running water because their spongelike caps often contain soil and grit.

SERVES 4

For the braised tomatoes

½ tbsp ghee, or clarified butter, for greasing

1½ cups ripe cherry tomatoes

salt and freshly ground black pepper

1 tbsp chopped fresh basil leaves, to garnish

For the frittata

scant 1oz (25g) dried morels, soaked in boiling water for 5 minutes to rehydrate, or 2½oz (75g) fresh morels, cleaned and finely chopped

3½oz (100g) shiitake mushrooms, sliced

3½oz (100g) crimini mushrooms, sliced

2 tbsp ghee

salt and freshly ground black pepper

2 tbsp finely chopped chives

8 large eggs, beaten

3 tbsp crème fraîche

1 Preheat the oven to 350°F (180°C). To braise the tomatoes, grease a baking sheet with the ghee, add the cherry tomatoes, season with salt and black pepper, and cook in the oven for 8–10 minutes, or until the tomatoes are cooked.

2 Meanwhile, place a large, nonstick skillet over medium heat and dry-fry all the mushrooms for 1–2 minutes to enhance their flavor, and allow them to release some of their moisture. Add 1 tablespoon of the ghee, let it melt, then sauté the mushrooms for 3–5 minutes, adding salt and black pepper to taste. Add half the chopped chives, reserving the rest to use as a garnish. Remove the mushrooms from the skillet and set aside.

3 Beat together the eggs and crème fraîche in a medium bowl with a little more salt and black pepper to taste. Melt the remaining tablespoon of ghee in the pan and pour in the egg mixture. Cook for 2–3 minutes over low heat until the base is firm, then add the mushrooms and cover to cook for 3–5 minutes, or until both the underside and top of the frittata are set.

4 To serve, scatter with the rest of the chives, divide among 4 serving plates, and add the braised cherry tomatoes. Garnish the tomatoes with the basil and serve immediately.

Buckwheat Pancakes With Nettles And Feta Cheese

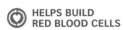 **HELPS BUILD RED BLOOD CELLS**   **HELPS ALLEVIATE DRY COUGHS** 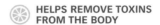 **HELPS REMOVE TOXINS FROM THE BODY**   **PROMOTES A HEALTHY COMPLEXION**

When combined, nettles and buckwheat enrich the blood, helping to increase red blood cells and restore metabolic balance. This dish is ideal for anyone with anemia, a dry cough, or a weak constitution. It can also aid those in need of a detox, or recovering from a long illness. Young nettles in spring are best, because they are small yet potent; wear gloves to gather them.

SERVES 4

For the pancakes

1–1¼ cups buckwheat flour

a pinch of salt

1 large egg

¼ cup milk

1 tbsp olive oil

1 tsp butter, plus extra for greasing

For the filling

3½oz (100g) young nettle leaves, finely chopped

3½oz (100g) feta cheese

3 large eggs

3½oz (100g) ricotta cheese

2 tbsp crème fraîche

a pinch of salt

1 Add the flour to a mixing bowl along with the salt, and make a well in the center. Crack the egg into the well and add the milk. Using a wooden spoon, stir the egg and milk, letting the flour gradually tumble in. Gradually add ⅓–½ cup water, little by little, stirring continuously until all the flour has been incorporated and the mixture is lump-free. If necessary, adjust the liquids or add a little more flour. If you have time, place the batter in the refrigerator to rest for 30 minutes to allow the milled grain to swell, which helps make the batter light and not heavy.

2 Preheat the oven to 350°F (180°C). Place the nettle leaves in a bowl and crumble in the feta cheese. Add the eggs, ricotta cheese, crème fraîche, and salt, combine all the ingredients together, and set aside.

3 To make the pancakes, heat the olive oil and butter in a medium skillet. When hot enough, add a ladle of the batter and swirl it around in the pan to make a thin pancake. Cook for 2–3 minutes, or until golden, then toss or turn the pancake and cook on the other side. Repeat until you have 8 pancakes.

4 Spread some of the filling over a pancake and roll it up. Repeat with the rest of the pancakes and the filling, then arrange all the pancake rolls in a buttered baking dish. Pour the remaining filling over the pancakes, and bake in the preheated oven for 20–25 minutes until cooked through and golden in appearance. The filling may ooze out of the pancakes during cooking, but this won't detract from the final look or flavor of the dish. Serve hot with a salad.

Buckwheat flour (p113) *is rich in natural antioxidants that help protect the heart.*

ARTICHOKES IN A SWEET SPICY SAUCE

 HAS A MILD DIURETIC ACTION

 HELPS LOWER CHOLESTEROL

SUPPORTS HEALTHY LIVER FUNCTION

PROMOTES A HEALTHY COMPLEXION

Globe artichokes are not only good to eat, they are a therapeutic herb—a bitter digestive remedy that helps stimulate and strengthen the urinary system and support the liver. Artichokes also help with fat metabolism and can reduce "unhealthy" (LDL) cholesterol levels in the blood. The hot sauce supports detoxification, which in turn can help improve the condition of the skin.

SERVES 4

4–8 artichokes

2 tbsp lemon juice

½ tsp salt

1 garlic clove, finely chopped

2 tbsp dry white wine

2 tbsp olive oil

2 cups quinoa, rinsed and soaked until sprouted (p204)

salt and freshly ground black pepper

3 tbsp pine nuts, toasted (optional)

3 tbsp fresh pomegranate seeds (optional)

For the dressing

¼ cup roasted sesame oil

⅔ cup Marsala wine

2 tbsp teriyaki sauce

3 tbsp fresh orange juice

2 garlic cloves, minced

1 medium-hot chile, seeded and minced

2 tbsp finely chopped flat-leaf parsley leaves

2 tbsp chopped lemon thyme leaves

1 Trim the artichoke heads by removing the tough outer scales to expose the paler, softer leaves, and cutting away the spiky leaves on the top. If the artichokes have their stems intact, peel off the stringy outer layer with a sharp knife. Slice each artichoke in half lengthwise and scrape away the furry choke with a spoon. Place the artichokes in a large bowl of water with the lemon juice to stop them from discoloring.

2 Bring a large saucepan of water to a boil. Turn the heat down, add the salt, garlic, wine, olive oil, and artichoke halves and poach gently for 20 minutes. Remove the artichokes from the water and drain.

3 Heat the sesame oil with 2 tablespoons of water in another large saucepan, and add the artichoke halves. Let them brown gently for 2–3 minutes, then remove and set aside.

4 Add the Marsala wine, teriyaki sauce, orange juice, garlic, and chile to the pan. Mix the ingredients briefly, then add the parsley and thyme, and remove the pan from the heat.

5 To assemble the dish, divide the sprouted quinoa among 4 serving plates and season with salt and black pepper. Swirl a spoonful of the sauce over the sprouted quinoa and arrange 1–2 artichoke halves on top of each portion. Spoon more sauce over the artichokes, sprinkle with toasted pine nuts and pomegranate seeds, if using, and serve.

TIP: Start to sprout the quinoa 1–3 days ahead, depending on how big you like the sprouts. Rinse and drain the quinoa every 8–12 hours.

***Artichokes** (p62) support immune function by detoxifying the liver and gallbladder.*

WILD RICE SALAD

 PROTECTS AGAINST FREE-RADICAL DAMAGE   **AIDS HEALTHY DIGESTION** 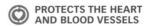 **PROTECTS THE HEART AND BLOOD VESSELS**

Black wild rice, which was once cultivated solely for China's emperors to consume, is a nutritious protein and antioxidant-rich grain with a nutty taste and chewy texture. Rice is classified as a sweet, neutral food in Chinese medicine, and is eaten to ease many stomach and digestive problems including diarrhea, indigestion, and constipation. Its fiber helps protect the heart.

SERVES 4

³/₄ cup black wild rice

1 cup vegetable or chicken stock

a pinch of salt

2 kaffir lime leaves

1 tsp orange zest

1 tsp lemon zest

¼ cup sun-dried tomatoes, chopped

1 large red pepper, seeded and diced

2 tbsp chopped cilantro leaves

For the dressing

2 tbsp basil oil

1 tbsp blackberry vinegar

a pinch of salt

1 Rinse the rice in cold water, drain, and transfer to a medium saucepan. Add the stock, salt, kaffir lime leaves, and citrus zest. Bring to a boil, then cover, reduce the heat, and simmer for 25–30 minutes, or until the rice is cooked and water has been absorbed.

2 Meanwhile, make the dressing. Place all the ingredients in a bowl or jar with a screwtop lid, add 1 tablespoon water, and mix well. When the rice is cooked pour the dressing over the rice while it is still hot, stir in the sun-dried tomatoes, and set aside until the rice has cooled.

3 When the rice is cold, mix in the chopped pepper. Garnish with the cilantro leaves, and serve.

FRESH CILANTRO LEAF PESTO WITH PASTA

 HELPS ELIMINATE TRACES OF METALS

 PROTECTS AGAINST NEURODEGENERATION

 AIDS HEALTHY DIGESTION

 PROTECTS THE HEART AND BLOOD VESSELS

This dish offers the detoxifying properties of fresh cilantro, which is a good chelating agent, helping to remove traces of heavy metals from the body. High levels of heavy metals are implicated in certain arthritic conditions, depression, memory loss, muscle pain, and weakness. Coriander seeds aid digestion, and pine nuts, cashews, and almonds help support heart health.

SERVES 4

a large bunch of organic cilantro leaves

1/3 cup olive oil

1 garlic clove

1/4 tsp ground coriander

2 tbsp blanched almonds

2 tbsp cashews

2 tbsp pine nuts

2 tbsp lemon juice

8oz (225g) fresh pasta, such as spelt spaghetti

1 scant cup sun-dried tomatoes in olive oil, drained and chopped

freshly ground black pepper

grated Parmesan cheese, to garnish

a small handful of chopped cilantro leaves, to garnish

1 Place the cilantro leaves and olive oil in a food processor or blender and purée until finely blended. Add the garlic, ground coriander, almonds, cashews, pine nuts, and lemon juice, and purée the ingredients to a paste. Alter the consistency and flavor of the pesto slightly, if you like, by adding a little more olive oil and/or lemon juice keeping to a 3:1 ratio of oil to juice.

2 Cook the pasta following package directions and drain. Immediately stir the pesto through the hot pasta so it melts, then add the sun-dried tomatoes, and toss the ingredients together. Season with black pepper. Scatter generously with grated Parmesan and cilantro leaves to serve.

PINE NUTS
Contain more vitamin K than other nuts, which helps protect arteries.

ALMONDS
Rich in monounsaturated oleic acid, a healthy fat that helps protect against heart disease.

CASHEWS
High in potassium, which helps you maintain a steady heartbeat.

HELP FIGHT HEART DISEASE
THREE ANTIOXIDANT-RICH NUTS SUPPORT ARTERIES, STRENGTHEN BLOOD VESSELS, AND LOWER BLOOD PRESSURE.

Braised Red Chicory And Celery Heart Salad

 AIDS DETOXIFICATION SYSTEM

 PROMOTES A HEALTHY DIGESTIVE TRACT

 HELPS MAINTAIN WATER BALANCE

 HAS NATURAL SEDATIVE PROPERTIES

A detoxifying meal with significant benefits for the body. Chicory, which has a bitter taste, stimulates digestion, improves both gallbladder and liver function, and cleanses the urinary tract. Celery helps regulate the body's water balance. Both vegetables are a good source of fiber and have important sedative and stress-relieving properties. This recipe makes a perfect side dish.

SERVES 4

1 tbsp olive oil

2 long (or banana) shallots, finely chopped

2 garlic cloves, minced

1 small chile, seeded and finely chopped

1 large bunch of celery, split into inner and outer stalks, with inner stalks finely chopped

8 heads of red chicory, halved lengthwise

1 tsp chopped lemon thyme leaves

salt and white pepper

1 Preheat the oven to 350°F (180°C). Heat the oil with a tablespoon of water in a medium saucepan over medium heat. Add the shallots, allow to soften, then add the garlic, chile, and chopped inner stalks of celery, or celery hearts, and cook for 2–3 minutes.

2 Meanwhile, juice the outer stalks and leaves of the celery in a juicer. Add the celery juice to the pan.

3 Arrange the chicory halves in an ovenproof ceramic dish with a lid. Pour the shallot and celery mixture over the chicory, cover, and bake in the oven for 20 minutes.

4 Transfer the chicory halves to a serving plate. Pour the celery mixture into a small saucepan, bring to a boil, add the lemon thyme, and boil for 3 minutes to reduce the liquid. Season with salt and white pepper to taste, pour the mixture over the chicory halves, and serve.

Red chicory (p73) is a variant of blanched white chicory. It contains high amounts of volatile oils that aid digestion.

MAIN MEALS

MAKE SURE YOUR MAIN MEAL FORMS A **HEALTHY** CENTERPIECE TO YOUR DAY, WHATEVER TIME OF DAY YOU EAT IT. **FRESH** INGREDIENTS BALANCED FOR FLAVOR, COLOR, AND TEXTURE—AND MOST IMPORTANTLY **HEALING POWER**—ARE KEY.

SPROUTED QUINOA WITH VEGETABLES

 EASY TO DIGEST AND GLUTEN-FREE

 HELPS BALANCE BLOOD SUGAR LEVELS

 MAINTAINS HEALTHY BLOOD VESSELS

 HELPS PROTECT EYE HEALTH

Sprouted seeds and grains are not just a pretty garnish. This gluten-free, fiber-rich dish is easy to digest and helps keep blood sugar levels stable. It's packed with vitamins, minerals, amino acids, and beneficial digestive enzymes that helps us extract maximum nutrition from food. Bell peppers, yellow squash, and green mango supply antioxidants to support cardiovascular and eye health.

SERVES 4

2 tbsp broccoli seeds

2⅓ cups quinoa

1 large red bell pepper, seeded and finely diced

1 large orange bell pepper, seeded and finely diced

1 fennel bulb, finely diced

1 yellow squash, finely diced

1 small unripe mango, peeled, seeded, and finely diced

1 garlic clove, minced

juice of 1 lime

3 tbsp extra virgin olive oil

salt and freshly ground black pepper

1 To sprout the broccoli seeds, place them in a large glass jar, pour in enough tepid water to liberally cover the seeds, fasten cheesecloth over the mouth of the jar with an elastic band, and set aside overnight. The next morning, pour the water out through the cheesecloth, pour in more water to rinse the seeds, and drain. Leave the jar upside down at an angle of 45 degrees, away from direct sunlight, so the excess water can drain away. Repeat the rinsing process every morning and evening for 3–5 days depending on the room temperature and how quickly the seeds sprout. Once sprouted, store the seeds in a glass jar sealed with a lid in the refrigerator and consume within 1–2 days.

2 To sprout the quinoa, place the seeds in a large glass jar, pour in enough tepid water to liberally cover the seeds, fasten cheesecloth over the mouth of the jar, and set aside for 2 hours. Pour the water out through the cheesecloth, pour in more water to rinse the seeds, and drain. Leave the jar upside down at an angle of 45 degrees, away from direct sunlight, so the excess water can drain away. Repeat the rinsing process the following day and you may find that little shoots are already breaking through. The quinoa is ready when most of the seeds have sprouted.

3 To assemble the dish, combine all the sprouts and diced peppers, fennel, yellow squash, and mango in a large bowl.

4 In a small bowl, mix together the minced garlic, lime juice, and olive oil, and add a pinch of salt. Pour this dressing over the ingredients in the bowl, mix well, and add black pepper. Taste and adjust the seasoning if necessary before serving.

Yellow squash (p60) skin is rich in antioxidant carotenes, such as lutein, which promote healthy eyes.

SPICY RAW VEGETABLE SPAGHETTI

 HAS A DIURETIC ACTION   **PROMOTES CLEAR SKIN**   **HELPS EASE CONSTIPATION**   **PROMOTES DETOX AT CELL LEVEL**

Raw vegetables provide more enzymes, vitamins, and other essential nutrients than if cooked, and the combination of ingredients used here has a cleansing effect on the body. A spiralizer is a gadget that turns the vegetables into lovely spaghetti-like strands, which changes their texture—the root vegetables in particular taste surprisingly light and vibrant.

SERVES 4

a handful of pine nuts

2 tbsp furikake, or 1 tbsp each of black and white sesame seeds

2 carrots, peeled

2 medium beets, peeled

1 zucchini and 1 yellow squash, stalks removed

3 small radishes

a large bunch of fresh cilantro leaves, large stalks removed, and finely chopped

For the dressing

juice of 3 celery stalks (about ¼ cup)

1 tbsp hemp oil

2 tbsp pumpkin seed oil

1 tbsp fresh lemon juice

2 tsp tahini

salt and freshly ground black pepper

1 To make the dressing, combine all the ingredients together in a food processor or blender, then set aside.

2 To toast the pine nuts and sesame seeds, heat a small skillet over medium heat, add the pine nuts and seeds, and dry-fry, stirring until lightly golden.

3 Put the carrots, beets, zucchini, yellow squash, and radishes through a vegetable spiralizer to turn them into long, thick spaghetti-like strips. Or, use a vegetable peeler and cut them into long thick ribbons.

4 Place all the vegetable strips, except the beets, in a serving bowl and toss with the chopped cilantro leaves (adding the beets separately stops the whole salad from turning pink). Distribute among 4 serving plates, add the beets, pour over the dressing, scatter each portion with a few of the pine nuts and furikake or sesame seeds, and serve.

Furikake is a Japanese seasoning of sesame seeds, seaweed, and other flavorings. Sprinkling a little over a salad, rice, or noodles is a great way of increasing the nutrient density of a dish.

Mung Bean And Purple Broccoli Rabe Stir-fry

 SUPPORTS HEALTHY LIVER FUNCTION

 PROMOTE BOWEL REGULARITY

 HAS A DIURETIC ACTION

This dish is bursting with ingredients to strengthen the liver, which helps the body to eliminate toxic substances, clear blood vessels, and enhance bowel movements and urine output. Both Belgian endive and artichokes are known as remedies for issues relating to the liver; in traditional Chinese medicine, sour foods and leafy green foods are thought to help strengthen and cleanse the liver.

SERVES 4

¼ cup vegetable stock

1 tbsp tamari soy sauce

1 tbsp olive oil

¾in (2cm) piece of fresh ginger, peeled and julienned

1 small chile, seeded and julienned

2 medium carrots, peeled and julienned

14oz (400g) purple broccoli rabe, trimmed and chopped into florets

2½ cups mung bean sprouts

1 small green mango, seeded and julienned

4 large heads of Belgian endive, leaves separated

1 tbsp black sesame seeds

For the dressing

juice and zest of 1 lime

2 tbsp pumpkin oil

1 tsp whole grain mustard

1 tsp honey

1 To make the dressing, in a pitcher, combine the lime juice and zest, pumpkin oil, mustard, and honey, and set aside.

2 Place the vegetable stock in a wok and heat gently. Add the tamari soy sauce, olive oil, ginger, and chile, and stir. Add the carrots and broccoli, stir again, and add the mung bean sprouts and mango, and sauté for 1 more minute.

3 Divide the Belgian endive leaves among 4 serving plates, arranging them in a rosette. Spoon a small amount of stir-fried vegetables into the middle of each rosette. Drizzle with the dressing and scatter with black sesame seeds. Serve with boiled rice.

Purple broccoli rabe *(p51) is packed with immune-boosting antioxidants. Stir-frying it lightly, as here, will help retain all its benefits.*

MARINATED TUNA STEAKS

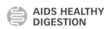 **AIDS HEALTHY DIGESTION**

PROTECTS THE HEART AND BLOOD VESSELS

Tuna steaks have an astringent quality and are traditionally used in Asia to soothe the digestive tract, while capers enhance this effect. This fish is a healthy choice for the heart if you want a substitute for red meat; its substantial flavor is deepened here by the addition of Japanese tamari soy sauce, which has more complex undertones than Chinese soy sauce.

SERVES 4

3 tbsp olive oil

2 tbsp tamari soy sauce

1 tbsp capers, rinsed

¼ cup Marsala wine or sweet sherry

1 tbsp whole grain mustard

2 garlic cloves, crushed

4 thin slices of lemon

4 tuna steaks

1 Place the olive oil, tamari soy sauce, capers, Marsala wine, mustard, garlic, and lemon slices in a ceramic baking dish and mix well. Add the tuna steaks and coat them in the marinade. Cover the dish with a lid or foil and leave in the fridge for 1 hour to marinate.

2 Preheat the oven to 350°F (180°C). Place the covered dish of tuna steaks in the oven and bake for 15–25 minutes. Cook the steaks lightly, turning them over after 10 minutes; thinner steaks will cook more quickly. To test if the fish is cooked, slice through a small section with a sharp knife; the center of the steak should still be slightly pink. Serve with steamed rice and salad or steamed vegetables.

Lemon (p40) aids good digestion and, with its antibacterial properties, also helps maintain a healthy urinary tract.

Sea Bass With Spinach And Mango

 HELPS COMBAT ANEMIA   **HELPS PROTECT EYE HEALTH**   **AIDS HEALTHY DIGESTION**   **HAS A DIURETIC ACTION**

This dish of firm-textured oily fish and iron-rich spinach helps lower blood pressure and prevent recurring headaches and dizziness. Antioxidants in the mango support healthy vision. The cooling effect of the spinach is balanced by the heat of chile, garlic, and ginger—all of which promote healthy circulation and digestion, and also help remove excess water from the body.

SERVES 4

4 sea bass, about 9oz (250g) each

a pinch of salt

3 tbsp finely chopped fresh ginger,

2 small chiles, seeded and minced

4 garlic cloves, minced

1 lemon, cut in half, with one half thinly sliced and the other half juiced

2 heaped tsp whole grain mustard

generous ⅓ cup olive oil

½ cup white wine

7oz (200g) spinach leaves

For the sauce

1 medium mango, peeled, seeded, and roughly chopped

2 tsp lime juice

1 tbsp olive oil

1 If you have time, soak the fish in a large bowl of salted water (1 tablespoon of salt to 3½ cups water) half an hour before cooking to clean them thoroughly. Preheat the oven to 350°F (180°C). Pat the fish dry with paper towel and place in a large ceramic baking dish. Sprinkle with the salt and pack the insides of the fish with the ginger, chile, and garlic. Arrange a few lemon slices on top of each fish. Blend the mustard, lemon juice, olive oil, and the wine (or ½ cup water) in a bowl and pour over the fish. Cover with foil and bake for 25–35 minutes, or until the fish flakes easily when you test it with a fork.

2 Meanwhile, prepare the sauce. Put the mango flesh, lime juice, and olive oil in a food processor or blender, pulse briefly, and set aside.

3 Boil a large saucepan of water, add the spinach, and cook for 30 seconds or until it wilts. Drain away the hot water, quickly rinse the spinach in cold water to halt the cooking process, then drain again very thoroughly. Place the sea bass on 4 serving plates. Divide the spinach into 4 portions, arranging it around the edge of each fish if you like. Drizzle a little of the mango sauce over the sea bass and serve the rest of the sauce in a small bowl on the side.

STUFFED PEPPERS

 HELPS STRENGTHEN THE IMMUNE SYSTEM   **HELPS IMPROVE CIRCULATION**

This vegetarian recipe is a substantial meal, with satisfying flavors equal to any meat dish. Bell peppers provide a broad range of antioxidant and anti-inflammatory nutrients that help improve circulation and build red blood cells, among other things. With the addition of mushrooms, garlic, and black pepper, this dish also helps enhance your resistance to seasonal infections.

SERVES 6

heaped ⅓ cup pine nuts

3½oz (100g) crimini mushrooms, finely diced

1 yellow squash, finely diced

1 small eggplant, finely diced

5 shallots, finely diced

3 garlic cloves, minced

1 red chile (optional, depending on how spicy you want the dish to be)

scant ½ cup brown or white rice, rinsed

2 tbsp quinoa

1 tbsp olive oil

a large sprig of flat-leaf parsley, finely chopped

2 tsp hot smoked paprika

salt and freshly ground black pepper

8 bell peppers of the same color, or a mixture of yellow, green, orange, and red bell peppers

1 tbsp chopped flat-leaf parsley leaves, to garnish

1 Preheat the oven to 375°F (190°). Dry-fry the pine nuts in a skillet until they are lightly golden. Place the finely diced vegetables in a large mixing bowl and add the pine nuts, rice, quinoa, olive oil, and parsley. Sprinkle in the hot smoked paprika and season, then combine the ingredients well.

2 Using a sharp knife, carefully remove the stalk and the "seeded heart" from each pepper so they remain whole. Stuff each pepper with the vegetable mixture, making sure that each pepper is packed full (the vegetables in the stuffing have a tendency to shrink during cooking).

3 Stand the stuffed peppers in a deep baking dish or casserole dish. Pour enough hot water into the dish to cover the bottom third of the peppers. Bake in the oven for about 50 minutes. Once the skin on the peppers turns slightly brown on top, cover the dish with a lid or foil. To check whether the filling is cooking, test the rice and quinoa. If it feels or looks dry, pour a splash of water inside each pepper to aid cooking. When the peppers are cooked, garnish with chopped parsley and serve with a side dish of hot mashed sweet potatoes.

BEANS BAKED IN A PUMPKIN POT

 HELPS REMOVE TOXINS FROM THE BODY   **HELPS LOWER CHOLESTEROL**   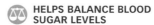 **HELPS BALANCE BLOOD SUGAR LEVELS**

This combination of okra, peppers, mushrooms, and spices works synergistically to support nearly every body system and aids the removal of waste and toxins, while eating legumes, such as lima beans, is a particularly good way to lower cholesterol and help balance blood sugar levels. Presenting the beans in a pumpkin adds extra nutrition, flavor, and a "wow" factor at the table.

SERVES 4

2 tbsp olive oil, plus extra for greasing

8 shallots, finely chopped

1 tsp coriander seeds, coarsely crushed in a mortar and pestle

1 red or green chile, seeded and minced

1 red bell pepper, seeded and diced

1 yellow bell pepper, seeded and diced

3 garlic cloves, minced

1 level tsp hot smoked paprika

14oz (400g) can organic lima beans, drained

salt and freshly ground black pepper

5½oz (150g) shiitake mushrooms, sliced

3½oz (100g) small whole okra, stems removed

1 bay leaf, fresh or dried

1 large or 2 medium pumpkins or winter squash (optional)

a small handful of roughly chopped cilantro leaves, to garnish

1 Preheat the oven to 350°F (180°C). Gently warm the olive oil with a spoonful of water in a medium saucepan over low heat. Add the shallots and stir until they turn translucent and golden. Add the coriander seeds and chile, stir, and add the diced peppers, garlic, and hot smoked paprika. Add the beans and stir well to coat them in the spices. Season with salt and black pepper and then add the shiitake mushrooms, okra, and bay leaf to the pan.

2 If you don't want to use a pumpkin, simply transfer the bean mixture to a shallow ovenproof dish with a lid. Add a dash of water, cover, and bake in the oven for 45–50 minutes. Remove from the oven, scatter with cilantro leaves, and serve.

3 If you want to bake and serve the baked beans in a pumpkin "pot," cut the top off the pumpkin and reserve. Remove the soft center and seeds, and scrape out a little of the flesh if necessary; the thicker the pumpkin wall, the longer it will take for the dish to cook.

4 Smear the inside of the pumpkin with a little olive oil, season with a little salt, and add the bean mixture and a dash of water. The pumpkin itself will add some liquid to the dish. Cover with the pumpkin "lid," place on a baking pan, and bake in the oven for 1 hour, or until the pumpkin is cooked through.

5 Remove the pumpkin lid and lift out the bay leaf and discard it. Scatter the beans with the fresh cilantro, and bring the pumpkin to the table. To serve, dig the serving spoon into the pumpkin flesh so that each portion contains a mixture of both pumpkin flesh and beans.

Lima beans (p114) *contain iron and fiber to support a healthy heart and circulation.*

KALE WITH BUCKWHEAT NOODLES

 HELPS LOWER CHOLESTEROL   **CONTAINS ANTICANCER SUBSTANCES**   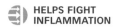 **HELPS FIGHT INFLAMMATION**

This dish of buckwheat noodles and kale benefits the heart. Kale is the ultimate leafy vegetable, full of antioxidants, omega-3 fatty acids, and natural substances that give it anti-inflammatory properties and can help reduce the risk of estrogen-related cancers. Any type of kale will do for this quick, easy dish, and it is best cooked lightly for a minimal amount of time.

SERVES 4

14oz (400g) soba (buckwheat) noodles

2 tbsp walnut oil, plus extra for sprinkling

1 red chile, seeded and minced

2 garlic cloves, crushed

2 tbsp tamari soy sauce

1¼lb (600g) fresh kale, cut into strips with the stalks removed

2 tbsp fresh orange juice

¼ cup walnut pieces, toasted, to garnish

1 Cook the soba noodles following package directions. Add a dash of walnut oil and a pinch of salt to the water before you add the noodles, if you like.

2 Meanwhile, place a large, heavy saucepan with a lid over medium heat and add the walnut oil along with 2 tablespoons of water. When the oil has warmed through, add the minced chile and crushed garlic, and stir. Add the tamari soy sauce, followed by the kale, and stir to coat the leaves in the other ingredients.

3 Add the orange juice, cover, and let the kale steam for 2–3 minutes, or until it is just cooked. Stir occasionally while it cooks, to stop it from sticking to the bottom of the pan, and add a dash of water if necessary. Remove from the heat. Arrange the soba noodles on a warmed serving dish, pile the kale on top, and scatter with the toasted walnuts. Sprinkle the dish with a few drops of walnut oil to serve.

VEGETABLE HOT POT

 PROMOTES A SENSE OF WELL-BEING   **HELPS REMOVE TOXINS FROM THE BODY**   **HELPS FIGHT INFLAMMATION**   **AIDS OPTIMAL DIGESTIVE HEALTH**

Dishes such as this medley of vegetables and spices, cooked slowly over low heat, are warming, sustaining, and uplifting for the mind and body. Sweet potato helps remove toxins and calm inflammation, while cabbage and garlic are antiparasitic and help improve digestion. The art of this dish lies in carefully layering the ingredients, so each diner receives a little of all the vegetables.

SERVES 4–6

5½oz (150g) shallots, quartered

1 tbsp ghee or clarified butter

¾ cup vegetable stock

½ cup dry white wine

1lb 5oz–1¾lb (600–800g) white cabbage, outside leaves removed, and cut into 8 segments

1 medium (7oz/200g) sweet potato, peeled and cut into 6 segments

2 small carrots, peeled and sliced

6 garlic cloves, minced

2 small chiles, seeded and chopped

4 inner celery stalks and leaves, chopped (discard stringy outer stalks)

9oz (250g) baby plum tomatoes

6 bay leaves

1 tsp ground coriander

1 tsp freshly ground black pepper

2 tsp smoked paprika

1 tbsp olive oil

salt

a small handful of chopped cilantro leaves, to garnish (optional)

1 Place half the shallots in a Dutch oven, add half the ghee, and a splash of vegetable stock and wine, and mix. Add some of the cabbage segments, sweet potato, and carrots, half the garlic, 1 chile, half the chopped celery and tomatoes, 3 bay leaves, and a dash of the spices to create a layer of ingredients. Repeat with the rest of the ghee, vegetables, and spices to create another layer.

2 Drizzle the olive oil over the top. Mix the stock and wine, season with a little salt, and pour two-thirds of the liquid into the pot. Bring it to a simmer on the stove top, cover with a lid, and simmer on low heat for 1 hour, occasionally adding more wine and stock blend. Remove the lid for the last 15 minutes of cooking time to allow any excess stock to evaporate. Remove from the heat, fish out the bay leaves, if possible, and discard, and serve. Garnish each portion with cilantro leaves, if using.

Marinated Tofu With Shiitake And Noodles

 HELPS FIGHT INFLAMMATION　　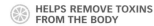 **HELPS REMOVE TOXINS FROM THE BODY**　　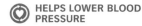 **HELPS LOWER BLOOD PRESSURE**

Soy is a traditional remedy for inflammatory conditions of the lungs and gut. Its phytoestrogens (plant hormones) can also help protect the heart and lower blood pressure. In small amounts, unfermented soy can help neutralize toxins in the body—helpful if you have a hangover—though high, regular consumption can lower the absorption of some minerals in food.

SERVES 6

10oz (300g) organic tofu, cut into bite-sized cubes

¼ cup sunflower oil

a pinch of salt

approximately 10oz (300g) medium noodles (egg or rice) for 6 people

10oz (300g) fresh shiitake mushrooms, halved or quartered

1 carrot, julienned

9oz (250g) mung bean sprouts, rinsed and drained

9oz (250g) snow peas, cut in half

3½oz (100g) baby corn, halved

1–2 tbsp tamari soy sauce

1 tbsp black sesame seeds

a small handful of cilantro leaves, chopped, to garnish

For the marinade

3 garlic cloves, crushed

1½in (3cm) piece fresh ginger, grated

1 small chile, seeded and minced

3 tbsp mirin sauce

2 tbsp toasted sesame oil

3 tbsp teriyaki sauce

3 small shallots, finely sliced

1 Arrange the tofu in a flat dish. Mix together the marinade ingredients and pour over the tofu cubes, making sure they are thoroughly coated. Cover the dish and let marinate overnight in the refrigerator. Turn the cubes over at some point to allow the flavors to infuse completely.

2 Remove the tofu cubes from the marinade and drain for a moment to let the juices drip away. Reserve the marinade.

3 Heat 2 tablespoons of the sunflower oil with 2 tablespoons of water in a wok over medium heat. Add the tofu cubes and fry until lightly browned on all sides, turning them gently so they don't break. Remove from the wok and transfer to a warm dish.

4 Meanwhile, bring a large saucepan of water to a boil, add a pinch of salt, and cook the noodles following package directions. Drain the noodles and rinse in cold water to stop them from cooking any more.

5 Scrape off any burned remnants of tofu in the bottom of the wok and add another tablespoon each of sunflower oil and water. Add the shiitake mushrooms and stir-fry for 2–3 minutes, then transfer to a warm dish. Add the carrot, mung bean sprouts, snow peas, baby corn, and tamari soy sauce, and stir-fry briefly. Then transfer to the warm dish of mushrooms.

6 Wipe the wok down again, and heat the last tablespoon of oil. Add the reserved marinade, let it heat through, then add the cooked noodles and stir-fry them briefly. Return all the vegetables to the wok and mix them into the noodles. Add the tofu and mix it in gently. Sprinkle the black sesame seeds on top, then transfer to 6 warmed noodle bowls. Scatter each portion with the chopped cilantro leaves to serve.

Mung beans *(p115) produce the thick, juicy sprouts that are popular in Asian cuisine. They are renowned for their detoxifying properties.*

STIR-FRIED SPRING VEGETABLES

 FEEDS GOOD BACTERIA IN THE GUT

 HELPS FIGHT INFLAMMATION

 HELPS LOWER BLOOD PRESSURE

 HELPS BALANCE BLOOD SUGAR LEVELS

Eating plenty of fresh, young, green vegetables in spring is a good way to cleanse the body after the dark days of winter. Asparagus stimulates the digestion by acting as a prebiotic. It also contains compounds that have an anti-inflammatory effect, so it is beneficial if you have high blood pressure and blood sugar imbalance. Young mint and chives gently invigorate the body.

SERVES 4

2 tbsp olive oil

¾lb (350g) asparagus, cut into 2in (5cm) pieces

9oz (250g) snow peas

5½oz (150g) wild garlic leaves, chopped

7oz (200g) small spinach leaves

1 tbsp raspberry vinegar

2 tbsp chopped mint leaves

2 tbsp finely chopped chives

1 Heat the olive oil and a dash of water in a wok over high heat. Add the asparagus and snow peas and stir-fry for 3 minutes, then add the wild garlic leaves and spinach and stir until they wilt.

2 Remove the wok from the heat and add the raspberry vinegar, mint, and chives. Combine and serve while hot with steamed rice or quinoa.

Asparagus *(p77) contains antioxidants that help fight free-radical damage and has a mild laxative effect—perfect for a spring detox.*

SQUAB BREASTS WITH GOJI BERRIES

 HELPS MAINTAIN ENERGY LEVELS

 ENHANCES VIGOR AND A SENSE OF WELL-BEING

 REPLACES IRON LOST IN MENSTRUATION

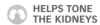 **HELPS TONE THE KIDNEYS**

Squab meat is lean, tender, and nutritious. In China, it is regarded as an excellent kidney tonic, but it is most commonly eaten to help combat male and female infertility by boosting blood circulation and improving energy levels. It also helps build iron levels after substantial blood loss, such as at childbirth or heavy menstruation. Goji berries are added to give a metabolic boost.

SERVES 4

4 whole squab

scant 1oz (25g) dried shiitake mushrooms

2 medium carrots, halved lengthwise

1 medium onion, peeled and quartered

1 medium red chile, whole

4 garlic cloves in their skins

½ tsp black peppercorns

a pinch of salt

4 tsp cornstarch

2½ tbsp goji berries

a dash of olive oil

cilantro leaves, chopped, to garnish

1 Remove the breast meat in whole pieces from each bird and reserve. Place the filleted birds in a large Dutch oven and add the mushrooms, carrots, onion, chile, garlic, black peppercorns, and salt. Pour in just enough water to cover, bring it to a boil, and simmer over low heat for 1½ hours, skimming off any impurities from the top of the stock as necessary. Watch the liquid level and add more water if needed. Toward the end of the cooking time, you should have approximately 2 cups or more of stock remaining.

2 Strain the stock, reserving the cooking liquid, shiitake mushrooms, garlic cloves, and some of the peppercorns. Discard the rest of the ingredients, including the squab meat, bones, and skin. Shred the mushrooms and squeeze the softened garlic cloves from their skins. Set the garlic paste aside.

3 Return the stock to the Dutch oven, reserving ¼ cup in a bowl, and set over medium-high heat. Thicken the liquid by mixing the cornstarch with the reserved stock in the bowl and adding it to the pot. Add the goji berries, shredded mushrooms, and the garlic paste and simmer the stock for 10–20 minutes until it thickens to the consistency of heavy cream. Adjust the seasoning if required.

4 Add a dash of olive oil to a skillet and warm over medium heat. Add the reserved squab breasts and pan-fry for 2 minutes on each side until just cooked through. Transfer to the Dutch oven and cook for 2–3 minutes.

5 Arrange the breasts on a warm serving plate, spoon over a little of the sauce, and garnish with the cilantro leaves. Serve with the remaining sauce and some boiled rice.

Goji berries (p36) are rich in pyridoxine (vitamin B₆), which supports efficient metabolism.

GINGER CHICKEN

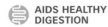 **PROTECTS AGAINST COLDS AND FLU**

 AIDS HEALTHY DIGESTION

SUPPLIES OXYGEN TO CELLS

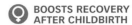 **BOOSTS RECOVERY AFTER CHILDBIRTH**

The marinade in this chicken dish contains fresh ginger, which is one of the most important foods for helping prevent and treat common colds. Its warming nature is enhanced here with lime, garlic, and honey—all known to help boost the immune system. This dish is ideal if you need to increase your resistance to seasonal bugs or build your strength after an illness.

SERVES 4

1 organic free-range chicken, approximately 3¼lb (1.5kg), cut into 8 pieces

1 tbsp ghee or clarified butter

2¼lb (1kg) potatoes, peeled and thinly sliced

½–1 tsp salt

1 tbsp paprika

½ tsp freshly ground black pepper

For the marinade

¼ cup tamari soy sauce

1 heaped tbsp finely chopped fresh ginger

3–5 garlic cloves, crushed

zest and juice of 1–2 limes

3 tbsp honey

1 Prepare the marinade by mixing the tamari soy sauce, ginger, garlic, lime juice, and honey in a large plastic container with a lid. Add the chicken pieces and marinate for 8–12 hours or overnight in the refrigerator.

2 Preheat the oven to 425°F (220°C). Grease a large ovenproof dish with the ghee. Arrange the sliced potatoes in thin layers in the dish and sprinkle with salt, paprika, and black pepper. Place the chicken pieces on top of the potatoes. Pour any remaining marinade on top and season with a little more salt and black pepper. Bake in the oven for 45–50 minutes, or until the chicken juices run clear when the meat is pierced with a sharp knife, and the potatoes are cooked. Serve with a salad.

Ghee (p120) is a good source of lauric acid, a healthy fat with antibacterial and antifungal properties.

QUINOA AND VEGETABLE STACK

 HELPS MAINTAIN ENERGY LEVELS

 SUPPORTS TISSUE GROWTH AND REPAIR

 EASY TO DIGEST AND GLUTEN FREE

 HELPS STRENGTHEN THE IMMUNE SYSTEM

High in protein and fiber, quinoa contains all the essential amino acids the body needs to sustain energy levels and support healthy tissue growth and repair. It is also gluten free, which makes it a good choice for anyone with gluten sensitivity. The sauerkraut brings multiple benefits for immunity and gut health and a selection of colorful fresh vegetables add valuable nutrients.

SERVES 4

5 small shallots or small red onions, finely sliced

1 medium-hot chile, minced

2 large red Romano peppers, or other red bell pepper, halved lengthwise, seeded, and sliced into ½in (1cm) strips

3 medium yellow squash, cut into ¼in (5mm) slices

3½oz (100g) shiitake mushrooms, stalks removed, sliced

2 garlic cloves, crushed

sea salt and freshly ground black pepper

2 tbsp olive oil

1¾ cups quinoa

a sprig of parsley, chopped, to garnish

a drizzle of extra virgin olive oil

½ cup sauerkraut, to serve (optional)

1 Pour in enough water to cover the bottom of a medium saucepan. Add the shallots and cook gently over low heat with the lid on until tender, adding more water if necessary. Add the chile and sauté gently. Add the peppers and let soften, then add the squash. Finally, add the shiitake mushrooms and garlic, season to taste with a pinch of sea salt, stir for a minute, and drizzle in the olive oil. Stir the mixture, replace the lid, then turn off the heat and leave the pan on the stove top to keep warm.

2 Cook the quinoa following package directions, drain, and set aside.

3 When you are ready to serve the food, take a serving dish, place a large cook's ring on it, and fill with a 1in (2.5cm) layer of the quinoa. Spoon a layer of vegetables on top of the quinoa and scatter with some chopped parsley. Remove the ring and repeat with 3 more stacks of quinoa, vegetables, and parsley. Season the stacks with black pepper and a drizzle of extra virgin olive oil, and serve with some sauerkraut arranged around the base of the stacks.

4 If you don't have a cook's ring, use a dome-shaped small bowl brushed with olive oil. Fill the bottom half of the bowl with the vegetables, top with quinoa, place the serving dish face down on the bowl, turn both upside down, and gently remove the bowl. Scatter with the parsley, season, drizzle with the extra virgin olive oil, and serve with the sauerkraut.

Sauerkraut Parcels

 PROMOTES A HEALTHY DIGESTIVE TRACT   **CALMING AND COMFORTING**

Fermented cabbage, or sauerkraut, is rich in vitamin C and contains a type of lactic acid that aids digestion by clearing harmful bacteria and combating toxins, food stagnation, and wind. Some nutritionists also maintain that it is an effective preventive food for cancer and degenerative diseases. Whole sauerkraut leaves can sometimes be found in Polish or Italian delicatessens.

SERVES 4

salt and freshly ground black pepper

2 tbsp wine vinegar

6 black peppercorns

16 whole sauerkraut leaves, or large cabbage leaves, stem and leaf veins removed

1 tbsp olive oil

2 medium onions, finely diced

3 garlic cloves, crushed

1lb 2oz (500g) ground meat (pork, beef, or a mixture of the two)

⅔ cup white or brown rice, rinsed

2 tsp paprika

2 tbsp chopped flat-leaf parsley leaves

1½ cups sauerkraut

7oz (200g) smoked rib of pork or smoked bacon, chopped

For the sauce

1 tbsp olive oil

3 tsp all-purpose flour

a pinch of salt

a few black peppercorns

2 tbsp tomato paste

1 small chile, seeded and minced

1 cup crème fraîche

1 If using fresh cabbage leaves instead of the whole fermented sauerkraut leaves, bring a large saucepan of water to a boil and add a pinch of salt, the wine vinegar, and black peppercorns. Place the leaves into the water, 2 at a time, and blanch for 2–3 minutes. Watch them carefully and remove as soon as they begin to wilt. Set aside to dry on paper towels.

2 Heat the olive oil in a skillet and sauté the onions and garlic until soft and translucent. Add the ground meat and cook for 10–15 minutes, or until it is lightly browned. Add the rice, paprika, and parsley, stirring well for 2–3 minutes. Remove from the heat and set aside until cool enough to handle.

3 Place a ball of the stuffing in the center of a sauerkraut or cabbage leaf. Fold in the sides of the leaf and roll it up to form a closed parcel. Repeat with the rest of the stuffing and cabbage leaves.

4 Arrange a layer of sauerkraut in the bottom of a large saucepan with a lid, followed by the cabbage parcels, loose ends facing down, and topped with the smoked pork or bacon. Carefully add hot water to the pan until it half-covers the contents of the pan. If necessary, weigh the parcels down with a small heatproof plate. Cover and simmer over low heat for 2 hours, or until cooked, making sure the water doesn't evaporate. The water should remain at the same level, half-covering the contents of the pan, throughout the cooking time.

5 Meanwhile, make the sauce. Heat the olive oil in a small saucepan, add the flour, and allow to brown slightly, then add the salt, black peppercorns, tomato paste, chile, crème fraîche, and enough water to make a sauce with the consistency of light cream. When the sauerkraut parcels are cooked, divide between 4 serving plates and pour some of the hot sauce over each portion.

TIP: Try making your own sauerkraut leaves by using the recipe on p330.

SAVOY CABBAGE PARCELS

 HELPS MAINTAIN ENERGY LEVELS   **HELPS BUILD MUSCLE**   **ENHANCES VIGOR**   **CALMING AND COMFORTING**

This dish is great comfort food, but it is also packed with healthy ingredients that boost energy levels. It is a good choice for men of all ages, because quinoa provides protein and essential amino acids that help the body build muscle, while walnuts can help improve men's fertility and are heart-healthy. This also makes an ideal complete meal for vegetarians and vegans.

SERVES 4

1¾ cups quinoa

½ cup walnuts, roughly chopped

⅓ cup sun-dried tomatoes, chopped

2 garlic cloves, minced

1 medium red onion, finely chopped

4 small shallots, finely chopped

scant ½ cup chopped parsley

¾ cup fresh or dried unsweetened cranberries

2 tsp ground allspice

½ tsp ground coriander

2 level tsp Italian herbs seasoning

Himalayan salt and freshly ground black pepper

1 large Savoy cabbage, leaves removed

4 bay leaves

2 tsp all-purpose flour, arrowroot, or kudzu (a popular Asian thickener)

thick plain yogurt, to serve

1 To make the stuffing, wash the quinoa grains, allow to drip-dry in a sieve, then add to a mixing bowl along with the walnuts, tomatoes, garlic, onion, shallots, parsley, and cranberries. Season with the allspice, ground coriander, Italian seasoning, and salt and black pepper. Stir to combine all the ingredients thoroughly.

2 Choose 10–12 tender medium-sized cabbage leaves and blanch in boiling water for 1–2 minutes, removing them as soon as they wilt. Reserve the cabbage cooking water. Allow the leaves to cool for a moment, then cut away the thick vein at the back of each leaf.

3 Place a spoonful of stuffing in the center of a cabbage leaf. Fold in the sides of the leaf and roll it up to form a closed parcel. Repeat with the rest of the stuffing and cabbage leaves.

4 Tightly arrange the parcels, loose ends facing down, in the bottom of a medium saucepan with a lid. Layer the parcels if necessary, adding the bay leaves as you work.

5 Add the reserved cabbage water to the pan, making sure that the bottom of the pan is covered but that the parcels are only partially covered with liquid. Bring to a boil, reduce the heat, cover, and simmer gently for 30 minutes.

6 Dissolve the flour in a little water in a bowl and whisk it into the pan. Simmer for another 15 minutes, or until the sauce has thickened and the parcels are cooked. Serve accompanied with a spoonful of thick yogurt.

Savoy cabbage *(p52) is a source of sulfur, essential for healthy bones, cartilage, tendons, and skin.*

CHANTERELLES AND CHILES WITH PASTA

 HELPS STRENGTHEN THE IMMUNE SYSTEM

 PROMOTES HEALTHY SKIN

 HELPS PROTECT EYE HEALTH

Like many mushrooms, chanterelles are rich in the amino acids that are essential for building protein in the body. They also contain vitamin A and so benefit eye health. Kamut is an ancient grain closely related to modern wheat. Even though it contains gluten, it has been found to be more easily digestible for people with allergies or intolerances to wheat.

SERVES 4

14oz (400g) fresh chanterelle mushrooms, sliced

4 tsp olive oil

2–3 garlic cloves, crushed

1–2 small chiles, seeded and finely chopped

⅓ cup sour cream

salt and freshly ground black pepper

1lb 2oz (500g) pasta, such as tagliatelle or spaghetti, made from kamut wheat

1 tbsp finely chopped flat-leaf parsley leaves, to garnish

1 Place the mushrooms in a medium saucepan and dry-fry them over low heat, shaking the pan gently, until their juices run. Then, turn the heat up so the liquid evaporates and the mushrooms are soft, but reasonably dry. Add 3 teaspoons of the olive oil to coat the mushrooms, then add the garlic, chiles, and sour cream. Let the mixture simmer over low heat for 2–6 minutes. Season with salt and black pepper.

2 Meanwhile, cook the pasta following package directions until it is al dente, adding the last teaspoon of olive oil to the cooking water to prevent it from boiling over and to enhance the flavor of the pasta. Drain and transfer to a warmed serving dish. Spoon the sauce over the pasta, garnish with the parsley, toss the ingredients well to combine, and serve with a green salad.

Chanterelle mushrooms (p91)
contain vitamins D and K, which work
together to protect the heart and bones.

SALMON WITH DILL AND TAMARI SAUCE

 HELPS MAINTAIN ENERGY LEVELS

 EASY TO DIGEST

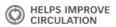 **HELPS IMPROVE CIRCULATION**

This simply baked salmon dish is paired with fresh dill for a classic combination of flavors. Salmon is considered a good food to eat if you are feeling debilitated or are recovering after an illness, because it helps improve energy levels and is easily digested. It is also rich in omega-3 fatty acids and selenium, which promote heart health and support healthy aging.

SERVES 4

4 salmon fillets, approximately 10oz (300g) each

¼ cup tamari soy sauce

a generous dash of lemon juice

¼ cup olive oil

4 garlic cloves, minced

4 thin slices of lemon

2 tbsp chopped dill leaves

1 Preheat the oven to 350°F (180°C). Place the salmon fillets in a ceramic baking dish. Blend the tamari soy sauce, lemon juice, olive oil, and a dash of water in a small bowl, add the garlic, combine the ingredients together well, and pour over the fish.

2 Arrange the lemon slices on top of the fish and sprinkle with the dill. Cover with foil and bake for 20–25 minutes. Carefully insert a sharp knife into the center of one fillet to check if the fish is cooked; the flesh should be opaque. Serve either hot or cold.

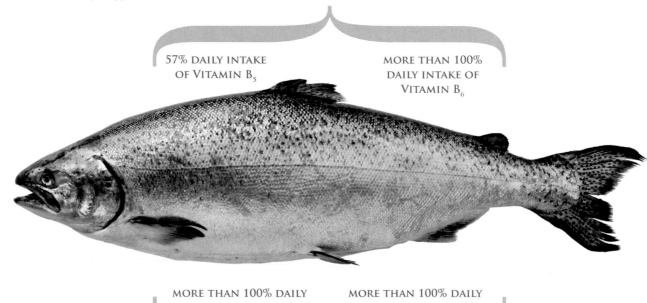

57% DAILY INTAKE OF VITAMIN B_5

MORE THAN 100% DAILY INTAKE OF VITAMIN B_6

MORE THAN 100% DAILY INTAKE OF VITAMIN B_{12}

MORE THAN 100% DAILY INTAKE OF VITAMIN D

BOOST YOUR VITAMIN INTAKE

EACH LARGE SALMON FILLET PROVIDES EXCELLENT QUANTITIES OF VITAMIN D AND AN ARRAY OF KEY B VITAMINS.

MARINATED DUCK WITH MANGO SALSA

 HELPS MAINTAIN ENERGY LEVELS

 HAS A DIURETIC ACTION

 SOOTHES AND TONES THE DIGESTIVE TRACT

 ENHANCES SPERM QUALITY

Duck meat is considered an empowering food in traditional Chinese medicine: it provides the body with energy and helps to increase stamina levels. Its diuretic properties help to reduce water retention and, coupled with a sweet and sour mango salsa, it benefits the digestive system and can help to alleviate nausea. It is also thought to boost men's sperm count.

SERVES 4

3 kaffir lime leaves

1 tsp honey

zest of 1 orange and juice of 2 oranges

1 tbsp tamari soy sauce

¼ tsp five-spice powder

4 duck breasts, without skin

¾ cup jasmine rice

4 fresh figs (optional) to garnish

For the mango salsa

2 medium mangoes, peeled, seeded, and diced

3 scallions, finely chopped

1 small green chile pepper, seeded and minced

1 small red chile pepper, seeded and minced

¼ cup chopped cilantro leaves

3 tbsp chopped basil leaves

1 small cucumber, seeded and finely diced

1 large tomato, seeded and finely diced

1 tbsp balsamic vinegar

2 tbsp extra virgin olive oil

salt and freshly ground black pepper

1 Place the kaffir lime leaves in a large mixing bowl, cover with ¼ cup boiling water, and leave to infuse for 15 minutes. Add the honey and stir until it dissolves. Add the orange zest and juice, tamari soy sauce, and five-spice powder and blend well. Immerse the duck breasts in the marinade to ensure they are well coated. Let marinate for 30 minutes.

2 Meanwhile, bring a medium saucepan of water to a boil and cook the jasmine rice following package directions.

3 Heat a heavy skillet over high heat. Remove the duck breasts from the marinade and transfer them to the pan to brown on both sides. Lower the heat, strain the marinade juices, and add them to the pan. Cook the duck breasts for a further 5–6 minutes, turning them frequently so they don't stick to the bottom of the pan or burn. Test to see how well cooked the meat is by carefully cutting into the center of the breast with a sharp knife. The center of the meat should still be pink after this time, so let it cook for a little longer if you prefer it well done. Remove the pan from the heat and set aside briefly. Make 2 deep cuts at right angles in the top of each fig, if using, and open out the 4 tips to create a flower-petal effect.

4 Transfer the duck breasts from the pan to a cutting board and slice diagonally into thin slices. Add all the mango salsa ingredients to the pan with the marinade juices and stir to mix and warm through. To assemble the dish, place a cook's ring in the center of each serving plate, half-fill with cooked jasmine rice, top off with some of the warm mango salsa, and carefully remove the ring. Arrange a sliced duck breast on each portion, position a fig "flower" on top of the duck, and serve.

VENISON CASSEROLE WITH CRANBERRIES

 HELPS RELEASE CELLULAR ENERGY　　 **HELPS INCREASE LIBIDO**　　 **STRENGTHENS THE REPRODUCTIVE SYSTEM**　　 **FIGHTS URINARY TRACT INFECTIONS**

Colder months are the time for this warming venison stew, best eaten at lunchtime to benefit from its energizing properties; iron-rich venison is traditionally eaten to help combat fatigue, as well as impotence and infertility. Cranberries are both astringent and antibacterial, and are commonly used to help prevent infections in the urinary tract, kidneys, and bladder.

SERVES 6

1 tbsp vegetable oil

2¼lb (1kg) lean venison shoulder, chopped into 1in (2.5cm) cubes

2 tbsp all-purpose flour, seasoned

1 tsp whole coriander seeds, coarsely crushed

7oz (200g) small shallots, quartered

3½oz (100g) crimini or brown button mushrooms, sliced

¼ cup dried apricots (without sulfur), roughly chopped

1 cup fresh or frozen cranberries

3 kaffir lime leaves

1 tbsp cacao nibs or dark chocolate (optional)

1½ cups red wine

salt and freshly ground black pepper

1 Preheat the oven to 350°F (180°C). Heat the vegetable oil in a Dutch oven on medium-high heat. Toss the venison cubes in the flour and brown in the pan in small batches. Set aside the browned meat, reduce the heat, and add the coriander seeds, followed by the shallots and mushrooms, to brown. Add a little water if necessary.

2 Add the apricots and gently stir them in. Return the meat to the Dutch oven together with all the juices, and add the cranberries and kaffir lime leaves. Stir in the cacao nibs and red wine. Stir everything thoroughly, cover, and place in the oven.

3 Let the stew cook for 1–1½ hours or until the meat is tender and the juices have thickened. Remove the kaffir lime leaves, add salt and black pepper to taste, and serve with boiled rice.

TIP: If you can't find fresh or frozen cranberries, substitute with ¾ cup fresh blueberries and ½ cup of dried cranberries instead.

Mediterranean Vegetable Medley

 HELPS STRENGTHEN THE IMMUNE SYSTEM   **HELPS IMPROVE CIRCULATION**   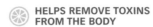 **HELPS REMOVE TOXINS FROM THE BODY**

This summer dish is full of vegetables with antioxidant and anti-inflammatory phytonutrients that help protect the body at a cellular level. Try to cut the peppers, eggplant, and tomatoes the same size to improve the appearance and cooking time of this simple dish. The zucchini is best left in larger cubes. It cooks quickly and its nutrients can be lost if overcooked.

SERVES 4

1 tbsp olive oil

4 shallots, minced

salt and freshly ground black pepper

a pinch of oregano or marjoram

2 red bell peppers, seeded and chopped

2 yellow bell peppers, seeded and chopped

1 medium eggplant, chopped

1 medium zucchini, chopped

4 tomatoes, skinned (optional), and chopped

2 garlic cloves, crushed

2 tbsp olive oil

¼ cup finely chopped parsley leaves, plus leaves to garnish

1 Heat the olive oil in a large, heavy saucepan over medium to low heat. Add the shallots and a pinch of salt, and stir until the shallots begin to turn translucent. Add a dash of water to bring the temperature down and to add moisture to the pan. After 2–3 minutes add the oregano or marjoram and the peppers. Cook until the peppers have softened.

2 Add the eggplant and the zucchini, and when the liquid in the pan has reduced, add the tomatoes. Let the mixture simmer for 15 minutes over low heat, taking care not to let the vegetables stick to the bottom of the pan and burn.

3 Add the garlic and a little more olive oil for added flavor and cook for a further 5 minutes. Stir in the chopped parsley and season with salt and black pepper to taste. Serve on a bed of brown basmati rice with some parsley scattered on top.

Eggplants (p64) have the ability to help remove harmful toxins from the body.

YELLOW WAX BEAN STEW

 AIDS HEALTHY DIGESTION

 HELPS BALANCE BLOOD SUGAR LEVELS

 HAS A DIURETIC ACTION

This blend of vegetables enhances digestion, balances blood sugar levels, and helps remove excess fluid from the body. Fresh beans also have a diuretic effect. Tender, golden-yellow, wax beans are best for this recipe, although any fresh beans will taste good. Look for young, succulent beans that aren't stringy and snap easily if you bend them in half.

SERVES 4

2 large tomatoes

2 large potatoes, peeled and diced

2 tbsp olive oil

1 onion, finely chopped

2 carrots, sliced into thin rounds

1 chile, seeded and minced (optional)

1¾lb (800g) tender, yellow wax beans, trimmed and sliced into 1¼in (3cm) pieces

3 garlic cloves, chopped

salt and freshly ground black pepper

1 tbsp chopped dill leaves, plus a few extra leaves to garnish

1 Cut a cross on the top of each tomato, dip in boiling water for 20 seconds, remove, and when cool enough to handle, peel off the skin and finely chop the flesh.

2 Place the potatoes in a saucepan, cover with cold water, bring to a boil, reduce the heat, and simmer until the potatoes are cooked.

3 Meanwhile, heat the olive oil in a large frying pan with a lid over medium heat. Add the onion and sauté until soft and translucent. Add the carrots and chile (if using), stir, and sauté for 2–3 minutes. Stir in the beans, then lower the heat, cover, and let the beans sweat for 1–2 minutes. Add the garlic and tomatoes and allow them to cook in the vegetable juices for 2–3 minutes. Add 1–2 tablespoons of water if the vegetables are beginning to stick to the bottom of the pan.

4 When the beans are al dente (cooked, but still slightly crunchy), add the cooked potatoes and a small amount of their cooking water. Add some seasoning and the dill, combine with the other ingredients, and cook for a further 2–3 minutes. Remove from the heat, transfer to 4 serving bowls, and garnish with dill leaves.

Red tomatoes (p65) enhance the cleansing effect of this recipe and are a good source of heart-friendly lycopene.

BROILED MACKEREL WITH CHARD

 PROTECTS THE HEART AND BLOOD VESSELS   **HELPS FIGHT INFLAMMATION**   **HELPS BALANCE BLOOD SUGAR LEVELS**   **HELPS BUILD STRONG BONES**

Mackerel is beneficial for cardiovascular health, and here it is combined with Swiss chard, which is known for its anti-inflammatory, antioxidant, and detoxifying properties. In addition, Swiss chard helps balance blood sugar levels, protect the body from chronic oxidative stress, and support bone health. Choose young leaves with narrow stems for an even cooking time.

SERVES 4

4 whole mackerel, filleted

2 celery stalks, chopped

2 garlic cloves, chopped, plus 2 garlic cloves, crushed

1 chile, seeded and chopped

a bunch of parsley leaves, roughly chopped

juice of 1 lemon

2 tbsp olive oil

1lb 2oz (500g) Swiss chard, chopped, with stems removed and finely chopped

1 tbsp blackberry vinegar (p334) or the juice of ½ lemon

salt and freshly ground black pepper

For the dressing

juice of 1 lemon

2 tbsp teriyaki sauce

1 tsp finely grated fresh ginger

2 tbsp olive oil

1 tsp honey

salt and freshly ground black pepper

1 With a sharp knife, make several diagonal scores through the skin along the length of each mackerel fillet to stop them from curling up while being broiled. Place the fillets in a shallow dish.

2 Place the celery, chopped garlic, chile, parsley, and lemon juice in a blender or food processor, add ½ cup water, and blend. Pour this marinade over the mackerel fillets, ensuring they are thoroughly coated, and set aside to marinate for 1 hour. Meanwhile, prepare the dressing by blending all the ingredients together.

3 Heat the broiler to high. Remove the mackerel from the marinade and place the fillets, skin-side up, on the broiler pan. Cook for 4–5 minutes or until the skin is crisp and the flesh is cooked through and flakes when tested with a fork.

4 Meanwhile, heat the olive oil and ¼ cup water in a large heavy saucepan over medium heat. Add the 2 crushed garlic cloves and chard leaves and stems, and stir thoroughly. Cook until the leaves wilt, then sprinkle with blackberry vinegar and remove from the heat. Add seasoning to taste and a dash more of the vinegar, if you like.

5 Transfer the mackerel fillets to 4 warm serving plates, pour the dressing over each portion, and place a serving of chard beside it.

Mackerel (p128) is abundant in healthy fats and nutrients that help support the cardiovascular and nervous systems.

GRILLED SARDINES WITH TOMATO SALSA

HELPS IMPROVE CIRCULATION

SUPPLIES OXYGEN TO CELLS

HELPS STRENGTHEN TENDONS AND BONES

HELPS CALM THE NERVES

Salty-sweet sardines boost circulation and help build red blood cells, which in turn increase the flow of oxygen around the body, and strengthen tendons and bones. Here, they are cooked with flavorsome ingredients including basil, which has a soothing and supporting action on the mind and cognitive processes, and rosemary, which has anti-inflammatory properties.

SERVES 4

6–8 large sprigs of rosemary

8 fresh sardines

1–2 tbsp olive oil

sea salt and freshly ground black pepper

1–2 lemons, cut into quarters, to serve

For the salsa

8 tomatoes, skinned, seeded, and finely diced

1 red chile, seeded and minced

3 scallions, finely chopped

2 tbsp chopped basil leaves

1 garlic clove, finely chopped (optional)

2 tbsp raspberry vinegar, or red wine vinegar

¼ cup olive oil

sea salt and freshly ground black pepper

1 To make the tomato salsa, combine all the ingredients together well in a bowl and season to taste.

2 Preheat the broiler to medium. Arrange the large rosemary sprigs on a broiler pan and lay the sardines on top. Drizzle with the olive oil and season with sea salt and black pepper.

3 Broil the sardines for 3–5 minutes on each side, or until cooked (they should be opaque, but still firm).

4 Divide the sardines and salsa among 4 serving plates, place 1–2 lemon quarters on each plate, and serve with a green salad and boiled new potatoes.

Rosemary *(p101) is rich in the compound borneol, which acts as an energizing tonic for the nervous system.*

Vegetable Moussaka

 **HELPS STRENGTHEN
THE IMMUNE SYSTEM**

 **HELPS EASE
CONSTIPATION**

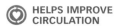 **HELPS IMPROVE
CIRCULATION**

This layered vegetable dish is full of flavor and health benefits. The combination of ingredients supports immune health, helps relieve constipation, and improves blood circulation. If you are vegan, omit the creamy topping and marinate 1½–2 cups of walnuts in 2 tablespoons of tamari soy sauce instead and scatter over the moussaka before the final stage of baking.

SERVES 6

4 medium-sized red bell peppers, halved and seeded

2 tbsp olive oil, plus extra for greasing

14oz (400g) sweet potato, peeled and thinly sliced lengthwise

1 tsp smoked paprika

salt and freshly ground black pepper

2 medium eggplant, thinly sliced lengthwise

4 garlic cloves, crushed

4 medium yellow zucchini thinly sliced lengthwise

3 tbsp chopped parsley leaves

14oz (400g) tomatoes

8 shallots, minced

¼ cup chopped basil leaves

1 large egg, beaten

2 tbsp sour cream

¾ cup home-made kefir cheese (p332), or store-bought organic ricotta cheese

1 Preheat the oven to 400°F (200°C). Place the peppers on a lightly greased baking sheet and bake for 20–25 minutes or until their skins blister and begin to blacken. Remove from the oven, transfer to a bowl, cover with plastic wrap, and set aside to sweat and cool. When cool enough to handle, peel their skins off.

2 Heat the broiler to medium-hot. Broil the sweet potato slices on both sides until golden, then transfer to a bowl, add the smoked paprika and some seasoning, mix, and set aside.

3 Broil the eggplant slices on both sides, then transfer to a bowl and add 2 of the crushed garlic cloves, mix together, and set aside to infuse. Broil the zucchini slices on both sides, transfer to a separate bowl, add the parsley, mix well, and set aside.

4 Cut a cross in the top of each tomato, dip in boiling water for 20 seconds, remove, and when cold enough to handle, peel off and discard the skin. Finely chop the flesh.

5 To prepare the sauce, heat 2 tablespoons of olive oil in a saucepan over medium heat, add the shallots, and cook until they turn translucent. Add the remaining 2 garlic cloves, the tomatoes, and ¼ cup water, and cook for 15 minutes. Add salt and black pepper to taste, stir in the basil leaves, then remove the pan from the heat.

6 Arrange the seasoned sweet potato slices in an even layer in the bottom of a square baking dish. Spread a thin layer of the sauce over them and arrange the zucchini slices on top, making sure you include all the chopped parsley. Spread another thin layer of sauce over the zucchini, followed by a layer of red peppers. Repeat with another thin layer of sauce, followed by the eggplant. Pour the rest of the sauce on top and bake in the oven for 30–40 minutes.

7 Meanwhile, combine the beaten egg, sour cream, kefir cheese or ricotta, and seasoning in a bowl to make a creamy sauce. Remove the vegetable dish from the oven, pour the white sauce over the vegetables, return to the oven, and bake for a further 20 minutes. The moussaka is cooked when the edges are bubbling and the surface is golden. Cut into 6 squares and serve with a salad on the side.

LAMB CASSEROLE WITH VEGETABLES

 HELPS COMBAT FATIGUE　　 **HELPS COMBAT ANEMIA**　　 **SUPPORTS HEALTHY KIDNEY FUNCTION**

If you need help overcoming exhaustion, this recipe is a tonic for the whole body. Lamb meat is traditionally considered a blood-nourishing and stimulating food, and it also helps to strengthen the kidneys, alleviating numbness in the lower limbs and relieving lower backache and other signs of kidney deficiency. Slowly cooking this dish in a low oven enhances its tonifying quality.

SERVES 6

4 tomatoes

1 tbsp ghee or clarified butter

2¼lb (1kg) boneless lamb shoulder, diced

1 tbsp all-purpose flour, seasoned with a little salt

8 small shallots, diced

1 small red chile, seeded and cut into strips

1 tsp coriander seeds, crushed

1 tsp paprika powder

1 medium white cabbage, core removed, and cut into 8 segments

3 bay leaves

6 garlic cloves, with skins on

3 medium potatoes, peeled and quartered

2 medium carrots, peeled and diced

1 fennel bulb, core removed, and cut into 6 segments (optional)

½ tsp white peppercorns

1 Preheat the oven to 325°F (160°C). Cut a cross in the top of each tomato, dip in boiling water for 20 seconds, remove, and when cool enough to handle, remove the skin. Finely chop the flesh, then set aside.

2 Heat the ghee in a Dutch oven over high heat. Toss the lamb in the seasoned flour and add a few pieces at a time to the hot ghee. Brown on all sides, then remove and set aside. Repeat with the rest of the meat. Reduce the heat, add the shallots, and cook for 2–3 minutes, or until they turn translucent. Add the chile, coriander seeds, and paprika and cook for 1–2 minutes, or until they release their aromas. Return the meat with the tomatoes to the Dutch oven and stir well to mop up the spices.

3 Nestle half the cabbage segments in between the meat, then add 2 of the bay leaves and half the garlic, potatoes, carrots, and fennel, followed by a second layer of cabbage and the rest of the vegetables. Add the final bay leaf and sprinkle in the peppercorns.

4 Add 1¼ cups water to the Dutch oven. Cover and bake in the oven for 1½–2 hours. Once cooked, allow to rest for 10 minutes, then spoon onto 4 serving plates, ensuring everybody gets enough meat and a helping of vegetables. Spoon some of the juices onto each portion to serve.

Fennel (p79) contributes to the kidney-toning effect of this recipe with its gentle diuretic properties.

Barlotto With Chestnut Purée

 HELPS MAINTAIN ENERGY LEVELS

 HELPS IMPROVE CIRCULATION

 PROMOTES BOWEL REGULARITY

 HELPS STRENGTHEN LOWER LIMBS

Barlotto is a version of risotto made with barley instead of short-grain rice. Barley is a good source of soluble fiber and together with sweet chestnuts assists the digestive and urinary systems. Black barley, an ancient grain that hasn't been hulled, is even more of a healing, energizing food, if you can find it. Toasting the barley first gives it a fragrant, nutty flavor.

SERVES 4

1¼ cups pearl barley
¾oz (20g) dried shiitake mushrooms
1 tsp sea salt or other unrefined salt
1 tbsp ghee, or clarified butter
8 small shallots, finely diced
1 medium carrot, diced
1 fennel bulb, cored and thinly sliced
2 garlic cloves, minced
¼ tsp freshly ground white pepper
¾ cup chestnut purée
1 large glass of dry white wine

For the vegetable stock
¼oz (10g) astragalus root (optional)
1 large carrot
2 celery stalks
6 thin slices of fresh ginger
3 thick slices of celeriac
3 shallots, quartered
4 small garlic cloves, with the skin left on
1 tbsp coriander seeds
a small handful of parsley leaves

1 To toast the barley, preheat the oven to 350°F (180°C), arrange the grains in a thin layer on a baking sheet, and place in the oven for 10–12 minutes. Toast the barley until it turns light golden, agitating it occasionally so it toasts evenly.

2 Put all the stock ingredients in a large stockpot and cover with 10½ cups water. Simmer on a low heat until the liquid reduces by roughly one-third. Strain through a colander into another pan and discard the stock vegetables, except the garlic. Squeeze the cooked garlic from its skin and add the paste to the strained stock.

3 Add the dried shiitake mushrooms and salt to the stock in the pan, and bring it back to a boil. Lower the temperature and simmer for 15 minutes to ensure the mushrooms have reconstituted fully.

4 Strain, reserving the stock, and mince the mushrooms. Place a heavy skillet over medium heat and add the ghee. Once the ghee has melted, add the shallots, cook for 2–3 minutes, then add the carrots, minced shiitake mushrooms, fennel, garlic, and white pepper, and cook for 10 minutes or until the vegetables have softened.

5 Stir in the toasted barley, making sure all the grains are well coated in the vegetable juices. Add a ladle of the hot stock and stir constantly until it is absorbed, then repeat with more stock. After 10 minutes of cooking, stir in the chestnut purée, and after 25 minutes, add the white wine. Cook for a further 5–15 minutes, or until the barley is cooked through, but still al dente (slightly firm to the bite). Remove from the heat and serve with a green salad.

GRIDDLED VEGETABLE ROLL WITH CASHEW AND BRAISED GARLIC CREAM

 HELPS LOWER CHOLESTEROL

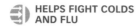 **HELPS FIGHT COLDS AND FLU**

 AIDS HEALTHY DIGESTION

These lightly cooked summer vegetables are bursting with nutrients that support the heart and blood vessels, and also enhance immunity and digestion. A sauce laced with a powerful combination of garlic and cashews enhances these tasty rolls' ability to lower blood cholesterol, and protect against viruses, colds, and the flu.

SERVES 4

2 tbsp olives in brine, drained and chopped

2 tbsp sun-dried tomatoes in oil, drained and chopped

1 red bell pepper, halved and seeded

1 yellow bell pepper, halved and seeded

a dash of olive oil

2 eggplants, sliced thinly lengthwise

2 zucchini, thinly sliced

2 small fennel bulbs, trimmed and quartered

2 marinated artichoke hearts in oil, drained and quartered

For the cashew and braised garlic cream

2 large garlic bulbs

¼ cup olive oil

1 small sprig of rosemary

⅓ cup cashews

a pinch of salt

1 tbsp finely chopped parsley leaves

1 garlic clove, minced

1 To make the braised garlic cream, preheat the oven to 350°F (180°C). Place the garlic bulbs, olive oil, and rosemary sprig in a small baking dish, cover with foil or a lid, and bake for 30–40 minutes or until the cloves are soft and just beginning to brown. Remove from the oven and, when cool enough to handle, squeeze the softened garlic from its skins into a small bowl.

2 Place the cashews and ⅓ cup of the braised garlic purée in a food processor or blender, add ½ cup water, and purée until smooth and sticky. Slowly add another ½ cup water or more until the consistency is like heavy cream and pourable. Add the salt to taste and purée again. Stir in the parsley leaves and garlic and set aside.

3 Increase the oven temperature to 375°F (190°C). Mix the olives and sun-dried tomatoes in a small bowl and set aside. Place the halved peppers on a rimmed baking sheet and bake in the oven for 15–20 minutes, or until their skins start blistering and turning slightly brown. Remove from the oven, transfer to a bowl, cover with plastic wrap to sweat and let cool. Once cool enough to handle, remove the skins and cut the flesh into quarters.

4 Brush a grill pan (or barbecue grill) with the olive oil and place over high heat. Add the eggplant slices in batches and grill for 2–3 minutes on each side. Repeat with the zucchini and fennel.

5 To assemble the vegetable rolls, place an eggplant slice on a cutting board, cover with 1 or 2 slices of grilled zucchini, and place a slice each of red and yellow pepper on top. Place an artichoke quarter on top of the layered vegetables at one side and a fennel quarter next to it. Carefully roll up the layered eggplant slice and fasten with a toothpick. Repeat with the rest of the ingredients. Arrange the vegetable rolls on a serving plate, scatter the olives and sun-dried tomatoes around them, drizzle the cashew and braised garlic cream on top, and serve with a kamut and pine nut salad, if you like.

Fragrant Rice And Millet

AIDS HEALTHY DIGESTION

PROMOTES A SENSE OF WELL-BEING

HAS ANTIFUNGAL PROPERTIES

This fragrant blend of brown rice, millet, vegetables, nuts, and herbs is a great dinner party dish. Cinnamon, cardamom, and coriander are all warming, digestive stimulants, and cardamom is also thought to help stimulate the mind and spirit. Millet is a diuretic, but it is also known to have antifungal properties and is often used in the treatment of candidiasis.

SERVES 4

4oz (115g) mixed walnuts and hazelnuts, halved

¾ cup long grain brown rice

heaped ½ cup millet

1 tbsp olive oil

⅓ cup finely chopped red onion

1 medium leek, sliced

20 coriander seeds, crushed

6 cardamom pods, crushed

a pinch of ground cinnamon

3½ cups vegetable or chicken stock

8oz (225g) mixed bell peppers, halved and seeded

2 tbsp chopped cilantro leaves

salt and freshly ground black pepper

For the dressing

1 tsp tamari soy sauce

juice of 1 lime

2 tbsp chicken stock

1 Soak the mixed nuts in water for 30 minutes. Preheat the oven to 350°F (180°C).

2 Rinse the nuts in fresh water and leave to drain for 2–3 minutes. Then scatter onto a baking sheet and toast in the oven for 30 minutes, shaking or stirring them every 6–10 minutes until dry and light brown in color. Remove the nuts from the oven as soon as they are toasted and increase the temperature to 375°F (190°C).

3 Meanwhile, rinse the rice and millet in fresh water and drain. Heat the olive oil in a medium saucepan over low heat and cook the onion, leek, and spices in the pan for 2 minutes. Add the rice, millet, and stock and simmer for 30 minutes, or until all the liquid has been absorbed and the grains are soft. Avoid stirring the rice mixture while it cooks, because this will release starch and alter the texture.

4 Transfer the mixture to a serving bowl, remove the cardamom pods, if possible, and let cool.

5 Put the mixed peppers on a rimmed baking sheet and bake for 15–20 minutes, or until their skins start blistering and turning slightly brown. Remove from the oven, transfer to a bowl, cover with plastic wrap to sweat, and let cool. Once cool enough to handle, remove the skins and dice the flesh.

6 Mix together all the ingredients for the dressing. Combine the peppers, nuts, and cilantro leaves with the cooled grains, pour over the dressing, adjust the seasoning to taste, and serve.

Cardamom (p116) is an excellent spice to aid digestion, and even boasts of antibacterial properties.

SWEET TREATS

WE ALL NEED A **LITTLE SWEETNESS** IN OUR LIVES. WHETHER HOT OR COLD, DESSERTS WITH FRESH FRUITS, NUTS, AND SEEDS AT THEIR CORE SUPPLY THE **ANTIOXIDANTS**, PHYTONUTRIENTS, HEALTHY OILS, AND **FLAVORS** THAT CAN UPLIFT AND HEAL.

FRESH FIG DELIGHT WITH PEAR AND RED WINE SAUCE

 SUPPORTS HEALTHY LUNG FUNCTION

 PROMOTES BOWEL REGULARITY

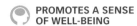 **PROMOTES A SENSE OF WELL-BEING**

 HELPS FIGHT INFLAMMATION

This impressive dessert combines a fig-filled sponge cake with a crisp almond base. It benefits the lungs and large intestine, 2 organs whose functions are closely related. Pears and almonds are cooling and uplifting and help lubricate the lungs, alleviating dry coughs, and also benefit the skin. Figs help to relieve constipation, alleviate inflammation, and build muscle.

SERVES 8

For the base

2 cup ground almonds

3 tbsp superfine sugar

4 tbsp butter, melted

pinch of salt

For the cake

12 tbsp butter, softened, plus extra for greasing

⅔ cup granulated sugar

4 large eggs, beaten

grated zest of 1 organic lemon

1 tsp vanilla extract

1 cup all-purpose flour

2 tsp baking powder

¼ cup whole blanched almonds

8–10 figs, quartered

For the sauce

3 soft pears, peeled, cored, and finely chopped

¼ cup red wine

¼ tsp ground allspice

1 tbsp maple syrup

freshly ground black pepper

1 Preheat the oven to 350°F (180°C). First, make the almond base. Mix together the ingredients for the base in a mixing bowl, combining well. Press the almond mixture evenly onto the base of a 9in (23cm) springform cake pan. Bake for 10 minutes, or until crisp, then transfer to a wire rack to cool. Reduce the oven temperature to 300°F (150°C).

2 Next, make the cake batter. Beat the softened butter and granulated sugar together in a clean bowl until pale and creamy. Then beat in the eggs, lemon zest, and vanilla extract until thoroughly combined. Sift in the flour and baking powder and fold into the wet ingredients until the cake batter is smooth. Finally, fold in the whole almonds. Smear a little butter around the inside of the springform pan.

3 Arrange the quartered figs all over the almond crust and cover with the cake batter. Bake in the oven for about 60 minutes, or until the top is golden and the sides of the cake have pulled away slightly from the inside of the pan. Remove from the oven and unclip the side of the springform pan, leaving the cake on its base. Let cool on a wire rack.

4 For the sauce, add the pears, red wine, and ground allspice to a medium saucepan, bring to a simmer, cover, and cook over low heat for 20 minutes, or until the pears are soft. Transfer to a blender or food processor and purée until smooth. Add the maple syrup and a pinch of black pepper. Purée again. Add more maple syrup to taste, if liked.

5 Place a slice of the cake on a serving plate and drizzle it with a little of the sauce to serve.

ALMOND AND RASPBERRY CAKE

 HELPS CLEAR CONGESTION

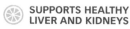 **SUPPORTS HEALTHY LIVER AND KIDNEYS**

 HELPS CALM NERVES

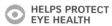 **HELPS PROTECT EYE HEALTH**

This dense, gluten-free cake is made with ground almonds instead of flour. Almonds soothe and support the respiratory system, helping to remove phlegm. Raspberries have a tonic effect on the liver, and a calming effect on the mind. Rich in antioxidants, they also support healthy vision. In traditional Chinese medicine, raspberries are used to treat impotence and infertility in men.

SERVES 6

18 tbsp butter, plus extra for greasing

1 cup superfine sugar

5 large eggs, separated

3 cups ground almonds

1 tsp vanilla extract

1⅓ cups raspberries

1 Preheat the oven to 275°F (140°C). Grease a 10in (25cm) springform cake pan with the butter and line the base with parchment paper, making sure the paper is exactly the same size as the base.

2 Cream the butter and sugar in a large bowl. Add an egg yolk, mix well, then add a little of the ground almonds and stir well. Repeat until all the yolks and almonds have been added to the mixture. Add the vanilla extract and combine well.

3 In a separate, clean large bowl, beat the egg whites to stiff peaks with an electric hand mixer. Gently fold the egg whites into the cake mixture with a metal spoon to keep the mixture as fluffy and light as possible. Reserve 6–12 raspberries to use as decoration later. Transfer half the mixture to the prepared cake pan, arrange half the raspberries on top, then add the rest of the cake mixture and finish with the rest of the raspberries. Don't stir the raspberries into the cake mixture, because they will break up and discolor the cake.

4 Bake in the oven for 45 minutes–1 hour, or until cooked through. To test if the cake is cooked, insert a clean skewer into the center. If the skewer is clean when you take it out, remove the cake from the oven. If not, bake for a little longer and test again.

5 Transfer the cake to a wire rack and let cool. Once cool, carefully remove the springform pan and parchment paper. Decorate the cake with the reserved raspberries to serve.

ELDERBERRY AND BLACKBERRY NUTTY CRISP

 HELPS FIGHT COLDS AND FLU

HAS A MILD DIURETIC ACTION

PROTECTS THE HEART AND BLOOD VESSELS

The best time to make this crisp is when elderberries are fully ripened and blackberries are just beginning to ripen on the bush. They are both worth foraging for, because they enhance immunity, especially against colds and flu. They also have a mild diuretic action, and help maintain healthy blood vessels. If elderberries are no longer in season, use blueberries instead.

SERVES 4–6

1¼lb (550g) apples, peeled, cored, and sliced

1½ cups fresh elderberries

1¾ cups fresh blackberries

For the topping

1 cup all-purpose flour

7 tbsp organic butter

2¼ cups ground almonds

2 tbsp molasses sugar, or other dark brown sugar

½ cup walnuts, finely chopped

crème fraîche, to serve

1 Preheat the oven to 350°F (180°C). To make the topping, place the flour in a mixing bowl, add the butter, and rub it into the flour with your fingertips. Add the ground almonds and molasses sugar and mix together well until the mixture resembles breadcrumbs. Add the chopped walnuts and mix them in well.

2 Add the apples along with a little water to a large saucepan over low heat and simmer for 10 minutes. Transfer the softened apples to a large, deep baking dish and add the berries. Completely and evenly cover the fruit mixture with the topping, pressing it down lightly. Bake in the oven for 35–40 minutes, or until golden on top, then serve either hot or warm with the crème fraîche.

Elderberries *are a good source of antioxidant anthocyanins, which help fight free-radical damage.*

Nutty Sugar Loaf

 PROMOTES A SENSE OF WELL-BEING

 PROMOTES BOWEL REGULARITY

 HELPS KEEP JOINTS SUPPLE

Containing walnuts, chestnuts, hazelnuts, and sprouted spelt, this is a deeply satisfying dish that helps to improve digestion and bowel regularity, and also to strengthen and improve movement in muscles and joints. This recipe, great for a party, requires some advanced preparation, because the spelt grains need 3–4 days to sprout.

SERVES 6–8

1½ cups spelt grains

1 cup hazelnuts

1 cup walnuts

¾ cup fresh sweet chestnuts, cooked, peeled

⅓ cup raw sugar

1 tbsp vanilla extract

mascarpone cheese, to serve

1 To sprout the spelt grains, start soaking them 3–4 days before you need them. Soak a heaped ½ cup of the grains for 8–12 hours in clean water in a large, clean, wide-mouthed glass jar covered with cheesecloth, securing the cloth in place with a rubber band. Strain the water from the grains, rinse the grains in fresh water, drain, then set the jar aside, out of direct sunlight. Rinse and drain the grains again 8–12 hours later. It usually takes 2–3 rinsing cycles for the spelt to sprout; the grains are sprouted when most of them have a tiny rootlet just pushing through. They are ready to use 8 hours later.

2 Preheat the oven to 350°F (180°C). To toast the hazelnuts, put them on a baking sheet and place in the oven for 15 minutes, keeping an eye on them and shaking the sheet occasionally so they don't burn, or they will taste bitter. Transfer to a bowl and cover with plastic wrap to let the nuts sweat for 2–3 minutes. Transfer a small batch of nuts to a piece of paper towel and rub them roughly to remove the majority of the skins. Repeat with the rest of the hazelnuts. Transfer to a blender or food processor and pulse briefly until coarsely chopped.

3 To toast the walnuts, soak in 2 cups water for 30 minutes, then drain. Transfer to a baking sheet and place in the oven for 25–30 minutes, turning them regularly until they become dry and light brown in color. Set aside to cool.

4 Cook the remaining spelt in plenty of water for 1 hour 20 minutes, or until soft, and set aside to cool.

5 Use a coffee grinder, hand grinder, or a powerful blender to grind the cooked spelt, walnuts, and chestnuts, and transfer the ground ingredients to a mixing bowl. Add the whole sprouted spelt grains, raw sugar, and vanilla extract, combining all the ingredients well.

6 Using your hands, mold the dry mixture into a sugar loaf shape on a serving plate (if you find the mixture too dry, blend a small quantity in a blender or food processor to bind it together, and use as a base on which to build the other ingredients). Alternatively, press into individual serving bowls and turn out before serving. Cover with the toasted, coarsely ground hazelnuts. To serve, cut a slice from the sugar loaf and serve with a spoonful of mascarpone cheese.

WARM FRUIT SALAD IN SWEET WINE SAUCE

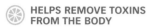 **HELPS REMOVE TOXINS FROM THE BODY**

 HAS AN UPLIFTING EFFECT

HELPS EASE CONSTIPATION

 HELPS LOWER BLOOD PRESSURE

The subtle flavors and textures of warmed fresh fruits, tossed in a sweet wine syrup, result in a deliciously different twist on a classic fruit salad. This combination of soft and crunchy fresh fruits and pistachio nuts is detoxifying, uplifting, and has a tonic effect on the whole body. The abundant fiber in the fruit supports healthy digestion and potassium helps lower blood pressure.

SERVES 4

3 tbsp butter

3 tbsp superfine sugar

1¼ cup sweet Marsala wine

1 ripe pear, cored and quartered

4 figs, halved

2 peaches, quartered, with pits removed

2 nectarines, quartered, with pits removed

1 apple, cored and quartered

¾ cup pistachio nuts, shelled and roughly chopped

1 Preheat the oven to 400°F (200°C). Melt the butter in a small saucepan, add the sugar and Marsala wine, and cook over low heat for 5–10 minutes, or until the mixture has a syrupy consistency. Remove from the heat and set aside to cool.

2 Place all the fruits in a bowl, add the pistachio nuts, and pour in two-thirds of the cooled Marsala syrup. Gently toss everything together to coat the fruit. Turn the fruit mixture out into a shallow baking dish and bake in the oven for 25–35 minutes, or until the fruit is warmed through, but not completely cooked.

3 Remove from the oven and spoon the warm fruit salad onto individual plates. Mix the remaining Marsala syrup with the juices from the baking dish, drizzle it over the fruit portions, and serve.

Nectarines (p22) of all types, including the white-fleshed variety, can help remove excess water from the body.

CHERRY STRUDEL

 PROTECTS AGAINST FREE-RADICAL DAMAGE   **PROTECTS THE HEART AND BLOOD VESSELS** **HELPS EASE JOINT INFLAMMATION** **HELPS RELIEVE INSOMNIA**

The tart morello cherries in this recipe are particularly rich in antioxidants, which help protect the heart and fight free-radical damage and inflammation, especially in the joints. They also contain melatonin, which aids restful sleep. If you can't find morello cherries, choose a sweet variety and marinate in the zest of an orange and the juice of half a lemon for a sharper flavor.

SERVES 4

scant ½ cup fresh breadcrumbs

¼ cup superfine sugar

¼ cup ground almonds

¼ cup ground walnuts

5 sheets store-bought filo pastry

2 tbsp unsalted butter, melted, plus a little extra for brushing

½ tsp ground cinnamon

11oz (325g) fresh morello cherries, pitted

3 tbsp sliced almonds (optional)

confectioner's sugar, for dusting

1 To make the filling, mix the breadcrumbs, superfine sugar, and ground almonds together in a bowl and set aside.

2 Preheat the oven to 375°F (190°C). If you can't find ground walnuts, grind some walnut pieces briefly in a food processor or blender. Arrange a sheet of parchment paper on a flat surface. Place a sheet of filo pastry on the parchment, with one of the longer edges of the pastry rectangle facing you. Brush the surface of the pastry with some of the melted butter and dust with a little of the cinnamon. Repeat with the rest of the pastry sheets, butter, and cinnamon. Scatter the breadcrumb filling over the pastry stack, leaving a 2in (5cm) border around the edge (this will help when you fold the pastry edges over to prevent the filling from escaping). If you want to make 2 strudels, cut the pastry in half, leaving a 4in (10cm) space in the middle. Scatter the ground walnuts over the filling and heap the cherries in a thick strip along the center of the pastry, leaving a 2in (5cm) gap at either end.

3 Fold in the short edges of the pastry rectangle. Then, using the parchment paper, fold over the long edge of the pastry rectangle nearest you, and roll up the pastry to enclose the filling and create a long roll. Brush the surface of the rolled pastry with more melted butter and scatter with the sliced almonds, if using.

4 Lift the parchment paper with the strudel, seam-side down, onto a large cookie sheet and bake in the oven for 30 minutes, or until the pastry is golden. Allow to cool for about 10 minutes, then dust with confectioner's sugar and serve.

Morello cherries (p20) are colored brightly with red pigments that produce a greater pain-relieving effect than aspirin.

Baked Quince

 SUPPORTS HEALTHY LIVER FUNCTION   **HELPS IMPROVE CIRCULATION**   **HELPS RELIEVE JOINT AND MUSCLE PAIN**   **SOOTHES UPSET STOMACHS**

Quince is a well-regarded medicinal fruit and a liver remedy in traditional Chinese, Tibetan, and Bhutanese medicine. It helps increase blood circulation to the muscles and tendons, and is used in the treatment of rheumatic pain and cramp in calf muscles. It is also used to treat deficiency in the spleen and the associated symptoms of vomiting, diarrhea, and dyspepsia.

SERVES 4

4 small or 2 large quince, peeled, cored, and quartered

½ tsp cardamom pods

1 tbsp soft brown sugar

¼ cup sweet dessert wine, plus a little for drizzling (Marsala or Muscat are good choices)

¼ cup mascarpone cheese

1 Preheat the oven to 350°F (180°C). Put the quince in a baking dish, scatter with the cardamom pods and sugar, and drizzle with half the dessert wine and 2 tablespoons water. Bake in the oven for about 1 hour, or until cooked through and golden in color. Check the quince occasionally to make sure it doesn't dry out and add more wine or water if needed.

2 Mix the rest of the sweet wine and the mascarpone in a bowl. Transfer the quince to 4 small serving bowls. Drizzle with the cooking juices and add 1 tablespoon of the flavored mascarpone to each portion to serve.

ROSE PETAL AND WHITE WINE SORBET

 HELPS RELAX AND UNWIND THE MIND

 HELPS IMPROVE CIRCULATION

 HELPS EASE MENSTRUAL CRAMPS

Roses have a deeply calming effect on the nervous system. Here they are combined with a small amount of sweet wine, which helps relax blood vessels and boosts their beneficial effect on circulation. Roses are also a good remedy for menstrual cramps and premenstrual symptoms. Highly perfumed roses (*Rosa damascena* or *Rosa gallica*) are best for this recipe.

SERVES 4

10 fresh red rose heads or a large handful of red rose petals, plus extra petals for decoration

1¼ cups sweet dessert wine (Marsala or Muscat are good choices)

1 cup superfine sugar

2 tsp agar flakes

juice of 1 lemon, strained

juice of 1 orange, strained

1 Combine half the roses and the sweet dessert wine in a pitcher or bowl and refrigerate. Infuse the rest of the roses in 1³/₄ cups boiling water and set aside to cool.

2 Strain the infused liquid and discard the petals. Transfer the liquid to a saucepan and add the sugar. Set the pan over gentle heat and stir frequently until the sugar has dissolved. Bring to a boil and boil (at 230°F /110°C, if you have a sugar thermometer) for 5–8 minutes, or until you have a light syrup. Remove from the heat and set aside to cool.

3 Melt the agar flakes in ¹/₄ cup hot water and add it to the syrup. Stir, transfer to a bowl, and then refrigerate until completely cold.

4 Combine the chilled dessert wine and fresh rose petal mixture with the rose syrup. Stir in the strained lemon and orange juices and pour the mixture into an ice cream maker. Process the sorbet for 20–30 minutes, or until it is cold and the right consistency. Spoon the ingredients into a freezerproof container and freeze if not serving immediately. If you don't have an ice cream maker, pour the wine and syrup mixture into a freezerproof container and place in the freezer. Take it out every hour to give it a stir until the mixture is completely frozen.

CALM YOUR MOOD

A SMALL AMOUNT OF WHITE WINE RELAXES YOUR BLOOD VESSELS. INFUSED WITH ROSE PETALS— TRADITIONALLY USED TO TREAT NERVOUS TENSION— IT WILL ALSO HELP TO INCREASE YOUR SENSE OF WELL-BEING.

Banana And Cranberry Ice Cream

 HELPS EASE CONSTIPATION **HELPS LOWER BLOOD PRESSURE** **FIGHTS URINARY TRACT INFECTIONS**

Ice cream without any cream—ideal for those who are allergic to cow milk. Ripe bananas promote bowel regularity and can help lower blood pressure, while cranberries have antibacterial properties that treat urinary tract infections (UTIs). In traditional Chinese medicine, cold food is thought to disrupt healthy digestion, so keep frozen foods for occasional treats.

SERVES 4

4 ripe bananas, sliced

2 cups cranberries

1 tbsp superfine sugar

1 tsp vanilla extract

scant ½ cup pistachio nuts, shelled and chopped

1 Put the bananas and cranberries in the freezer and remove when semifrozen. If they are completely frozen, allow to thaw slightly for about an hour. Place them in a blender or food processor and pulse until the fruits are coarsely combined and still have some texture. Divide among 4 freezerproof serving bowls (such as enamel bowls, which are freezerproof) and place in the freezer for 3 hours. Alternatively, freeze the ice cream in a clean plastic container.

2 Meanwhile, place the sugar in a small saucepan over low heat and add just enough water to wet the sugar. When the sugar has dissolved completely, add the vanilla extract and stir in the pistachios, then remove from the heat and allow to cool.

3 Remove the bowls, or container, from the freezer, let sit at room temperature for a short while, then use an ice-cream scoop to divide the ice cream among 4 serving bowls. Drizzle the sugar solution and nuts over each portion to serve.

TIP: If you have a weak digestive system, you may like to add a few drops of freshly squeezed ginger juice, instead of water, to the sugar to dissolve it (grate fresh ginger, wrap in a piece of cheesecloth, squeeze the cheesecloth, and collect the juice). Children may also benefit from ginger juice, because their digestive systems are still developing, but make sure they are familiar with, and enjoy the taste of, ginger before you include it. If you can't find fresh or frozen cranberries, use blueberries, which freeze well and taste just as good.

MEDITERRANEAN NUT SQUARES IN ROSE AND CARDAMOM SYRUP

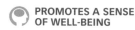 **PROMOTES A SENSE OF WELL-BEING**

 ENHANCES VIRILITY

 HELPS COMBAT FATIGUE

Also known as baklava, this "pick-me-up" from the eastern Mediterranean is a popular delicacy across Europe. Traditionally, walnuts and pistachios were considered beneficial to the mind, and to increase virility in men; here cardamom pods are added to enhance the rejuvenating benefits of these nuts. High-quality fresh walnuts are essential for this recipe.

MAKES 24 SQUARES

3 cups walnuts halves
1½ cups pistachio nuts, shelled
1 tbsp unsalted butter, melted
1lb 2oz (500g) filo pastry
⅔ cup walnut oil

For the syrup

1¼ cups raw sugar
3 tbsp rosewater
juice of 1 lemon
1 lemon, thinly sliced
10 green cardamom pods

1 Preheat the oven to 350°F (180°C). Roughly grind two-thirds of the walnuts into chunky pieces in a food processor or blender, and pulse the remaining walnuts until finely chopped; too many finely ground nuts will make the finished baklava heavy. Pulse the pistachios until finely chopped, then mix the walnuts and pistachios together in a bowl.

2 Use a rectangular baking pan a little smaller than the size of the sheets of filo pastry (to retain the filling) and brush it with some of the melted butter. Lay the first sheet of pastry in the pan, brush with a little walnut oil, and layer a second sheet on top; repeat with a third sheet and more walnut oil. Then spread a thin layer of chopped nuts on the pastry. Continue layering, alternating 1 layer of pastry with 1 layer of nuts, and brushing the pastry with walnut oil, until you have used all the nuts. Finish with 2 or 3 final layers of pastry, with a little walnut oil brushed in between them, and brush the top layer with melted butter.

3 With a sharp knife, slice lengthwise right through the pastry layers, all the way down to the bottom, at 1½in (4cm) intervals, to create strips of layered pastry. Rotate the baking pan by 60 degrees and repeat, cutting diagonally across the pastry strips at 1½in (4cm) intervals to make individual diamond-shaped portions. If the pastry starts lifting while you are cutting it, press it back in place. Bake for 25 minutes, then lower the temperature to 300°F (150°C) and bake for a further 25 minutes, or until the squares are crisp and golden.

4 Meanwhile, make the syrup by boiling the sugar with the rosewater, lemon juice, thinly sliced lemon, cardamom pods, and 1¼ cups water in a saucepan over high heat. Simmer uncovered for 10–15 minutes on medium heat. Remove from the heat and set aside to cool. Once cool, remove the cardamom pods and discard. When the squares are cooked, pour the syrup and sliced lemons over them and cover with a clean dish towel. Let cool a few hours or overnight. Baklava is best served the next day when the flavors have infused, and it will keep fresh for 4–5 days if stored in an airtight container in a cool place.

SESAME HEART COOKIES

 HELPS CLEAR CONGESTION

 PROMOTES BOWEL REGULARITY

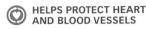 **HELPS PROTECT HEART AND BLOOD VESSELS**

 HELPS EASE LOWER BACK PAIN

A traditional tonic food, sesame seeds lubricate the lungs and intestines, relieving dry coughs and constipation, protecting the heart and easing rheumatic conditions and lower back pain. Soaking the seeds overnight and dry-frying them before grinding reduces their oxalic acid content (which prevents the absorption of other nutrients) and makes them more digestible.

MAKES 50–60 COOKIES

1¾ cups sesame seeds
8 tbsp butter
¼ cup sesame oil
1 cup superfine sugar
2 large eggs, beaten
2 tsp vanilla extract
1½ cups all-purpose flour
¾ cup self-rising flour

1 Place the sesame seeds in a bowl, cover generously with cold water, and let soak overnight. Drain the seeds, allow to drip-dry for 2–3 minutes, then lightly dry-fry them in a medium saucepan over low heat and set aside.

2 Preheat the oven to 350°F (180°C). Put the butter, sesame oil, sugar, eggs, and vanilla extract in a mixing bowl and beat together to a light, creamy consistency.

3 Place the sesame seeds in a blender or food processor, pulse briefly to crush them lightly, then beat into the butter and egg mixture. Sift the flours together and stir them into the mixture to make a dough.

4 Gather the dough together with your hands, pressing it gently into a round ball. Don't overwork the dough, because this will yield a cookie that is tough. Wrap the dough in plastic wrap and leave to rest for 30 minutes in the refrigerator.

5 On a lightly floured surface, roll out the dough until it is ¼in (5mm) thick, and cut out heart shapes using a small heart-shaped cookie cutter. Place on a baking sheet lined with parchment paper and bake for 7 minutes, or until the cookies turn golden. They burn easily, so watch them carefully. Remove from the oven, transfer to a wire rack to cool, and store in an airtight container. They will keep for 2–3 weeks.

Sesame seeds (p94) contain plant hormones that support cardiovascular health, making the heart shape of these cookies appropriate.

ALMOND AND PISTACHIO MACAROONS

 SUPPORTS LUNG FUNCTION

 PROMOTES A HEALTHY DIGESTIVE TRACT

 HELPS IMPROVE CIRCULATION

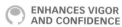 **ENHANCES VIGOR AND CONFIDENCE**

Almonds and pistachios are both good sources of protein and, together with cardamom, are beneficial for your respiratory system, circulation, and digestive health. They are also traditionally regarded as an aphrodisiac for both men and women. This recipe makes quite a number of macaroons, so halve the quantities if you like.

MAKES 45

3 large egg whites
1 cup superfine sugar
1 tsp crushed cardamom seeds
4 cups ground almonds
2 tbsp rose water
3 tbsp shelled whole pistachios

1 Preheat the oven to 300°F (150°C). Put the egg whites in a mixing bowl and beat into soft or stiff peaks with an electric hand mixer, gradually adding the sugar as you beat. When all the sugar has been incorporated, add the cardamom, ground almonds, and rose water and combine all the ingredients together.

2 Line a baking sheet with parchment paper. Wet your hands with water so the mixture won't stick to your fingers. Divide the mixture into small walnut-sized balls and arrange on the parchment paper, allowing sufficient space around each ball. Place a pistachio in the center of each.

3 Bake for 10–12 minutes, then transfer to a wire rack to cool. Store the macaroons in an airtight container. They will keep for up to 2 weeks.

Almonds *(p92) are rich in cholesterol-lowering monounsaturated fatty acids.*

POPPY SEED AND WALNUT ROULADE

 HELPS COMBAT FATIGUE   **PROMOTES A SENSE OF WELL-BEING**   **SUPPORTS HEALTHY KIDNEY FUNCTION**   **PROTECTS THE HEART AND BLOOD VESSELS**

The filling of walnuts and poppy seeds together deliver a revitalizing and physically strengthening boost in this sweet bread roulade. Poppy seeds have a balancing effect on emotions, while walnuts bring a sense of well-being and help strengthen the heart. Walnuts can also improve men's fertility, which may account for their traditional use as an aphrodisiac.

SERVES 8

For the dough

½oz (15g) fresh yeast

¼ cup sugar

1½ cups all-purpose flour, plus extra for sprinkling

a pinch of salt

3 tbsp butter, softened

½ cup milk

1 tbsp light rum

grated zest of 1 lemon

1 large egg yolk

1 tsp vanilla extract

oil, for greasing

1 large egg, beaten, for brushing

confectioner's sugar, for dusting

For the filling

2½ cups ground poppy seeds

½ cup chopped walnuts

¼ cup milk

grated zest of 1 lemon

a pinch of ground cinnamon

1 tbsp light rum

2 tbsp butter

¼ cup sugar

2 tbsp vanilla sugar, or ¼ tsp vanilla extract mixed with 2 tbsp superfine sugar

1 large egg, beaten

1 To make the dough, crush the yeast, add it to a medium bowl, and mix it with 1 tablespoon each of the sugar and flour. Add 1–2 tsp lukewarm water and stir it in with a fork until the yeast dissolves to form a thick paste. Cover and set aside in a warm place for about 15 minutes to rise.

2 Sift the remaining flour into a bowl and add a pinch of salt. Add the yeast paste mixture and gently rub it into the flour until the mixture resembles bread crumbs.

3 In a small saucepan, warm the butter gently to melt it. Remove from the heat and add the milk, remaining sugar, rum, lemon zest, egg yolk, and vanilla extract. Stir well and pour into the flour and yeast mixture. Mix together and knead gently until the dough is smooth and no longer sticks to the bowl. Knead the dough with a little flour if necessary to form a smooth dough. Sprinkle with flour, cover with a clean cloth, and set aside in a warm place for 20–30 minutes to rise.

4 Preheat the oven to 375°F (190°C). To make the filling, put all the ingredients in a large bowl and mix into a thick paste.

5 Turn the risen dough onto a well-floured wooden cutting board or work surface and roll it into a rectangle about 10in (25cm) x 7in (18cm), and ½in (1cm) thick. Cover the surface with the filling, leaving a border of about ½in (1cm), then fold one long edge of the dough over and roll carefully into a cylindrical shape. Place the dough roll on a well-greased baking sheet and set aside in a warm place for 20–30 minutes for the dough to rise again.

6 Brush the surface of the dough roll with the beaten egg and bake in the oven for 25–30 minutes. Remove from the oven and let cool on the baking sheet. Dust with confectioner's sugar, and cut into slices to serve.

TIP: To make your own vanilla sugar, put 2 cups of white sugar in an airtight container. Take 1 vanilla bean and split it and scrape out the seeds; add both bean and seeds to the sugar. Leave to infuse for 2 weeks before using.

Dried Fruit And Nut Roll

 HELPS EASE CONSTIPATION

 PROMOTES A SENSE OF WELL-BEING

Try this as a variation on a traditional fruit cake to grace your table during a festive celebration. It is high in fiber, which helps improve bowel regularity and enhances gut health. Prunes, figs, and dates also supply slow-release energy, while hemp seeds and walnuts are said to bring a sense of well-being and help strengthen the heart. You will need to start the recipe two days ahead.

SERVES 8–10

⅔ cup dried prunes, finely chopped

¾ cup dates, finely chopped

¾ cup dried figs, finely chopped

½ cup finely chopped fresh orange peel

1¼ cups walnuts, finely chopped

⅓ cup sugar

½ cup sweet Marsala wine

heaped ¼ cup cacao nibs, chopped

⅓ cup hemp seeds

confectioner's sugar, for dusting

1 Place all the ingredients except the confectioner's sugar in a medium saucepan. Heat gently over low heat, stirring until the sugar has dissolved and the mixture is thoroughly combined.

2 Dust a wooden cutting board or work surface with confectioner's sugar and transfer the fruit mixture onto it. Roll into a sausage shape, about 2in (5cm) thick and 12in (30cm) long, then wrap in a clean dish towel. Set aside in a cool place to dry out; it's best to let it stand for a few days. Cut into thin slices, about ¾in (2cm), to serve.

Dried figs (p26) are a fantastic source of fiber, which aids a healthy digestive system.

DRINKS

SOOTHING, **UPLIFTING**, AND NUTRITIOUS DRINKS
AND BEAUTIFUL BLENDS **DELIVER NUTRIENTS**
QUICKLY AND IN AN EASILY **ABSORBABLE** FORM—
WHETHER YOU OPT FOR REFRESHING COOL DRINKS
OR **NURTURING** HOT BROTHS AND TEAS.

HOT LEMONADE WITH GINGER AND HONEY

  HELPS FIGHT COLDS AND THE FLU   **AIDS HEALTHY DIGESTION**   **HELPS IMPROVE CIRCULATION**   **CONTAINS SLOW-RELEASE SUGARS**

Lemon juice, mint, and ginger are the perfect trio to help combat the symptoms of a cold. The thin skin and fibrous root of fresh ginger have anti-inflammatory properties that can lessen the aches and pains, while honey is a natural antibiotic and lemon and mint have antibacterial benefits. Drink this healing tea as soon as you feel the first signs of a cold coming on.

SERVES 2

1in (3cm) piece fresh ginger, grated
zest and juice of 1 lemon
1 tbsp honey
1 tbsp chopped mint leaves

1 Place the grated fresh ginger in a small saucepan, cover with 1½ cups water, and bring to a boil. Turn the heat down to low and simmer for 15 minutes.
2 Pour the mixture through a strainer into a pitcher, add the lemon juice and zest, stir in the honey and mix well. Add the mint leaf and serve in heatproof glasses. Drink the tea and eat the chopped mint leaves.

ALOE AND HONEY HOT TODDY

 HELPS STRENGTHEN THE IMMUNE SYSTEM   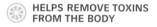 **HELPS REMOVE TOXINS FROM THE BODY**

Honey and aloe are known to help the body detoxify and to strengthen the immune system, which in turn enables all the major organs to function more efficiently. Traditionally, the variety of aloe known as *Aloe arborescens* (which produces red flowers when in bloom) is used for this recipe; it has a high concentration of complex sugars and other phytonutrients that work synergistically.

SERVES 2

5½oz (150g) aloe leaves
½ cup honey
3 tbsp grappa or Cognac

1 Clean the fresh aloe leaves with a damp cloth, cut off and discard the spines, chop the leaves, and put them in a blender or food processor. Add the honey and grappa or Cognac and purée. Add a dash of water if you want to dilute the flavor slightly. Pour into 2 heatproof glasses and serve. If using as a therapeutic drink, allow to cool, transfer to a dark glass bottle, seal, and store in the refrigerator for up to 1 week. Take 1–2 tablespoons a day.

BLACKBERRY LEMONADE

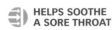 **HELPS SOOTHE
A SORE THROAT**

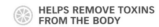 **SUPPORTS HEALTHY
KIDNEY FUNCTION**

**HELPS REMOVE TOXINS
FROM THE BODY**

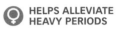 **HELPS ALLEVIATE
HEAVY PERIODS**

Blackberries are a great medicine if you have a painful or swollen throat, mouth, or gums. Their antioxidant, kidney-toning, and detoxifying properties make them a must-have when in season. Collect the leaves too, because a blackberry-leaf infusion enhances the anti-inflammatory effects further. Serve with ice, or as a warm drink, if you have a throat condition.

SERVES 2

4 tsp dried blackberry leaves, or 12 fresh leaves

2 cups blackberries, rinsed

2 lemons, juiced, plus a few thin slices for decoration (optional)

3 tbsp maple syrup

1 To make an infusion with the leaves, boil 1¼ cups water, pour over the leaves, and let it infuse for 10 minutes. Strain the mixture, reserving the liquid to use in the lemonade. Discard the leaves.

2 Place the blackberries in a food processor or blender and purée to a pulp. If you don't like the gritty texture of the seeds in your drink, strain the pulp through a fine mesh strainer and collect the smooth juice.

3 Pour the lemon juice, blackberry juice, and 1 cup of the blackberry leaf infusion into a pitcher, add the maple syrup, and stir well. Pour into large glasses, decorate each with a slice of lemon, and serve.

BARLEY GRASS AND BARLEY LEMONADE

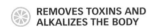 **REMOVES TOXINS AND
ALKALIZES THE BODY**

 **FIGHTS URINARY
TRACT INFECTIONS**

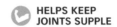 **HELPS KEEP
JOINTS SUPPLE**

This juice combines the benefits of the dry barley grain with those of the fresh barley juice to provide a powerful, alkalizing, anti-inflammatory, and purifying drink. It helps support healthy joints and benefits the intestines, urinary system, and skin, all of which eliminate waste materials from the body. It also helps revitalize and energize the body and slows signs of aging.

SERVES 4

½ cup whole, nonhulled barley (optional)

½ cup pearl barley

1in (2.5cm) lemon peel, cut into 4 strips

⅓ cup lemon juice

2 tbsp honey, or more as desired

⅓ cup barley grass juice

4 lemon slices, to garnish

1 If you want to grow your own barley grass, soak the nonhulled barley in a bowl of water overnight. Drain and arrange the soaked barley on a seed tray filled with organic propagation mix. Gently press the grains down into the soil and leave to germinate. Mist twice daily until it grows to 5–6in (12–15cm) high, when it is ready to harvest (about 10 days).

2 Place the pearl barley into a fine mesh strainer, pour boiling water over it, and allow to drain. Transfer to a medium saucepan, add the lemon peel and 4 cups water, and bring to a boil. Reduce the heat to low and simmer for 25 minutes. Remove from the heat and strain into a clean container. Add the lemon juice and honey to taste, mix well, and refrigerate until chilled. Juice the barley grass (if you have grown it yourself) just before serving and stir into the lemonade or simply add the store-bought barley grass juice. To serve, pour into tall glasses, add a slice of lemon to each glass, and stir.

Blackberry Lemonade ▶

Sour Cherry Drink

 AIDS RECOVERY AND MUSCLE STRENGTH   **HELPS PROMOTE PEACEFUL SLEEP**   **HELPS WITH FAT AND SUGAR METABOLISM**

A popular drink in eastern Europe and western Asia where sour cherries commonly grow, this is a must-have remedy for building strength after a hard day's work, aiding recovery from a tough workout, and relaxing your mind to get a good night's sleep. Cherries also help balance blood sugar, and assist the liver in metabolizing fat after a meal.

SERVES 4

1 cup dried sour cherries, pitted

³/₄ cup sugar

1 tbsp vanilla extract

1½lb (675g) sour cherries, pitted

maple syrup to taste (optional)

1 lime, thinly sliced, to garnish (optional)

1 Rinse the dried cherries, transfer to a bowl, cover with water, and stir to remove some of the oil they are coated in. Drain and repeat. Transfer to a large bowl, cover with water, and soak for 6 hours or overnight to reconstitute. Drain, set aside the cherries, and reserve the soaking water.

2 Measure the soaking water and add enough fresh water if necessary to make ³/₄ cup. Transfer to a small saucepan, add the sugar, set over low heat, and let the sugar dissolve. Bring to a boil, turn the heat down, simmer for 10 minutes, and add the soaked cherries. Simmer for 20–30 minutes, or until the cherries are soft and the syrup has thickened. Strain the mixture, return the syrup to the pan, and discard the fruit. Bring the syrup back to a boil, remove from the heat, and stir in the vanilla extract. Set aside to cool while you juice the fresh sour cherries.

3 Mix 1³/₄ cups each of cherry juice and syrup in a pitcher and dilute with water. Add maple syrup to taste, and lime slices, if using. Store any unused syrup in a sterilized glass bottle in the refrigerator for 1–2 weeks.

Elderberry Syrup

 PROTECTS AGAINST COLDS AND THE FLU   **HELPS CLEAR CONGESTION**   **HELPS MAINTAIN WATER BALANCE**   **HELPS EASE CONSTIPATION**

Pungent, bitter-sweet, ripe elderberries are rich in antioxidants that help prevent and treat colds, coughs, and the flu by promoting sweating, strengthening the lungs, maintaining water balance and bowel regularity, and shifting mucus. Use this syrup as a quick flu remedy or in cooking.

SERVES 2

10oz (300g) elderberries

1¾in (4cm) fresh ginger, grated

1¼ cups superfine sugar

juice of 2 lemons

1 Put the berries and ginger into a medium saucepan and add 1¼ cups water. Bring to a boil, cover, turn the heat down, and simmer over low heat for 20–30 minutes, or until the fruit is soft.

2 Strain the fruit through some cheesecloth or a very fine sieve into a clean saucepan. Discard the fruit and ginger left behind after straining.

3 Add the sugar to the pan and allow it to dissolve over low heat, stirring constantly. When it has dissolved, add the lemon juice and increase the heat. Bring to a boil and boil for 10–15 minutes, or until the liquid becomes syrupy. Transfer to a heat-sterilized bottle, seal, label, and date. Store in the refrigerator and use within 6 weeks.

WINTER PICK-ME-UP JUICE

 PROTECTS AGAINST COLDS AND FLU

 HELPS MAINTAIN ENERGY LEVELS

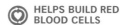 **HELPS BUILD RED BLOOD CELLS**

There is usually a brief window in the fall when wild rosehips, blackberries, and blueberries can be harvested at the same time. The high antioxidant levels of these wild berries help boost your immunity and energy levels, and traditionally they are considered to be a blood tonic. Cinnamon is rich in antioxidants too, and is also an effective aid in the treatment of colds and the flu.

SERVES 2

4oz (115g) rosehips, halved and seeded
³/₄ cup blackberries
³/₄ cup raspberries
³/₄ cup blueberries
¼ tsp cinnamon
2 tbsp elderberry syrup (left)
coconut water, to dilute

1 Put all ingredients except the coconut water in a food processor or blender and blend until smooth. Add coconut water until you achieve the desired consistency.

BLUEBERRIES

ROSEHIPS

BLACKBERRIES

RASPBERRIES

FIGHT THE COLD

THIS JUICE IS THE PERFECT WINTER GUARD. ANTIOXIDANT-RICH BERRIES ENHANCE YOUR IMMUNITY AND FIGHT COLDS AND FLU. THIS QUANTITY OF ROSEHIP ALONE ACCOUNTS FOR MORE THAN 1½ TIMES YOUR RECOMMENDED DAILY INTAKE OF VITAMIN C.

HEALTH BOOST JUICE

 PROTECTS AGAINST COLDS AND THE FLU   **HELPS REMOVE TOXINS FROM THE BODY** **AIDS HEALTHY DIGESTION**

This juice is a beneficial tonic, especially in the winter. Red kuri squash, which has a mild sweet flavor, supplies anti-inflammatory and antioxidant properties, while fragrant ginger can improve digestion. Tart grapefruit helps ward off common colds, improves liver function, and treats gallstones, and salty-tasting celery has a diuretic action that helps detoxify the body.

SERVES 2

3½ oz (100g) Red kuri squash

1 small piece fresh ginger, skin on

1 large grapefruit, peeled and pith removed

2 celery stalks and leaves, roughly chopped

1 Cut the squash in half, scoop out all the seeds, and discard or reserve them to roast later and use as an ingredient in other recipes (such as Presoaked Barley Breakfast, p190), or as a topping for salads and soups. Leave the skin on the squash to benefit from its nutrients and chop the flesh if necessary, so it fits through the hopper of your juicer.

2 Juice all the ingredients and combine in a pitcher. Strain through a sieve to remove the grapefruit seeds and serve immediately in tall glasses.

COOLING, SOOTHING JUICE

 PROMOTES A HEALTHY DIGESTIVE TRACT   **HELPS REMOVE PARASITES IN THE GUT** 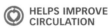 **HELPS IMPROVE CIRCULATION**

Aloe vera has a cooling, anti-inflammatory effect on the gut; it helps relieve constipation and can help clear intestinal parasites. Turmeric has a similarly soothing effect on the gut, relieving pain and tension, and also helps improve circulation. Fresh ginger tones and stimulates the digestive tract, but it can raise blood pressure; if you suffer from high blood pressure, omit the ginger.

SERVES 2

¾in (2cm) piece fresh turmeric

¾in (2cm) piece fresh ginger

1 green apple

2 celery stalks

2 small leaves of aloe vera

coconut water, to dilute

1 Using a juicer, juice the fresh turmeric, fresh ginger, apple, and celery and combine the juices in a pitcher.

2 Using a sharp knife, remove the spine from each aloe vera leaf, slice the leaves open lengthwise, and scrape out the gel. Add the gel to the juices in the pitcher and mix thoroughly. Pour into 2 tall glasses. To serve, dilute with coconut water until the juice is your preferred consistency.

STAY SUPPLE JUICE

 HELPS FIGHT INFLAMMATION   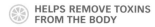 **HELPS REMOVE TOXINS FROM THE BODY**   **HELPS COMBAT FATIGUE**

This pungent vegetable juice addresses the cause of joint problems. Cucumber, spinach, and turmeric combine to relieve joint inflammation and stimulate the circulation and, together with chile and ginger, they help expel accumulated toxins from the body by encouraging bowel movements, promoting sweating, and acting as a mild diuretic.

SERVES 2

1 small cucumber, skin on

2 cups spinach leaves

1½ in (4cm) piece fresh ginger, skin on

1½ in (4cm) piece fresh turmeric, skin on

4 celery stalks

2 green apples, skin on

½ fresh red chile, seeded

1 Using a juicer, juice each ingredient, transfer to a glass pitcher, stir to mix well, and serve. Consume immediately to avoid any loss of valuable nutrients.

FIVE-FLAVOR JUICE

 AIDS DETOXIFICATION SYSTEM   **SUPPORTS AND PROTECTS THE LIVER**   **PROMOTES HEALTHY SKIN**

Traditional Chinese medicine categorizes foods into 5 flavors—bitter, sweet, salty, sour, and hot. This recipe includes all 5 flavors to help keep the body in balance. In addition, hot black radish is a traditional Chinese remedy for liver conditions, while beets and carrots are both packed with antioxidants that increase oxygen and nutrient levels in the blood and benefit the skin.

SERVES 2

1 medium black radish or turnip

1 large beet

2 large carrots

8 celery stalks

4 small Seville oranges, with half the peel removed

1 Using a juicer, juice each ingredient, transfer to a glass pitcher, stir to mix well, and serve. Consume immediately to avoid any loss of valuable nutrients.

BUILD-ME-UP JUICE

 AIDS DETOXIFICATION SYSTEM　　 **HELPS RELEASE CELLULAR ENERGY**　　 **HELPS IMPROVE CIRCULATION**　　 **AIDS HEALTHY DIGESTION**

This particular blend of root vegetables is high in antioxidants and phytonutrients that help revitalize the blood by improving circulation and increasing oxygen levels. It also supports the health of major organs, such as the heart, liver, and kidneys, builds body tissues and fluids, and enhances the digestive process by promoting bowel regularity and general intestinal health.

SERVES 2

2 large carrots
1 large beet
4 celery stalks
½ celeriac, peeled
2 fennel bulbs
¾in (2cm) piece fresh ginger, skin on
1 small lemon, peel on
coconut water, to dilute

1 Using a juicer, juice each ingredient, transfer to a glass pitcher, stir to mix well, and add coconut water to taste. Serve in tall glasses and consume immediately to avoid any loss of valuable nutrients.

ALERT AND JOYFUL JUICE

 SUPPORTS HEALTHY LIVER FUNCTION　　 **HELP PREVENT URINARY TRACT INFECTIONS**　　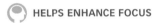 **HELPS ENHANCE FOCUS**

According to traditional Chinese medicine, sour flavors are said to tonify and enhance liver function, promote the elimination of waste products through the intestines and urinary system, calm emotions, improve your sense of well-being, and focus the mind. Adjust the flavor of this sour-based juice to your liking by adding some coconut water to modify its acidity.

SERVES 2

heaped ½ cup fresh or frozen cranberries
1 small Seville orange, peel on, and quartered
1 red bell pepper, seeded
3 celery stalks
1 small cucumber
¼ chile, seeded
½in (1cm) piece fresh ginger, skin on
coconut water, to dilute

1 Using a juicer, juice each ingredient, transfer to a glass pitcher, stir to mix well, and add enough coconut water to taste. Serve in tall glasses and consume immediately to avoid any loss of valuable nutrients.

ROSE SYRUP

 HELPS TO RELAX AND UNWIND THE MIND   **HELPS STRENGTHEN THE IMMUNE SYSTEM**

Mildly sedative and immune-enhancing rose syrup can be used to sweeten herbal infusions, poured over pancakes and ice cream, drizzled over fruit salads, used in a sorbet, or diluted with water and drunk as a cordial. Highly perfumed damask rose (*Rosa damascena*) or French rose (*Rosa gallica*) are best for this recipe. Keep the temperature low to preserve their benefits.

MAKES 2 CUPS

1 cup raw sugar
juice of 1 lemon
juice of 1 orange
3½oz (100g) dried red rose petals, or the petals of 10 fresh red rose heads

1 Dissolve the sugar in 1¼ cups water in a small saucepan over low heat without letting it boil (boiling will make the mixture cloudy).

2 Add the citrus juices, then turn the heat right down and simmer for 5 minutes. Over the next 15 minutes, gradually add the rose petals and stir thoroughly before adding more. Remove from the heat, let cool, and strain.

3 Meanwhile, sterilize a heatproof glass bottle and lid: wash them in hot soapy water; drain upside down; then place in a cool oven at 275°F (140°C) for 15 minutes. Pour the hot syrup into the sterilized glass bottle, seal, and label. Keep refrigerated and use within 6 weeks.

VALENTINE'S SPECIAL

 PROMOTES A SENSE OF WELL-BEING   **HELPS COMBAT FATIGUE**   **HELPS IMPROVE CIRCULATION**

This is a feel-good drink: nutritious, healthy, and life-enhancing. It contains antioxidant-rich soft fruits and coconut water, which help rehydrate the body and reduce feelings of fatigue, while the pistachio nuts, cardamom seeds, and concentrated rose in the rose syrup are said to keep love on your mind! If you prefer, add yogurt instead of the coconut water to make a smoothie.

SERVES 2

1 cup raspberries, washed
scant 1 cup blueberries, washed
a dash of rose syrup
¼ tsp cardamom seeds, crushed (no more than 10 pods)
2 tbsp pistachio nuts, shelled
1 cup coconut water

1 Put all the ingredients in a powerful food processor or blender and blend to a smooth consistency. If serving immediately, pour into tall glasses and serve. Otherwise, the drink will last for up to 2 days if stored in a tightly sealed bottle and refrigerated.

◄ Valentine's Special

Winter Wake Up

 SUPPORTS HEALTHY LIVER FUNCTION

 HELPS CLEAR CONGESTION

 HELPS IMPROVE CIRCULATION

Bitter Seville oranges add a fantastic cleansing element to this juice, benefitting liver function and enhancing bowel regularity. This effect is enhanced by fennel, which helps clear mucus in the lungs, and cilantro, which helps eliminate any traces of heavy metals in the body. Ginger boosts the circulation and carrots act as an anti-inflammatory and antiallergic agent.

SERVES 2

4 Seville oranges, 3 peeled
1 large fennel bulb
1 large carrot
1 small bunch of cilantro leaves and stalks
½in (1cm) piece fresh ginger

1 Using a juicer, juice all the ingredients and combine in a pitcher. Mix well and serve in tall glasses.

Party Aftermath

 AIDS DETOXIFICATION SYSTEM

 HELPS MAINTAIN WATER BALANCE

 AIDS DIGESTION, EASES CONSTIPATION

This is a juice to get you going the morning after. All these ingredients have strong detoxifying properties, that stimulate the digestive and urinary systems to eliminate accumulated waste. Sauerkraut, which is traditionally used to maintain a healthy digestive system, is also included to help combat a hangover, especially if accompanied by an upset stomach.

SERVES 2

1 cucumber
4 celery stalks
1 small bunch of flat-leaf parsley
1 small bunch of cilantro leaves
¼ lemon with peel on
¼ cup sauerkraut (p330)
1 tbsp milk thistle tincture
freshly ground black pepper, to garnish

1 Using a juicer, juice the cucumber, celery, parsley, cilantro, lemon, and sauerkraut and combine in a pitcher. Add the milk thistle tincture and mix well. Pour into tall glasses, sprinkle a dash of black pepper on top, and serve.

DEEPLY PURIFYING JUICE

 HELPS REMOVE TOXINS FROM THE BODY   **AIDS HEALTHY/OPTIMAL DIGESTION**   **PROTECTS AGAINST FREE-RADICAL DAMAGE**

This deeply nurturing juice strengthens the body's normal detoxifying processes because it is rich in chlorophyll, which enhances intestinal health and helps eliminate stored toxins. Barley grass and wheat grass supply valuable enzymes that support healthy digestion, help to regulate metabolism, and help protect vital tissues and organs from oxidative stress, and therefore premature aging.

SERVES 2

a bunch of wheat grass
a bunch of barley grass
1 bunch of flat-leaf parsley
8 large dandelion leaves
½ small cucumber
2 celery stalks
½in (1cm) piece fresh ginger

1 Using a juicer, juice all the ingredients and combine thoroughly in a pitcher. Pour into 2 glasses, add filtered water or springwater to adjust the taste if necessary, and serve.

A CUP OF HAPPINESS

 HAS AN UPLIFTING EFFECT   **HELPS COMBAT FATIGUE**

Plants can have as powerful an effect on our mind and emotions as they can on our bodies. The herbs in this blend have long been used to promote an improved sense of well-being and to alleviate feelings of melancholy, depression, and exhaustion. Drink this tea for a quick lift, especially if you are recovering from a long illness or long-term debilitation.

SERVES 2

1 tsp dried St. John's wort (*Hypericum perforatum*), chopped
1 tsp dried skullcap (*Scutellaria lateriflora*), chopped
1 tsp dried silk tree flowers (*Albizia julibrissin*), chopped

1 Place the dried herbs in a teapot and cover with 2 cups boiling water. Leave to infuse for 15 minutes, then strain and drink.

TIP: Silk tree flower can be sourced from Chinese herbalists.

MINT AND FRIENDS TEA

 AIDS HEALTHY DIGESTION

HELPS TO RELAX AND UNWIND THE MIND

The aromatic plants in this refreshing tea are useful digestive aids, helping to relieve stomach cramps and bloating. They may also relieve nervous tension headaches, because they generally help to relax the mind and ease tension. It's up to you how long you choose to infuse the herbs, according to your palate.

MAKE 2 CUPS

1 tbsp mint leaves, plus a few small leaves to garnish
½ tbsp fennel leaves
½ tbsp dill leaves
½ tbsp marjoram leaves

1 Remove the leaves from their stalks (although including a few odd stalks is not a problem, because they contain a lot of flavor). Chop each herb separately and transfer to a teapot.

2 Cover with hot, but not boiling, water (water at a temperature of 165–175°F/75–80°C is best for infusing the fine fragrant compounds in these plants).

3 Allow the herbs to infuse for 5 minutes or more, strain, and serve in heatproof glasses decorated with a few small mint leaves on top.

Sweet marjoram (p102) contains a natural analgesic that can ease abdominal cramps.

MARSHMALLOW AND LICORICE TEA

 HELPS TO RELAX AND UNWIND THE MIND

 HELPS TO REHYDRATE SKIN AND LUNGS

 PROTECTS AGAINST COLDS AND FLU

This is a refreshing, fragrant tea that is especially beneficial if you work in a crowded, centrally heated, stressful office environment. Together these herbs help calm, relax, and focus the mind. They also help protect against airborne microorganisms and provide relief from the effects of central heating by moistening and soothing the respiratory system and rehydrating the skin.

SERVES 2

1oz (30g) dried marshmallow root (*Althea officinalis*), chopped

¾oz (20g) dried marshmallow leaf (*Althea officinalis*), chopped

¾oz (20g) dried linden flower (*Tilia cordata*), chopped

¾oz (20g) dried vervain (*Verbena officinalis*), chopped

¼oz (10g) dried licorice (*Glycyrrhiza glabra*), chopped

1 Combine all the dried herbs thoroughly in a bowl, transfer to a dark container, metal tea caddy, or a cookie can, and label and date.

2 To make the tea, place ¾oz (20g) of the dried herbs in a small saucepan with a lid, cover with 2 cups of water and bring to a boil. Reduce the heat, cover with the lid, and let it simmer for 10 minutes. Remove from the heat, leave to infuse for 10 more minutes, strain, and serve. Alternatively, pour the strained tea into a resealable heatproof container and sip through the day.

3 To make an occasional drink, place 1 heaped teaspoon of the dried herbs, or an infuser ball filled with the herbal blend, in a mug. Cover with 1 cup boiling water, let stand for 10 minutes, strain, and drink.

Marshmallow root *(p99) soothes irritation and inflammation, and is particularly useful for treating gastric ulcers and irritable bowel syndrome.*

DEEP SLEEP TEA

 **HELPS PROMOTE
PEACEFUL SLEEP**   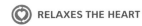 **RELAXES THE HEART**

Restful, refreshing sleep comes when we are able to switch off our minds fully and consciously let go of any physical tension in our bodies. This calming tea helps take the edge off ragged emotions, lowers stress levels, and releases any tension in your muscles. It also helps to naturally slow your heartbeat so you can and drift off to sleep easily.

SERVES 2

½oz (15g) dried valerian root (*Valeriana officinalis*), chopped

scant 1oz (25g) dried hawthorn flowers (*Crataegus sp.*), chopped

1oz (30g) dried passion flower leaf (*Passiflora incarnata*), chopped

20g (¾oz) dried schisandra berries (*Schisandra chinensis*), chopped

10g (¼oz) dried chamomile flowers (*Matricaria recutita*), chopped

1 Grind the valerian root briefly in a coffee grinder or blender if it is too thick to chop easily by hand.

2 Combine all the ingredients thoroughly in a bowl, transfer to a dark container, metal tea caddy, or a cookie can, and label and date.

3 Place ¾oz (20g) of the dried herbs in a small saucepan with a lid, cover with 2 cups water, and bring to a boil. Reduce the heat, cover, and let simmer for 10 minutes. Remove from the heat, leave to infuse for 10 more minutes, strain, and serve. Alternatively, pour the strained tea into a resealable heatproof container and sip through the day.

4 To make an occasional drink, place 1 heaped teaspoon of the dried herbs, or an infuser ball filled with the herbal blend, in a mug. Cover with 1 cup boiling water, let stand for 10 minutes, and strain. Add 1 tablespoon of Cherry Syrup (p308), if you prefer, because it is also an effective sleep aid; stir well and drink.

DEEPLY WARMING TEA

 **PROTECTS FROM COLDS
AND FLU**   **FIGHTS RESPIRATORY
INFECTIONS**

Drinking 1 or 2 cups of this immune-boosting tea a day provides extra health insurance in cooler weather because it helps strengthen the body's innate immunity against colds, the flu, and upper respiratory tract infections. It is particularly beneficial if you have chronic immune deficiency.

SERVES 2

scant 1oz (25g) astragalus root (*Astragalus membranaceus*), finely chopped

¾oz (20g) dried elderberries (*Sambucus nigra*)

¾oz (20g) dried echinacea root (*Echinacea purpurea*), chopped

½oz (15g) fresh ginger, finely chopped

¾oz (20g) dried elderflowers (*Sambucus nigra*), rubbed

1 Combine all the dried herbs thoroughly in a bowl, transfer to a dark container, metal tea caddy, or a cookie can, and label and date.

2 Place ¾oz (20g) of the dried herbs and the ginger in a small saucepan with a lid, cover with 2 cups water and bring to a boil. Reduce the heat, cover, and let simmer for 10 minutes. Remove from the heat, leave to infuse for 10 more minutes, strain, and serve. Alternatively, pour the strained tea into a resealable heatproof container and sip through the day.

3 To make an occasional drink, place 1 heaped teaspoon of the dried herbs, or an infuser ball filled with the herbal blend, in a mug. Cover with 1 cup boiling water, let stand for 10 minutes, strain, and drink.

DEEP CLEANSING TEA

 HELPS REMOVE TOXINS FROM THE BODY   **PROMOTES CLEAR SKIN**   **HELPS KEEP JOINTS SUPPLE**

This tea comprises herbs that have deep-cleansing properties and help remove toxic accumulations from the body while its antioxidant content improves skin tone. It can also benefit those who suffer from recurrent inflammatory arthritic conditions, such as gout. If you grow your own blackcurrants, harvest and dry the leaves to use throughout the year.

MAKES 5 DAYS' SUPPLY

¾oz (20g) dried blackcurrant leaves, chopped

¾oz (20g) dried red clover flowers, chopped

¾oz (20g) dried celery seeds, chopped

¾oz (20g) dried nettle leaves, chopped

¾oz (20g) dried dandelion leaves, chopped

1 Combine all the ingredients in a bowl, transfer to a sealed container, label, date, and store in a cupboard away from direct light.

2 To make the tea, put ¾oz (20g) of the dried leaves and 2½ cups water in a saucepan, cover, and bring to a boil. Lower the heat and simmer for 10 minutes. Remove from the heat, leave to infuse for 10 minutes, and strain the liquid into a heatproof resealable container. Sip throughout the day. To make a single drink, take 1 heaped teaspoon of dried herbs, or fill an infuser ball with the herb blend, cover with 1 cup boiling water, let stand for 10 minutes, strain, and drink.

DEEP NURTURE TEA

 HELPS PROTECT AGAINST POLLUTION   **PROTECTS AGAINST FREE-RADICAL DAMAGE**   **REMOVES ENERGY-DRAINING TOXINS**   **PROMOTES HEALTHY SKIN**

The antioxidant, antiaging nutrients in this tea help to protect the body against environmental pollutants; wild fruits supply unique antioxidants that aren't typically found in commercially grown fruits and vegetables. Adding wild fruits to your diet can help enrich your blood, which in turn supports your energy production, skin health, and benefits your overall well-being.

MAKES 5 DAYS' SUPPLY

¾oz (20g) dried rosehips, chopped

¼oz (10g) dried bilberries, chopped

¾oz (20g) goji berries, chopped

¾oz (20g) dried orange peel (p220, step 1), chopped

¼oz (10g) dried hibiscus flowers, chopped

½oz (15g) dried schisandra berries, chopped

⅛oz (5g) dried licorice root, chopped

1 Combine all the ingredients in a bowl, transfer to a container, seal, label, date, and store in a cupboard away from direct light.

2 To make the tea, put ¾oz (20g) of the dried leaves and 2½ cups water in a saucepan, cover, and bring to a boil. Lower the heat and simmer for 10 minutes. Remove from the heat, let infuse for 10 minutes, and strain the liquid into a heatproof resealable container. Sip throughout the day. To make a single drink, take 1 heaped teaspoon of dried herbs, or fill an infuser ball with the herb blend, cover with 1 cup boiling water, let stand for 10 minutes, strain, and drink.

RAINBOW VEGETABLE BROTH

 HELPS COMBAT FATIGUE   **HAS A MILD DIURETIC ACTION**   **HELPS STRENGTHEN THE IMMUNE SYSTEM**

This is an alkalizing broth that lifts energy levels by balancing the body's pH and fluid levels. Using vegetables in season assures a broad range of essential nutrients. Drink on its own at any time of day, or use as a base for stock for soup. Broths like this are excellent if you are recovering from an illness, and will fortify you against illness if you include them in your daily diet.

SERVES 2

½ leek, chopped
1 scallion, quartered
1 celery stick with leaves, chopped
1 carrot, chopped
1 potato with skin on, chopped
1 small beet with skin on, chopped
1 small radish with skin on, chopped
2 slices of fresh ginger
1 sprig of parsley
1 tsp coriander seeds
3½ cups mineral water
1 wakame seaweed, chopped (optional)

1 Place all the ingredients in a large saucepan, add the mineral water, and bring to a boil. Cover and simmer for 1½–2 hours over low heat.

2 Remove the pan from the heat and strain the liquid. Discard the vegetables. Pour the hot broth into a heatproof resealable container, add the chopped wakame seaweed, and seal. Drink glassfuls of the broth throughout the day.

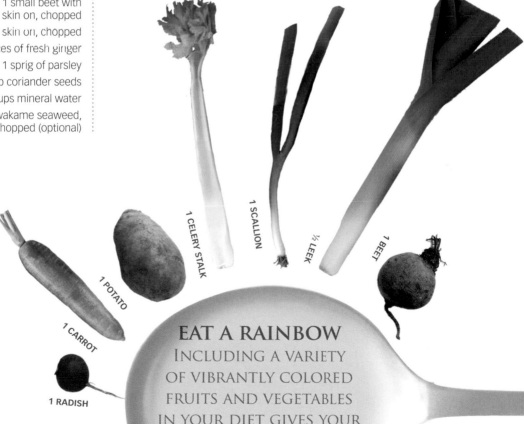

1 CELERY STALK
1 SCALLION
½ LEEK
1 BEET
1 POTATO
1 CARROT
1 RADISH

EAT A RAINBOW
INCLUDING A VARIETY OF VIBRANTLY COLORED FRUITS AND VEGETABLES IN YOUR DIET GIVES YOUR IMMUNE SYSTEM THE BENEFIT OF A RANGE OF ANTIOXIDANTS.

Astragalus And Schisandra Broth

 PROMOTES A SENSE OF WELL-BEING

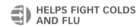 **HELPS FIGHT COLDS AND FLU**

 HELPS DETOX AND ALKALIZE THE BODY

We are so used to thinking of herbal teas and other plant essences as occasional or emergency "therapy" that we have almost forgotten the nutritional and health benefits they bring as part of a daily diet. You can also use all this broth as part of an individual detox treatment. Store it in a heatproof, resealable container and sip it through the day.

SERVES 2

⅛oz (6g) astragalus root
⅛oz (6g) schisandra berries
⅛oz (6g) wood ear mushrooms
6 thin slices of fresh ginger, peeled
4 garlic cloves, skins on
4 shallots, skins on
1 tbsp coriander seeds
½ tsp anise seeds
½ cup peeled chopped celeriac
1 large carrot, sliced
1 strand of kelp or wakame
10 black peppercorns

1 Place all the ingredients in a medium saucepan, cover with 2 cups water, and bring to a boil. Reduce the heat and simmer for 1½ hours, then strain.

2 If serving as a soup, transfer to 2 serving bowls. If using as a drink pour into 2 heatproof glasses and serve, or store the broth (see above) and sip through the day as a detox treatment.

Kelp (p131) has a high iodine content, which supports a healthy thyroid function.

Seaweed And Miso Broth

 HELPS LOWER CHOLESTEROL

 HAS A POWERFUL DIURETIC ACTION

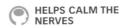 **HELPS CALM THE NERVES**

Traditionally, seaweeds are used to alkalize the blood and help lower blood cholesterol. They are also used for their diuretic properties, and to help protect against the effects of radiation. If using as a drink, pour into 2 heatproof glasses and serve. You can also use all this broth as part of an individual detox treatment. Store it in a heatproof, resealable container and sip it through the day.

SERVES 1 (MAKES 2 CUPS)

⅛oz (5g) wakame
⅛oz (5g) dulse
1 small blade of kelp
2 sticks of lemongrass
3 kaffir lime leaves
½ tbsp coriander seeds
½ cup peeled chopped celeriac
½in (1.5cm) piece fresh ginger, chopped
1 carrot, chopped
1 tbsp barley miso
1 tbsp chopped cilantro leaves

1 Rinse the seaweeds in a bowl of cold water to help remove some of their salty taste.

2 Place all the ingredients except the barley miso and cilantro leaves in a medium saucepan, cover with 2 cups of water and bring to a boil. Reduce the heat to a simmer and cook, covered, for 1½ hours on low heat.

3 Strain the liquid and pour it into a heatproof resealable container. Discard the ingredients in the sieve. Add the barley miso and allow it to dissolve, then add the cilantro leaves. Store the broth in the container and sip through the day.

Dulse (p131) is a good source of chlorophyll, which helps remove toxins from the body.

OILS, DRESSINGS, AND EXTRAS

IT'S THE LITTLE EXTRAS THAT MAKE A MEAL.
BEAUTIFUL BREADS AND "LIVING" FERMENTED
FOOD CONDIMENTS, DEEPLY **FLAVORED** OILS, AND
FRUITY VINEGARS ALL ADD VARIETY AND BRING
YOU THE BEST OF HEALTH.

FLATBREAD WITH SWEET POTATO AND CORIANDER

 HELPS KEEP JOINTS SUPPLE **SUPPORTS AND PROTECTS THE LIVER** **HELPS IMPROVE CIRCULATION**

This is a take on traditional Indian paratha, and is a versatile bread that tastes equally good freshly baked and spread with soft kefir cheese (p332) or eaten as an accompaniment to all sorts of hot dishes and salads. Its main ingredients are sweet potato, turmeric powder, and coriander, which together have anti-inflammatory benefits, support the liver, and help improve circulation.

MAKES 8–10

1 sweet potato

¾ cup all-purpose flour, plus extra for dusting

⅓ cup chickpea flour

½ tsp salt

2 tbsp ghee, or clarified butter

1 small red onion, finely chopped

1 garlic clove, minced

1 tsp coriander seeds, crushed

1 tsp turmeric powder

scant 1oz (25g) cilantro leaves, chopped

juice of ½ lime

1 Preheat the oven to 350°F (180°C). Wrap the sweet potato in foil and bake for 25 minutes, or until soft. When the potato is cool enough to handle, peel off the skin and discard, and chop the flesh finely.

2 Combine the 2 flours in a small bowl, add the salt, and mix well. Set aside while you heat 1 tablespoon of the ghee in a small saucepan. Add the chopped onion and cook over medium heat until it has softened. Add the garlic, coriander seeds, and turmeric powder, stir for 1 minute, then remove from the heat and add the cilantro leaves, sweet potato, and lime juice, and mix well.

3 Transfer the sautéed ingredients to a large bowl and mix thoroughly. When all the ingredients are combined, knead into a dough and let stand for 15 minutes.

4 Remove the dough from the bowl, place it on a lightly floured work surface, and shape into a long roll. Divide into 8 or 10 equal amounts and shape into small balls. Roll each ball out into an ⅛–¼in (3–5mm) thick round that will fit in a heavy skillet. Repeat with the rest of the dough balls. The thinner the flatbreads, the more quickly they will cook.

5 Place the skillet on medium heat and set a flatbread in it. Cook for about 3 minutes. Brush the surface of the flatbread with some of the remaining ghee before turning it over to cook on the other side for 3 more minutes. Keep in a warm place while you cook the rest of the flatbreads, then serve.

Sweet potato (p88), especially this dark-skinned variety, contains high levels of beta-carotene and can therefore help strengthen the immune system.

SOURDOUGH RYE BREAD

 HELPS MAINTAIN ENERGY LEVELS

 HELPS STRENGTHEN BONES

 PROMOTES HEALTHY SKIN AND HAIR

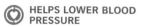 **HELPS LOWER BLOOD PRESSURE**

Good-quality bread is the ultimate slow food: taking time to make it means you get a flavorful loaf. Rye grain, commonly used to make sourdough bread, boosts energy levels, strengthens bones and fingernails, enhances the condition of hair, and is also thought to benefit the heart and circulatory system. Buy freshly milled whole grain rye flour that supplies the most nutrients.

MAKES 1 LOAF

For the sourdough starter

1½ cups whole grain rye flour

1½ cups springwater

For the bread

1lb (450g) sourdough starter

1 tbsp blackstrap molasses

2½–2¾ cups whole grain rye flour

1 tbsp sunflower seeds

2 tbsp pumpkin seeds

1 tbsp caraway seeds

a pinch of salt

1 tsp coriander seeds

a knob of butter, plus extra for greasing

1 To make the sourdough starter, mix ⅓ cup of the rye flour with ½ cup of springwater in a large clean jar, cover with a clean kitchen towel, and leave in a warm place for 24 hours. The ideal room temperature for the starter to ferment is 64–68°F (18–20°C). When the dough starter develops a bubbly texture and a fragrant sour smell, "feed" it with ⅓ cup more rye flour and ½ cup springwater. Stir, add a little more water or flour if necessary to keep it smooth, and leave for another 24 hours. It should now be bubbling, with a fruity sour taste. Add a further ¾ cup of flour and ¾ cup more springwater. Let rise overnight to become a fragrant, light dough.

2 Place 1lb (450g) of the starter dough in a large bowl, add ½ cup water and the blackstrap molasses, and stir. Add about 2 cups of the rye flour to begin with and work it in with your hands; it will be quite a sticky mixture. Add more flour if necessary until the dough is of a manageable consistency—neither too thin nor too thick—allowing for the fact that it is likely to thicken with standing, and that seeds will be added to it. Cover with a clean kitchen towel and let stand in the bowl in a warm place for a few hours; if the starter is vigorous enough, the dough should double in size within 8–12 hours.

3 Add the pumpkin, sunflower, and caraway seeds, and salt to the risen dough and mix in thoroughly using your hands. Heat a small skillet, add the coriander seeds, dry-fry until they release their aroma, then transfer to a mortar and pestle and crush to a powder. Grease the inside of a 2lb (900g) loaf pan with a little butter and sprinkle in the coriander powder, making sure it covers the insides of the pan evenly. Place the dough in the pan, smooth the top, dust with a little flour, cover with a clean kitchen towel, and leave in a warm place to rest for a few hours, or until it has visibly risen.

4 Preheat the oven to 410°F (210°C) and bake the loaf for 10 minutes. Lower the oven temperature to 350°F (180°C) and bake for a further 45 minutes. Remove the loaf from the oven, mix 2 tablespoons of boiling water with a knob of butter, and pour the liquid over the hot bread. Turn the oven off, return the loaf to the oven, and leave for 30 minutes, or until completely cold. Remove from the oven, cover with a linen cloth, and transfer to a wire rack to cool completely. The flavor of rye bread improves during storage. Wrapped in the linen cloth and stored in a wooden bread bin or a fabric bread bag, this loaf will last for 5–6 days.

SAUERKRAUT

 FEEDS GOOD BACTERIA IN THE GUT　 **HAS AN UPLIFTING EFFECT**　 **HELPS STRENGTHEN THE IMMUNE SYSTEM**　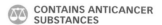 **CONTAINS ANTICANCER SUBSTANCES**

Preserving vegetables in a brine solution, known as lactofermentation, encourages the growth of gut-friendly bacteria. Homemade sauerkraut not only tastes better, it is richer in enzymes that support a healthy gut which, in turn, can improve both physical and emotional health. It also preserves the immune-boosting and cancer-fighting properties of cabbage.

MAKES 3LB (1.35KG)

5½–6½lb (2.5–3kg) hard white or red cabbage, or half red and half white cabbage

about 2oz (60g) coarse sea or rock salt (see method)

1 tbsp caraway seeds

1 Remove the outer leaves of the cabbage, slice in half, remove the cores, quarter, and shred finely in a food processor or using a sharp knife. Weigh the shredded cabbage and calculate the amount of salt you need: approximately 2oz (60g) of salt per 5½lb (2.5kg) of cabbage.

2 Place the cabbage in a large, clean bowl and scatter evenly with salt. Using your hands, work the salt thoroughly into the cabbage—imagine you are making pie dough—until it begins to feel wet. Leave for a few minutes for the salt to soften the cabbage and draw out its juices.

3 Pack into a very large sterilized crock or jar. Add 2in (5cm) of shredded cabbage at a time and scatter with the caraway seeds. Pack each layer down with a clean tamper, such as the end of a rolling pin, a large pestle, or a jam jar. Leave 3in (7.5cm) of space at the top of the jar. Add any juices from the bowl and cover with cold brine (1½ tbsp of salt to 3½ cups boiled cooled water) to cover the cabbage.

4 Place the jar on a tray, place clean cheesecloth over the cabbage, and place a snug-fitting plate or saucer on top. Place a large jar, or a sandwich bag filled with water and sealed well, on top of the plate.

5 Leave in a well-ventilated place at room temperature (the ideal temperature is 68–72°F/20–22°C). Check every day that the cabbage is submerged. Remove any scum regularly and replace the cheesecloth with a fresh clean piece, if necessary.

6 Fermentation is complete when all the bubbling has ceased; if the room temperature is ideal, the sauerkraut will be ready in 3–4 weeks. Transfer to sterilized jars, seal, and store in the refrigerator.

TIP: If the room temperature is below 55°F (13°C), fermentation will stop, and if it is higher than 76°F (24°C) it will spoil. If your sauerkraut develops a pinkish hue on its surface, turns dark, or is very soft and mushy, it has not fermented properly and shouldn't be eaten.

KIMCHI

 HELPS FIGHT INFECTION   **HELPS IMPROVE CIRCULATION**   **ENCOURAGES HEALTHY DIGESTION**   **CONTAINS ANTICANCER SUBSTANCES**

A traditional Korean cabbage dish, kimchi has numerous variations and this is one of the simplest. The mixture of spices in kimchi can help the body fend off bacterial and viral infections. The spices also have a strengthening effect on the circulation and digestion. Kimchi uses cabbage as its base, which means it also contains a range of cancer-fighting nutrients.

MAKES 1–1¼LB (450–600G)

1 small head Napa cabbage

2 tbsp sea salt

4 scallions, chopped

1in (2.5cm) piece fresh ginger, peeled and grated

1 garlic clove, crushed

¼ cup rice vinegar

1 tbsp Thai fish sauce (nam pla)

juice of 1 lime

2 tbsp sesame oil

2 tbsp toasted sesame seeds

2 tbsp sambal oelek chili paste

1 Cut the head of the Napa cabbage lengthwise into quarters, then into 2in (5cm) chunks. Place in a colander over a bowl. Add the sea salt, toss well, and let stand overnight at room temperature.

2 Wash the cabbage to remove the salt, tossing the leaves with your hands to rinse them thoroughly. Drain and dry on paper towels.

3 Transfer to a freezerproof container (large enough to hold up to 1¼lb/600g of Napa cabbage) with a lid. Add the remaining ingredients and toss together thoroughly.

4 Place the lid on the container, let stand at room temperature overnight to marinate, then transfer to the refrigerator for a few days to allow the flavors to develop. Store in the refrigerator and use within 2 weeks.

Napa cabbage is a good source of antioxidants and vitamin C, which can help to protect from certain kinds of cancer.

Kefir Milk

 FEEDS GOOD BACTERIA IN THE GUT   **HELPS STRENGTHEN THE IMMUNE SYSTEM**   **PROMOTES A SENSE OF WELL-BEING**

Milk cultured with kefir grains benefits the digestive system, which is closely linked to the immune, endocrine, circulatory, and central nervous systems. The smooth functioning of these internal systems in turn helps boost a feeling of well-being. For best results, use unpasteurized milk, otherwise use whole pasteurized nonhomogenized cow's, sheep's, or goat's milk.

MAKES 3½ CUPS

1 tbsp kefir grains

3½ cups unpasteurized or whole pasteurized nonhomogenized milk at room temperature

1 Put the kefir grains in a clean glass jar and add the milk. Cover with a clean kitchen towel and store in a dark place, such as a kitchen cupboard, for 18 hours–1 day.

2 Strain the milk through a clean plastic sieve. Reserve the kefir grains and add to a new batch of milk.

3 Store the kefir milk in a jug or a bottle in the refrigerator and use within 1 week, although it is best drunk fresh. It will continue to ferment at a lower rate during this time and have a consistency of thick milk.

Kefir Milk Cheese

 FEEDS GOOD BACTERIA IN THE GUT   **HELPS STRENGTHEN THE IMMUNE SYSTEM**   **PROMOTES A SENSE OF WELL-BEING**

Using kefir grains gives you a degree of control over the quality of dairy products you include in your diet. This soft, creamy cheese boosts immunity and digestion by enhancing intestinal health. Most of the lactose in kefir cheese is predigested by bacteria and yeasts before you ingest it, and some proteins are also broken down, so some lactose-intolerant people can tolerate it.

MAKES APPROXIMATELY 10OZ (300G)

1 tbsp kefir grains

3½ cups unpasteurized or whole pasteurized nonhomogenized milk at room temperature

1 Put the kefir grains in a clean glass jar and add the milk. Cover with a clean kitchen towel and store in a dark place such as a kitchen cupboard for 2–4 days or until the liquid separates into liquid whey and solid curds. The live kefir grains usually remain on the top layer of the curd; use a plastic spoon to remove as many of them as you can and reserve in the refrigerator to add to a new batch of milk, if you like.

2 Strain the curd and whey using a clean plastic sieve positioned over a large glass bowl. Retain the curd and use the whey for soups or as a drink, if you like. Store the cheese in a covered ceramic bowl in the refrigerator and use within 1 week on crackers or toasted rye bread.

3 If you want a smoother, denser soft cheese, wrap the curds in a piece of cheesecloth and hang it overnight or until the cheese is as firm as you like (the firmer you want the cheese, the longer you leave it to drain). If you want to add extra flavors, mix with cracked flaxseeds or other seeds and nuts, or fresh herbs, such as marjoram, basil, lemon thyme, and dill.

CORIANDER AND JUNIPER OIL

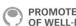 **PROMOTES A SENSE OF WELL-BEING**

 HELPS IMPROVE CIRCULATION

 PROMOTES PROSTATE HEALTH

An aromatic oil blend to liven up your life. The therapeutic action of this combination of seed oils and spices has a warming, strengthening, and energizing quality that can help enhance your sense of well-being and sex drive. Use it as part of a dressing for salads or on its own to flavor cooked rice, spaghetti, or noodles.

MAKES ¾ CUP

2 tbsp peppercorns
⅓ cup + 1 tbsp coriander seeds
2 tbsp juniper berries
¼–½ tsp chili flakes
⅔ cup sunflower oil

For the base oil
2 tbsp walnut oil
2 tbsp pumpkin oil
1½ tbsp hemp seed oil
1½ tbsp black seed oil

1 Put the dried ingredients in a mortar and pestle and crush roughly. Transfer to a clean heatproof glass jar and cover with the sunflower oil.

2 Preheat the oven to 120°F (50°C), then turn it off. Wrap the bottom of the jar in a cloth (to prevent the glass from cracking while standing on the hot metal rack) and place it, unsealed, in the oven. The dried ingredients need to infuse at a temperature of around 104°F (40°C) for 6–8 hours, so you may need to turn the oven on and then off again briefly every so often, to keep the mixture warm.

3 Strain the oil and discard the dried ingredients; you should have at least ⅓ cup of flavored oil. Pour into a sterilized dark glass bottle and add the walnut, pumpkin, and hemp and black seed oils. Seal, shake well, label, and date. Store in the refrigerator and use within 3 weeks.

ROSE AND FENNEL SEED OIL

 RELIEVES MENOPAUSAL AND PMS SYMPTOMS

 HELPS FIGHT INFLAMMATION

 PROMOTES HEALTHY SKIN

This is a rejuvenating oil blend to help us age beautifully. The body loses its ability to convert dietary fats into gamma-linolenic-acid (GLA) with age and, because this dietary oil blend contains significant levels of GLA, it may be helpful in age-related conditions resulting from GLA deficiency. It can also be useful for relieving menopausal symptoms and premenstrual syndrome.

MAKES ¾ CUP

3 tbsp dried thyme
1 tbsp fennel seeds
⅛oz (5g) dried rose petals
⅛oz (5g) dried marigold flowers
⅔ cup sunflower oil

For the base oil
3 tbsp evening primrose oil
2 tbsp borage oil
2 tbsp hemp seed oil
1 tbsp black seed oil

1 Put the dried ingredients in a mortar and pestle and crush roughly. Transfer to a clean heatproof glass jar and cover with the sunflower oil.

2 Preheat the oven to 120°F (50°C), then turn it off. Wrap the bottom of the jar in a cloth (to prevent the glass from cracking while standing on the hot metal rack) and place it, unsealed, in the oven. The dried ingredients need to infuse at a temperature of around 104°F (40°C) for 6–8 hours, so you may need to turn the oven on and then off again briefly every so often, to keep the mixture warm.

3 Strain the oil and discard the dried ingredients; you should have at least ⅓ cup of oil. Pour into a sterilized dark glass bottle and add the evening primrose, borage, and hemp and black seed oils. Seal, shake well, label, and date. Store in the refrigerator and use within 3 weeks.

ROSE AND RASPBERRY VINEGAR

 HAS A MILD DIURETIC ACTION

 ENHANCES DIGESTION OF FATS

 PROMOTES HEALTHY SKIN AND HAIR

 HELPS EASE MENSTRUAL CRAMPS

Infused vinegars are useful and versatile. This vinegar can be used as a flavoring for food, or drink 1 teaspoonful in a cup of warm water every morning to improve detoxification. For the best result, use the petals of fragrant roses, such as *Rosa damascena* or *Rosa gallica,* to benefit from their healing qualities, and choose a good-quality organic apple cider vinegar.

MAKES 1¼ CUPS

⅔ cup fresh raspberries

2 tbsp fresh rose petals

1¼ cups organic apple cider vinegar

1 Put the raspberries and rose petals in a clean glass jar, cover with the vinegar so the berries are completely submerged, and seal tightly with the lid. Leave in a dark cupboard to infuse for 2–3 weeks, then strain, pour the vinegar into a clean bottle, and seal, label, and date. Reserve the raspberries, if you like, and use in a smoothie. Use within 3 months.

BLACKBERRY VINEGAR

 HELPS FIGHT COLDS AND FLU

 PROMOTES A HEALTHY COMPLEXION

 HELPS IMPROVE CIRCULATION

If picked when fully ripe, blackberries are a perfect foraging food, with many health benefits: they contain anthocyanins, salicylic acid, ellagic acid, and fiber, which are good for skin and hair. Traditionally, blackberry vinegar is used as a gargle for sore throats, and as a drink to avert the onset of a cold or the flu. Choose a good-quality organic apple cider vinegar.

MAKES 1¼ CUPS

⅔ cup fresh blackberries

1¼ cups organic apple cider vinegar

1 Put the blackberries into a clean glass jar, cover with the vinegar so the blackberries are completely submerged, and seal tightly with the lid. Leave in a dark cupboard to infuse for 2–3 weeks, then strain, pour the vinegar into a clean bottle, and seal, label, and date. Reserve the blackberries, if you like, and use in a smoothie. Use within 3 months.

TURMERIC AND GINGER OIL

 HELPS FIGHT INFLAMMATION   **PROTECTS THE HEART AND BLOOD VESSELS**   **AIDS HEALTHY DIGESTION**

This is a blend of fine seed oils and anti-inflammatory medicinal plants. Together they make an oil that is particularly beneficial for arthritic and rheumatic conditions, and protects the heart and digestive tract. This warming, immune-enhancing oil is delicious as a salad dressing, or drizzle a spoonful or 2 onto steamed vegetables or yogurt, or add to smoothies.

MAKES 1¾ CUPS

⅓ cup dried oregano
2 tbsp dried sage leaves
1½ tbsp juniper berries
3 tbsp dried rosemary leaves
1 tsp ground turmeric
1 tsp ground ginger
1 cup sunflower oil
3 tbsp flaxseed oil
3 tbsp hemp oil
3 tbsp borage oil
3 tbsp rosehip oil

1 Place the oregano, sage leaves, juniper berries, and rosemary leaves in a blender or food processor, and pulse to reduce their volume. Place the herbs and ground spices into a glass jar and cover with the sunflower oil.

2 Preheat the oven to 120°F (50°C), then turn it off. Wrap the bottom of the jar in a cloth (to prevent the glass from cracking while standing on the hot metal shelves) and put it, unsealed, in the oven. The dried ingredients need to infuse at a temperature of around 104°F (40°C) for 6–8 hours, so you may need to turn the oven briefly on and then off again every so often to keep the mixture warm.

3 Strain the oil and discard the dried ingredients; you should have at least a scant ½ cup of flavored oil. Pour into a sterilized glass bottle and add the flax, hemp, borage, and rosehip oils. Seal well and shake. Label and date, store in the refrigerator, and use within 3–4 weeks.

BASIL OIL

 HELPS EASE BRONCHIAL COMPLAINTS   **HELPS ALLEVIATE PMS**   **PROMOTES A SENSE OF WELL-BEING**

Basil is beneficial for the respiratory, reproductive, and nervous systems. It is a good remedy for conditions that require relief from congestion, such as sinusitis, a loss of smell, and some bronchial conditions. Basil is traditionally known as an herb that awakens joy and courage because it helps restore vitality, enhance memory, and lift your mood.

MAKES 1 CUP

a small bunch of basil
½ cup extra virgin olive oil
½ cup grapeseed oil

1 Bring 2 cups water to a boil in a saucepan. Fill another small pan with cold water and add some ice cubes to it to make an ice-water bath. Holding the bunch of basil by its stems, immerse the leaves into the boiling water for 8 seconds. Plunge the wilted basil leaves into the ice-water bath to prevent them from discoloring and cooking further. Dry with paper towels, cut off the stems, and put the leaves into a blender or food processor. Add the two oils, and purée until smooth.

2 Use immediately, or if you want to store it for a few days in a refrigerator, leave to infuse for 1–2 hours, then strain the oils through a cheesecloth and discard the puréed basil leaves. Transfer to a sterilized bottle, seal, label, and date. Store in the refrigerator and use within 3–4 weeks.

◀ Turmeric and Ginger Oil

VITAMIN SUPPLEMENTS CHART

The better quality your food is, the more abundant it will be in the vitamins that are essential to your continued health and well-being. Processing, cooking, and storage, as well as soil-damaging pesticides and fertilizers can leave food nutrient poor. Supplementing at optimal levels can help fill the gap between what you need and what you often get—see p17 for details about ADI and Supplemental Range.

Nutrient	Functions	Rich Food Sources	Notes	Average Daily Intake/ Supplemental Range
Vitamin A and Carotenoids	**Vitamin A:** Antioxidant; vision and night vision; growth and reproduction; collagen production; moistness of mucosa. **Carotenoids:** Precursors to vitamin A; antioxidant; healthy heart and circulation; healthy mucosa.	**Vitamin A:** Fish-liver oils; animal liver; oily fish; egg yolks; whole milk; and butter. **Carotenoids:** Green and yellow fruits and vegetables; dark green leafy vegetables; sweet bell peppers; sweet potato; broccoli; carrots; dried apricots; prunes; kale; parsley; spinach; squash; and watercress.	Animal sources of Vitamin A may be much better absorbed than vegetable sources.	**Vitamin A—** ADI: 5,000–9,000IU SR: 10,000+ **Beta-carotene—** ADI: 5–8mg SR: 10–40mg
Vitamin B$_1$— Thiamin	Release of energy from carbohydrates; growth; appetite regulation; healthy digestion and nervous system.	Yeast extract; wheat germ; whole wheat flour; sunflower seeds; brown rice; brazil nuts; pecans; pork; beans; buckwheat; oatmeal; hazelnuts; rye; liver; cashews.	Unstable to light and heat e.g. milling flour causes 60–80% loss.	ADI: 1–5mg SR: 5–150mg
Vitamin B$_2$— Riboflavin	Combines with protein to regulate respiration; growth; healthy skin and eyes.	Yeast; animal liver; kidneys; almonds; wheat germ; wild rice; mushrooms; egg yolks; millet; wheat bran; oily fish; kale; cashews; sunflower.	Unstable to light.	ADI: 1.5–2mg SR: 10–200mg
Vitamin B$_3$— Niacin	Required for energy release and synthesis of steroids and fatty acids; healthy digestion, skin, and nervous system.	Yeast; wild rice; brown rice; whole wheat flour; peanuts; animal liver; turkey; trout; mackerel; chicken; sesame seeds; sunflower seeds; lean red meat; buckwheat; barley; almonds.	Relatively stable.	ADI: 15–20mg SR: 100–3,000mg
Vitamin B$_5$— Pantothenic Acid	Regulates carbohydrate and fat metabolism; resistance to stress; healthy immune system; digestion.	Yeast; animal liver; kidneys; peanuts; mushrooms; split peas; brown rice; soybeans; eggs; oatmeal; buckwheat; sunflower seeds; lentils; rye flour; cashews; oily fish; turkey; broccoli; avocados.	Unstable to heat (cooking), freezing and canning. Considerable loss when milling grains.	ADI: 5–10mg SR: 20–500mg
Vitamin B$_6$— Pyridoxine, Pyridoxal-5-phosphate	Metabolism of carbohydrate and protein; synthesis of hormones and fatty acids; healthy nervous system, hormone-balance growth, and skin.	Yeast; sunflower seeds; wheat germ; tuna; liver; soybeans; walnuts; oily fish; lentils; buckwheat flour; beans; brown rice; hazelnuts; bananas; pork; avocados; whole wheat flour; sweet chestnuts; egg yolk; kale; rye flour.	Unstable to light and cooking. Milling flour causes 75% losses.	ADI: 1.6–2.6mg SR: 10–150mg

Nutrient	Functions	Rich Food Sources	Notes	Average Daily Intake/ Supplemental Range
Vitamin B$_{12}$— Cobalamin	DNA synthesis; new red blood cells; lipid production; myelin sheath; healthy nervous system, blood cells, gut mucosa, skin.	Liver; shellfish; kidneys; oily fish; egg yolk; lamb; beef; cheese.	Plants do not contain bioactive forms of B$_{12}$ so vegans must supplement.	ADI: 2–50ug SR: 300–5000ug
Folic Acid	DNA and RNA synthesis; new blood cells; protein synthesis; growth; healthy digestion; nervous system; red blood cells.	Yeast; Black-eyed peas; soybeans; wheat germ; liver; kidney beans; mung beans; asparagus; lentils; walnuts; spinach; kale; beet greens; peanuts; broccoli; barley; whole wheat cereal; Brussels sprouts; almonds; oatmeal; cabbage; figs; avocado.	Unstable to heat and light. Storage and cooking causes losses. Supplementation may be advisable before and during pregnancy.	ADI: 400ug SR: 500ug–5mg
Vitamin C— Ascorbic Acid	Antioxidant; healthy immune system, bones, teeth, gums, cartilage, capillaries, connective tissue, healing; synthesis of steroid hormones, absorption of iron, regulating cholesterol.	Acerola cherry; sweet bell peppers; kale; parsley; leafy vegetables; broccoli; watercress; strawberries; papaya; oranges; grapefruit; cabbage; lemon juice; elderberries; liver; mangoes; asparagus; oysters; radishes; raspberries.	Unstable to heat and light. Cooking may cause 10-90% losses.	ADI: 75–125mg SR: 250–2,000mg
Vitamin D— Calciferol	Controls calcium absorption for healthy bones and teeth; healthy immune system and nervous system; cancer-protective; hormone-balance.	Fish liver oils; sardines (canned and fresh); salmon; tuna; shrimp; butter, sunflower seeds; liver; eggs; milk; mushrooms; cheese.	Synthesized by the action of sunlight on the skin. Supplementation may be advisable if not exposed to sunlight regularly.	ADI: 1–5mg SR: 5–150mg
Vitamin E— Tocopherol, etc.	Antioxidant; healthy immune system; heart and circulation; lipid balance; sex hormone regulator; fertility; gestation; growth.	Sunflower seeds; sunflower oil; safflower oil; almonds; sesame oil; peanut oil; corn oil; wheat germ; peanuts; olive oil; butter; spinach; oatmeal; salmon; brown rice; rye flour; pecans; wheat germ; whole wheat bread; carrots.	Losses caused by heat and light. Milling of flour causes up to 80% loss.	ADI: 30mg SR: 100–800mg
Vitamin K— Phylloquinone, Menaquinone	Blood clotting; calcium metabolism; blood sugar-balance; healthy lung tissue; heart and circulation; metabolism; bones; skin; bacterial synthesis in the gut.	Broccoli; lettuce; cabbage; liver; spinach; watercress; asparagus; cheese; butter; oats; peas; whole wheat; green beans; pork; eggs; kelp.	Unstable to light. If bowel microflora are healthy up to 50% of Vitamin K needs are manufactured in the gut.	ADI: 70–150ug SR: 1–20mg
Bioflavonoids— Citrin, Hesperidin, Rutin, Quercetin, etc.	Antioxidant; anti-inflammatory; healthy immune system; cancer-protective (Quercetin); healthy blood vessels (Rutin).	Apples; black and red berries; blackcurrants; buckwheat; citrus fruit; apricots; garlic; green-growing shoots of plants; onions; rosehips; cherries.	Some loss during cooking and processing.	ADI: N/A SR: 500–3,000mg
Essential Fatty Acids— Omega oils	Regulate inflammation; healthy blood coagulation; lipid balance; reproduction and growth; brain function; nervous system; eyes; skin; joints; metabolism; hormones; heart and circulation.	Fish liver oils; oily fish; milk; cheese; Flaxseed oil; hempseed oil; canola; soy oil; walnut oil; blackcurrant seed oil.	Hydrogenation, light, heat.	3–8% of calories

Mineral Supplements Chart

Just like vitamins, minerals are essential for our overall health and have specific roles to play in building bones, making hormones, and regulating heartbeat. Modern food production and farming methods remove important minerals from our food. The body cannot make its own, so it's essential to obtain minerals in adequate amounts from either food or good-quality supplements (find more on p17).

Nutrient	Functions	Rich Food Sources	Notes	Average Daily Intake/ Supplemental Range
Boron	Activates Vitamin D; bone and joint health.	Drinking water; almonds; apples; dates; nuts; beans; peanuts; prunes; soy.	Available from most plants grown where boron is present in the soil.	ADI: 2–3mg SR: 2–10mg
Calcium	Bone and teeth formation; regulates nerve and muscle function; hormones and blood pressure.	Kelp; seaweed; cheese; carob; molasses; almonds; yeast; parsley; corn; watercress; goats milk; tofu; figs; sunflower seeds; yogurt; beet greens; green leafy vegetables; wheat bran; cows milk; buckwheat; sesame seeds; olives; broccoli.	Water softeners remove calcium. Excess phytates (rhubarb, spinach, grains, and cereals) can decrease absorption.	ADI: 800–1400mg SR: 1000–2500mg
Chromium	Glucose metabolism; growth; insulin and cholesterol regulation.	Brewer's yeast; beef; liver; whole wheat bread; rye flour; chile; oysters; potatoes.	Refining flour causes up to 50% losses.	ADI: 50–200ug SR: 100–300ug
Copper	Synthesis of enzymes required for iron absorption; red blood cell formation; maintenance of skin, bone, and nerve formation; collagen synthesis.	Oysters; shellfish; nuts; brazil nuts; almonds; hazelnuts; walnuts; pecans; dried beans; split peas; liver; buckwheat; peanuts; lamb; sunflower oil; crab; copper water pipes.	Zinc and calcium are antagonists (high levels prevent absorption of copper).	ADI: 1–3mg SR: 2–10mg Metabolism of copper is highly individual.
Iodine	Synthesis of thyroid hormones.	Seaweed; kelp; clams; shrimp; haddock; shellfish; salmon; sardines; liver; pineapple; eggs; peanuts; whole wheat bread; cheese; pork; lettuce; spinach.	Often added to table salt but not sea salt.	ADI: 150ug SR: 100–1000ug
Iron	Red blood cell function; energy release; growth; bone regulation; healthy respiration, skin, and nails.	Kelp; yeast; molasses; wheat bran; pumpkin seeds; liver; sunflower seeds; millet; parsley; clams; almonds; prunes; cashews; red meat; raisins; nuts; chard; dandelion leaves; dates; cooked dried beans; eggs; lentils; brown rice; dried apricots; raw chocolate.	Vitamin C enhances iron absorption.	ADI: 10–20mg SR: 15–50mg

Nutrient	Functions	Rich Food Sources	Notes	Average Daily Intake/ Supplemental Range
Magnesium	Synthesis of proteins, carbohydrates, and lipids; DNA repair; energy production; modulation of muscle activity; homeostasis of calcium; heart and circulation health.	Kelp; seaweed; wheat bran and wheat germ; almonds; cashews; molasses; brewer's yeast; buckwheat; brazil nuts; nuts; millet; rye; tofu; beet greens; coconut meat; soy; spinach; brown rice; figs; apricots; dates; shrimp; sweetcorn; avocado.	Milling/refining of grains and cereals causes up to 90% losses.	ADI: 350mg SR: 300–800mg
Manganese	Antioxidant; enzyme activator; bone and ligament formation.	Nuts: pecans, brazil, almonds; barley; rye; buckwheat; split peas; whole wheat bread; spinach; oats; raisins; rhubarb; Brussels sprouts; avocado; beans.	Milling/refining of cereals causes 80–90% losses.	ADI: 2.5–7mg SR: 2–20mg
Molybdenum	Regulates iron, copper, and fat metabolism; teeth health; anticarcinogenic.	Lentils; liver, dried beans; cauliflower; wheat germ; spinach; kidney; brown rice; garlic; oats; eggs; rye; corn; barley; fish; chicken; beef; potatoes; onions; coconut.	Refining flour causes up to 80% losses.	ADI: 75–250ug SR: 100–1000ug
Phosphorus	Healthy bones; calcium homeostasis; RNA and DNA synthesis; energy metabolism and production; Vitamin B activator.	Brewer's yeast; wheat bran and wheat germ; pumpkin seeds; brazil nuts; sesame seeds; dried beans; almonds; cheese; rye; peanuts; cashews; liver; scallops; millet; barley; seaweed; chicken; brown rice; eggs; garlic; crab; mushrooms; milk.	Because phosphorus is so widespread in food, dietary phosphorus deficiency is extremely rare.	ADI: 800mg SR: 400–3000mg
Potassium	Blood pressure regulation; water balance regulation; hormone balance; muscle and nerve health.	Seaweed; sunflower seeds; wheat germ; almonds; raisins; nuts; dates; figs; yams; garlic; spinach; millet; dried beans; mushrooms; broccoli; banana; red meat; squash; chicken; carrots; potato.	Diuretics and certain medicines cause your body to lose potassium.	ADI: 4,500-5,100mg SR: 3–8g
Selenium	Antioxidant; detoxification of chemicals; anticarcinogenic; sperm health; reproductive system health; fertility; thyroid health; DNA repair.	Butter; herring; wheat germ; brazil nuts; cider vinegar; scallops; barley; lobster; shrimp; oats; chard; shellfish; crab; milk; fish; red meat; molasses; garlic; barley; eggs; mushrooms; alfalfa.	Milling/refining of cereals causes 40–50% losses.	ADI: 50–200ug SR: 200–800ug
Zinc	Antioxidant; anticarcinogenic; immune system regulator; antiviral; DNA and RNA synthesis; enzyme activator; wound healing; skin; hair; muscle and respiratory health; fertility; reproductive health; growth; insulin synthesis.	Oysters; ginger; red meat; nuts; dried beans; liver; milk; egg yolk; whole wheat; rye; oats; brazil nuts; peanuts; chicken; sardines; buckwheat; oily fish; shrimp; white fish.	Milling/refining of cereals causes 80% losses, freezing of vegetables causes 25–50% losses.	ADI: 15mg SR: 10–70mg

References for vitamin and mineral supplements charts: Osiecki, H., "*The Nutrient Bible 8th Edition*" (2010, Bioconcepts, Australia)
Liska et al, "*Clinical Nutrition: A Functional Approach*" (2004, The Institute for Functional Medicine, Washington USA)

INDEX BY HEALTH AREA

Beneficial foods are grouped under each specific health area.

INDEX

Index entries in italic are full recipes from the recipe section (pp176–337). In addition, the main source of information for each food gives suggestions about other culinary uses.

ACKNOWLEDGMENTS

The authors would like to thank Peter Kindersley whose tireless support for organic food and a natural lifestyle helped to create this book. Thanks also to Daphne Lambert for recipe inspiration and feedback, and for allowing us to reproduce her Almond and Raspberry Cake recipe on page 268; to Alex Savage for assisting with research; and to all at Dorling Kindersley for helping to steer this volume from concept to completion.

Dorling Kindersley would like to thank the great team at Neal's Yard Remedies.

Recipe photography Stuart West
Art direction Kat Mead
Food styling Jane Lawrie
Prop styling Liz Hippisley
Additional ingredients photography Ian O'Leary
Proofreading Sue Morony, Kokila Manchanda, and Neha Ruth Samuel
Indexing Marie Lorimer
Recipe testing Hülya Balci, Amy Carter, Francesa Dennis, Katy Greenwood, Clare Nielsen-Marsh, and Ann Reynolds
Editorial assistance Martha Burley
Design assistance Collette Sadler and Pooja Verma

Jacket images: Front: Dorling Kindersley: Stuart West bl, b, bc, br; Back: Dorling Kindersley: Stuart West tl, t, tc, tr

All other images © Dorling Kindersley
For further information see: **www.dkimages.com**

PUBLISHER'S NOTE
The recipes contained in this book have been created for the ingredients and techniques indicated. The Publisher is not responsible for your specific health or allergy needs that may require supervision. Nor is the Publisher responsible for any adverse reactions you may have to the recipes contained in the book, whether you follow them as written or modify them to suit your personal dietary needs or tastes.

DISCLAIMER: Every effort has been made to ensure that the information contained in this book is complete and accurate. However, the publisher is not engaged to provide professional advice or services to the individual reader, and the general suggestions made in this book are not intended as a substitute for individual medical advice. All matters regarding your health require medical supervision. The publisher cannot be held responsible for any loss or damage allegedly arising from any information or suggestion made in this book.